THE

# THERAPEUTICS

OF

# INTERMITTENT FEVER.

BY

H. C. ALLEN, M.D.,

UNIVERSITY OF MICHIGAN.

B. Jain Publishers (P) Ltd.
USA — Europe — India

**THE THERAPEUTICS OF INTERMITTENT FEVER**

9th Impression: 2019

> **NOTE FROM THE PUBLISHER**
> Any information given in this book is not intended to be taken as a replacement for medical advice. Any person requiring medical attention should consult a qualified practitioner or a therapeutist.

No part of this book may be reproduced, stored in a retrieval system or transmitted, in any form or by any means, mechanical, photocopying, recording or otherwise, without any prior written permission of the publisher.

© with the publisher

Published by Kuldeep Jain for
**B. JAIN PUBLISHERS (P) LTD.**
D-157, Sector-63, NOIDA-201307, U.P. (INDIA)
*Tel.:* +91-120-4933333 • *Email:* info@bjain.com
*Website:* www.bjain.com
**Registered office:** 1921/10, Chuna Mandi, Paharganj, New Delhi-110 055 (India)

Printed in India

ISBN: 978-81-319-1787-9

TO

THE FACULTY AND ALUMNI .

OF THE

HOMŒOPATHIC DEPARTMENT, UNIVERSITY OF MICHIGAN,

THIS

𝕸𝖔𝖓𝖔𝖌𝖗𝖆𝖕𝖍

IS

RESPECTFULLY AND GRATEFULLY INSCRIBED

BY THE

AUTHOR.

# PREFACE TO THE FIRST EDITION.

A NEED long felt in my own practice was supplied by Dr. Bell's admirable monograph on "Diarrhœa and Dysentery," and a desire for some better guide in the treatment of intermittent fever has been the inspiration which has induced me to undertake the labor of the present compilation. I have culled from the literature of our school —wherever a fact could be found or a principle deduced—and the indulgence of my professional colleagues is asked for the many omissions and imperfections. At the same time, I also ask their earnest co-operation in perfecting the work, so that should a future edition be found necessary, it may be made worthy the demands of the times and the possibilities of our law of cure. This can only be accomplished by united action; the experience of any one, no matter how extensive, will alone be insufficient. A somewhat extended personal acquaintance has convinced me that but comparatively few of our practitioners use a repertory in selecting the remedy; hence, a bracketed comparison has been substituted in its place, as more likely to meet the wants of the majority.

I cannot too strongly urge that marginal notes of omissions, corrections and clinical verifications may be made, that the future may produce a more perfect work on THE THERAPEUTICS OF INTERMITTENT FEVER.

H. C. ALLEN, M.D.

*Detroit, November,* 1879.

# PREFACE TO THE SECOND EDITION.

THE first edition, crude and imperfect as it was, met with such a demand that it was soon exhausted. In the present edition we have endeavored to erase misprints and correct, as far as may be, our former sins of omission and commission. The difficulty of mastering our voluminous and rapidly increasing symptomatology, has naturally led to the demand for monographs and repertories; hence to the bracketed comparison of the former edition have been added some leading characteristics of each remedy and a complete repertory.

The author is under many obligations to professional colleagues for valuable corrections and suggestions, to whom he again appeals for assistance in making a future edition still more complete.

H. C. ALLEN, M.D.

*Ann Arbor, Michigan,* 1884.

# INTERMITTENT FEVER.

"After he has found all the existing and appreciable symptoms of the disease, the physician has found the disease itself—he has a complete idea of it, and knows all he need know to cure it."—
*Hahnemann's Medicine of Experience.*

## THE CAUSE.

A PHYSICIAN is rarely to be met with who cannot at once and with apparent certainty, formulate *a theory* for the *cause* of intermittent fever. This universal knowledge is only equaled by the variety of theories entertained, and the failures inseparable from the attempt to treat *the theory of the cause*, and the *name of the disease*, instead of the totality of the symptoms—subjective and objective—presented by the patient. The natural result of this attempt to follow the teachings and practice of Allopathy, is the charge, so often made by our medical brethren of the opposite school, that "Homœopaths are not honest in their practice;" and this charge has been more frequently based upon what they have seen of our treatment of this disease, than of all other diseases combined. Allopathy affirms that Intermittent Fever cannot be cured without Quinine, because Quinine is the antidote of "Marsh Miasm," which is the *cause* of intermittent fever; and many homœopaths—departing from the law of cure, and neglecting their Materia Medica—honestly cherish a similar delusion.

The object of this work is to deal with therapeutic facts, not with speculative theories. The author has no theory to advance; and none to disprove except such as interfere with the successful homœopathic treatment of this *bête noir* of our profession. As yet we are unable to offer an intelligent explanation of the *cause* of sporadic or epidemic intermittent fever, that will bear the test of scientific investigation. Hahnemann's *one fact* is worth more at the bedside than all the theories that have ever been advanced.

The following is a brief notice of some of the prevailing theories and the treatment based upon them:

"Intermittent fever is a neurosis. Its phenomena, as chill and heat are distinct; their origin must also be distinct. The heat is due to the action on the sympathetic system; the chill to the spinal system."—*Lord, on Int. Fever.*

"We believe intermittent fever is a neurosis, whose seat is especially in the ganglionic system, and therefore only nerve remedies, and particularly such as act on the vaso-motor part, can cure."—*Wurmb and Caspar on Int. Fever.*

"Acute cases must always be treated by cerebro-spinal remedies; chronic cases by organic remedies."—*Burt's Characteristics.*

"Ague remedies may be divided into two classes, viz.: Quinine, Gelsemium, Eucalyptus, Nux vomica, Arsenic, and Cedron, which have the power of destroying protozoa, infusoria, and cryptogamic fungi; and Eupatorium, Cornus, Salicine, Arnica, Natrum mur. and Hydrastis which have not that power, yet correspond to the periodicity of the paroxysm."—*Hale's Therapeutics*, p. 609.

Bartlett, Salisberry, and others who maintain the cryptogamic theory, have many followers in our school; and here Carbolic acid, Salicylic acid, Sulphite of Soda, etc., must be used to destroy the germs.

Grauvogl's theory of splenic congestion and constitutional divisions, has many advocates. But it requires a Grauvogl to detect the constitution, and splenic congestion; or a Lord, or Wurmb and Caspar, to select the cerebro-spinal or sympathetic remedy; or a Burt. Hughes, Hale, or Kafka to classify the remedies.

## THE MALARIAL THEORY,

### (Marsh Miasm),

Is, however, most generally accepted. The evidence advanced in its support is the prevailing occurrence of epidemics, where this poison presumably exists. It is supposed to be the result of decaying vegetable and other organic matter, and is found along rivers with low, swampy, alluvial shores, subject to frequent overflow; near bodies of stagnant water; in the neighborhood of recently dug canals, cellars, or freshly plowed virgin soil; near marshes, particularly on leeward side of prevailing winds. It is confined near the earth, seems to spread in a horizontal direction; and its progress may be cut off by walls, hedges, high banks, and dense forests. Unlike the poison of Diphtheria,

Rubeola, Scarlatina, Variola, and Typhus, it is neither contagious nor infectious; but also unlike them, each attack only renders the system more liable to a subsequent one.

But, on the other hand, it has long been known that the fever may exist on a dry, or even on a sandy soil, and in rocky, mountainous regions where it is often more extensive and severe than in the adjoining low country. Ziemssen says: "On the Tuscan Appenines fevers are found at the height of 1,100 feet; on the slopes of mountains of Ceylon at 6,500 feet; on the Pyrenees at 5,000 feet; and on the Andes, in Peru, at 10,000 and 11,000 feet; while at the same time the neighboring plains are entirely free, or are only visited in a very mild form." There are large tracts of lands where all the conditions of malaria exist, and yet no intermittent fever; and other districts where no conditions of miasma are to be found, and yet ague is endemic every season. The fever occurs in a sporadic form where miasma never prevails, and the patients had never been in a malarial region. Moreover, the inhabitants of a valley where the disease prevails removing to a mountainous region where it is unknown, are often attacked with intermittent fever. The microscopist, with his most powerful lens, has never yet been able to detect the miasm; and chemical and spectral analysis are alike powerless to solve the problem.

A recent monograph by G. H. Wilson, M.D., of Meridan, Conn., member of the State Board of Health, presents some valuable and suggestive facts which go far towards clearing up the question of *malaria*, as one of the causes, at least, in the production of epidemic intermittent fever. The evidence, although negative in character, proves pretty conclusively what ague *is not*, if it do not prove what it is. If it can be shown that *malaria* is a phantom, it may prevent Quininism and drugging and lead to a more successful—the homœopathic—treatment of our patients.

"The movement of the present malarial epidemic in Connecticut and other parts of New England, is illustrated by a map with isochronal lines, showing the extent and direction of its annual progress during the past twenty-three years. The data upon which the article is based have been obtained from personal observations, reports of medical men and others in nearly every town in the three States of Connecticut, Massachusetts and Rhode Island, and are believed to be reliable.

"It will be seen that the course, as shown by the successive waves, and later, by the concentric lines of its annual progress, indicates an advance in one definite direction, independent of any known or recognized influence, whether atmospheric, telluric, magnetic, or climatic, and through the most diverse conditions of surface, soil, humidity, and temperature, general and local.

"We are unfortunately constrained by long usage to denominate the class of diseases under consideration malarial, and so in a sense endorse by word, what in the argument we must disown. Our inability to say what the cause of ague is, does not debar us, however, from proving what it is not. In fact, if the question can be cleared of the halo of error, which has hitherto surrounded it, the truth may more readily appear; and the object of this paper is to show, how little its conclusions agree with the favorite opinions of laymen and physicians, from Lancisi down, regarding the cause of ague, and its future in Connecticut.

"In this epidemic we may be sure that ague is not produced by "heat, moisture, and decay," arising from ponds, reservoirs, swamps, or low grounds, overflowed by freshets, or exposed by evaporation; for new cases arise at any and all seasons of the year, and upon the highest land, as it has done in one-third of the towns in the State; nor by uncovering lately submerged lands, for in most towns no such lands exist. Not only does the disease not appear under the conditions appropriate to the paludal theory, but it does not confine itself to, or remain in, the alluvial tracts, even when established upon them.

"Not from 'disturbance of earth,' by grading, ditching, or railroad building in the country, or by laying down sewers, or gas or water pipes in towns; for these operations have been going on for ages, while no ague came because of them, and it appeared at the same relative time in territory whose surface had or had not been disturbed. Not from the 'transportation of clay, manures, or other decaying and fermenting substances, from New Jersey and New York,' or of sawdust in the river beds, floated down from the mills of the north; for in several towns so affected none of these things have been introduced to this day, and in others, the disease failed to appear at the time called for by the theory.

"Not from 'stagnant, or even foul water,' no matter how offensive to smell or taste, for water with these qualities has always existed in many towns free from ague; and, on the other hand, many tracts of dry and sandy soil have been its favorite haunts. Not from *bacillus malariæ* in the water, which would be carried *with* the current; while ague moves up stream, and *against* the current of every principal river in Connecticut. It cannot be from germs carried by winds; for the direction for the year, in the State, and in New England generally, is north of west, and is very rarely, and for a short time only, in the direction of the ague movement.

"Probably no error is so common among the people of towns, as that it may be caused by imperfect drainage, by the filth of houses. Doubtless bad conditions lower the vitality and decrease the resisting power of the system, and promote the liability to suffer from exposure to specific influence, but no amount of filth or degree of debility will produce one case of ague *de novo*.

"Ague is specific, and can only be produced by its own cause. That ague is found in all these conditions is fortunate for the handy hypothesis of local influence, and the daily use of talkative laymen and lazy physicians; but *post hoc* is not *propter hoc*. These alleged causes of ague might have been left to the defence of their inventors, and not have burdened this paper, but for the benefit of the contrast which the lessons and conclusions of the map presept to the unsettled condition of thought on that subject.

"In its invasion of this State the ague crossed, diagonally but decidedly, every one of our main rivers. Starting on the coast, west of the Housatonic, it crossed its valley the next year, but did not ascend it, more than about fifteen miles, in as many years. It next crossed the Naugatuck, within five miles of its mouth. The Quinnipiac, it first reached and crossed, in South Meriden, sixteen miles from East Haven; the Connecticut at Middletown, twenty-five miles from the Sound; and the tributaries of the Tames in Coventry, forty miles from the sea.

"I would mention that in Rhode Island, also, it entered at Westerly, and passed through the State to the north-east, leaving the south-east and north-west portions unaffected. \* \* \* \* \*

"In conclusion, it appears that New England is now suffering from an epidemic of intermittent, which has moved from the first, and is still moving, north-easterly, with an irregular front, continuous in time, but sometimes interrupted in manner. It is not too much to suppose, that it came over from Long Island and New Jersey, and possibly further south, as well as from the same region over Westchester County, N.Y.; that its front extends from the Hudson on the west, to Buzzard's Bay on the east; that it has moved a hundred miles north and east, and still reaches out its favors to those belated northmen and downeasters, who have hitherto mocked us."

On such evidence—quite as strong against as in favor of the malarial theory—we may be pardoned if we doubt the existence of such an agent in the production of intermittent fever. And when we are asked to abandon the *certainties* of our *law of cure,* and accept a treatment based upon the antidoting of an unknown poison, as homœopaths, we should respectfully decline. We know quite as much of the nature of those poisons which produce scarlatina, diphtheria and typhus as we do of that which produces intermittent fever; yet the success of the antidotal treatment so-called is not such as would warrant any homœopath in abandoning the teaching of his Materia Medica for it. This search after a hypothetical cause, and the adoption of a treatment based upon its supposed discovery, have been the fatal "Scylla" upon which has stranded many a homœopathic success. The element of accuracy once removed, our practice degenerates into empiricism.

It would, no doubt, be a great satisfaction to be able to explain *the cause* of intermittent fever; and it would be equally gratifying to be able to tell **why all persons, subjected to the same exposure, are not attacked**; just as it would be a satisfaction to be able to explain the cause of many phenomena in physical science existing all about us. Such knowledge might aid us in a sanitary way in preventing the disease or modifying its severity; but it could never be of the slightest benefit in its homœopathic treatment. When once we depart from Hahnemann's method of individualizing each case, we enter upon the sea of doubt and uncertainty upon which our allopathic brethren, without a compass, have ever sailed. "If our school ever gives up the strict inductive method of Hahnemann, we are lost, and deserve only to be mentioned as a carricature in the history of medicine."—Constantine Hering.

Hale—in condemning the indiscriminate use of Quinine—says: "Unless the physician is absolutely certain that the attack is due to miasmatic poisoning, he should wait until the disease shows its true character." How is it possible for the physician to be "absolutely *certain*" that he is dealing with miasmatic poisoning? And how can that knowledge change the symptoms presented by the patient, or enable us with more ease, or greater certainty, to select the remedy? There is a very nice distinction between *certain* and *sure*. I am *certain* the sun will rise; I am *sure* it has risen. The successful treatment of intermittent fever requires that the physician should not only be *certain*, but *sure*. I am *sure* I have a sick man to treat who presents certain symptoms; but I am not *certain* that he has been poisoned with miasma, or has been within a hundred miles of it; and I am quite *uncertain* whether the "cerebro-spinal" or "sympathetic" is affected; or *whether* to select, or *how* to select, a cerebro-spinal or organic remedy.—There are many remedies which affect both nervous systems; my patient requires but *one*. *But of this, I am sure, that the objective and subjective symptoms of which he complains are in every respect similar to those produced on the healthy subject by Cinchona.* For me and my patient this simple fact is all-sufficient. It approximates a mathematical demonstration. There are no doubts or uncertainties about it. My patient does not have to wait until I can demonstrate the truth or falsity of some favorite theory, which, whether right or wrong, could never change the characteristics of his case, so far as the selection of the remedy is concerned.

## EXAMINATION OF THE PATIENT.

The first step in individualization—the keystone of the homœopathic arch—begins with an examination of the patient. It is impossible to examine a patient *in general;* and prescribe for him *in particular*. Before we can select a remedy for a given case we must first ascertain the particular symptoms of which the patient complains, which form the picture of the disease; and this is often a most difficult task.

Hahnemann says: "The totality of the symptoms which characterize a given case, being once committed to writing, the most difficult part is accomplished."

Dunham says: "Do you say that this is an easy matter? Gentlemen, it is the most difficult part of your duty. To select the remedy after a masterly examination and record of the case is comparatively easy. But to *take* the case requires great knowledge of human nature, of the history of disease, and, as we shall see, of the "*Materia Medica.*"

"Make haste slowly" never had a better illustration in medical science than in this advice; as no disease demands a closer observance of instructions, or a more strict adherence to principle for its successful treatment, than intermittent fever.

The symptoms occurring before and during the *chill, heat, sweat* and *apyrexia;* the *time* of occurrence of paroxysm; the *parts* of the body in which the chill first makes its appearance; the *regularity* of its stages; the *degree* or *absence* of *thirst,* and *time* of its appearance; as well as the constitutional ailments aroused by the fever, are all to be carefully noted.

"Till the present time, pathology has only been acquainted with one single *intermittent fever*, which has been called *ague*. It admits of no other difference than the interval which exists between the paroxysms; and upon this are founded the particular denominations, quotidian tertian, quartan, etc. But, besides the variety which they present in regard to the periods of their return, the intermittent fevers exhibit yet other changes that are much more important. Among these fevers there are many which cannot be denominated agues, because their attacks consist solely of heat; others are characterized by cold only, succeeded or not by perspirations; while yet others freeze the body of the patient, and inspire him notwithstanding with a sensation of heat, or even create in him a feeling of cold, although he seems very warm to the touch; in many, one of the paroxsysms is confind to shivering or cold, which is immediately succeeded by a comfortable sensation, and that which comes after it consists of heat followed by perspiration or not. In one case, it is heat which manifests itself first, and cold succeeds; in another, both the cold and heat give place to apyrexia; while the next paroxysm, which sometimes does not occur before an interval of several hours, consists merely of perspiration; in certain cases no trace of perspiration is perceptible; while in others the attack is composed solely of perspiration, without either heat or cold, or of perspiration that flows during the heat alone. There exist, likewise, innumerable differences relative to the accessory symptoms, the particular kind of headache, the bad taste in the mouth, the stomach sickness, the vomiting, the diarrhœa, the absence or degree of thirst, the kind of pains felt in the body and·limbs, sleep, delirium, spasms, changes of the temper, etc., which manifest themselves before, during, or after the cold, hot, or sweating stages, without taking into account a multitude of other deviations. These are usually intermittent fevers that are very different from one another, each of which demands naturally that mode of homœopathic treatment most appropriate to it individually. It must be confessed that they may almost all be suppressed (a case that so frequently occurs) by large and enormous doses of Cinchona or Quinine —that is to say, Cinchona prevents their periodical return and destroys the type. But where this remedy is employed in intermittent fevers, where it is inappropriate (as is the case with all epidemic intermittents, which pass over whole countries, and even mountains), the patient is not at all cured, because the character of the disease is destroyed; he is still indisposed, and often much more so than he was before; he suffers from a peculiar chronic bark complaint, often incurable, and yet this is what physicians term a cure."—Note to § 233, Organon.

The physician of the "rational" (?) school searches only for general conditions. To be able to diagnose *ague* and its quotidian, tertian, or quartan form is enough for him; it satisfies the supposed demands of science, and enables him to prescribe some preparation of Cinchona (see Organon, p. 195). Either the ready facility of this generalizing practice with the entire absence of consistency in its application, or a praiseworthy, yet unsuccessful attempt to utilize the pathological theories of Allopathy, have induced many very excellent men of our school to abandon if they ever possessed a knowledge of Hahnemann's inductive method, for this "short cut" to success. This can be better illustrated by the following comparison of

| GENERALIZING. | INDIVIDUALIZING. |
| --- | --- |
| **Arsenicum.** | **Cinchona.** |
| If the paroxysm varies widely from the typical form; if there is no chill or no sweat; if there are unusual gastric, hepatic, intestinal or cerebral disturbances; well-marked capillary congestion, and the patient is half sick during the apyrexia; we may be sure that the malarial poison has made a profound impression on the sympathetic ganglia. Arsenic, not Quinine, the typical remedy for this state.--W. H. HOLCOMBE, *U. S. M. & S. J.*, Jan., 1872. | The paroxysm is preceded by headache, nausea, hunger, anguish and palpitation of the heart. Thirst before the chill and during the sweating stage Chills alternating with heat, skin cold and blue, headache, nausea and absence of thirst. During hot stage, dryness of the mouth and lips, red face and headache. After the heat, *thirst* and *profuse sweat*. Ringing in the ears, with dizziness and a feeling as if the head was enlarged. Pain in the region of the liver and spleen when bending or coughing. Sallow complexion.—*Johnson's Key.* |

There are many remedies that would fulfill the requirements of Dr. Holcombe's Arsenic case. Each one of Dr. Burt's organic remedies is apparently well indicated. On the other hand, there is but a single remedy that will meet the requirements of Dr. Johnson's. It does not aid us in finding the remedy to know that the paroxysm is not of the typical form, or that gastric or cerebral disturbance be present, or that malarial poison has profoundly impressed the sympathetic ganglia, or even to know that he feels as he did in his former attack. We want a statement of the case in graphic figurative language, not in the abstract terms of science. We want a clear statement of the objective and subjective phenomena which precede, accompany or follow the various stages of the paroxysm.

### Quinine.

A simple, fresh, uncomplicated case of intermittent fever, with distinct cold, hot, and sweating stages, and perfect apyrexia, is promptly cured by moderate doses of Quinine.—W. H. HOLCOMBE, *U. S. M. and S. J.*, Jan., 1872.

### Arsenicum.

Tertian intermittent fever; first chill, then heat, then perspiration. Thirst during the whole paroxysm, *drinks often, but little at a time;* during cold stage, pain in the small of the back and lower limbs; tongue blue; great prostration and debility after the paroxysm. Arsenic cured.—B. F. JOSLIN, *Hom. News.*

"A simple, fresh, uncomplicated case of intermittent fever," etc., may be promptly cured by twenty-five or thirty other remedies as well as Quinine; but Arsenic, alone, will cure that of Dr. Joslin's. To know that Quinine, or any other remedy, has cured intermittent fever *is of no value to the homœopath*; unless he be given the particulars in which *this fever*, cured by Quinine, *differed from other similar fevers;* and generalization can never give him this knowledge.

"There are diversities in the form in which intermittent fever appears in different persons and in different epidemics; that these forms require different remedies, and that thus there is a form which is capable of being cured by Arsenic, and by nothing else; a form capable of being cured by Quinine and by nothing else; and so of other drugs. In this view, when a case of intermittent fever presents itself, the question can never be: Is Arsenic a better remedy for this disease than Quinine is? Does it offer greater chances of a cure? There can be no better or worse. The question is between right and wrong; suitable and not suitable.

The question should be always: Which remedy corresponds to this particular case, and is therefore, indicated in it?"—*Dunham*, Vol. II, p. 201.

## THE GENUS EPIDEMICUS.

As the prevailing cough which occurs during epidemic whooping-cough is relieved by the genus of the epidemic; or the acute angina occurring when diphtheria is prevalent is also most readily controlled by the remedy which controls the epidemic; so also may our attention be directed to the curative remedy in intermittent fever by carefully observing the character of the prevailing disease. This is especially the case in sea-side intermittents which so often find their similimum in Arsenicum, Gelsemium, or Natrum Muriaticum. Where the epidemic breaks out after an overflow of a river, Bryonia, Capsicum or Rhus tox. may frequently be called for; or during epidemic dysentery occurring in autumn Colchicum may relieve every case. Cinchona, Eucalyptus, Eupatorium, Ipecacuanha and other drugs are often thought of in this connection, when a careful study will lead to the remedy required.

Hahnemann calls attention to this feature of disease in the following: "Epidemics of intermittents occurring in places where such fevers are not epidemic, partake of the nature of chronic diseases, and are composed of a series of acute attacks. Each epidemic possesses a peculiar uniform character, common to all individuals attacked by the epidemic disease. By observing the complex of symptoms peculiar to all patients, this common character will be found to point out the homœopathic (specific) remedy for all cases in general. This remedy will also usually relieve patients who, previous to this epidemic, had enjoyed good health, and who were free from developed psora.

## WHEN TO ADMINISTER THE REMEDY?

Although this has never been a question of much controversy, yet the prevailing practice has been to administer Aconite, Gelsemium, Veratrum viride, or some other favorite during the paroxysm, for the double purpose of "doing something" and "controlling the fever." Every observing physician who has had much experience in the treatment of intermittent fever will testify that this plan rarely has any perceptible effect upon the paroxysm, unless it be to render it more obscure. This "doing something" can be successfully accomplished with sac. lac., if it be absolutely necessary to do anything. The easiest, safest, most satisfactory and scientific method is that of Hahnemann, and no cause for regret will ever follow its adoption.

Hahnemann says, Organon, § 236: "In these cases, the medicine is generally most efficacious when it is administered a short time after the termination of the paroxysm, when the patient has partially recovered from it. During the intermission the medicine will have time to develop its curative effect in the organism, without violent action or disturbance; while the effect of a medicine, though specifically adapted to the case, given just before the next paroxysm, would coincide with the renewal of the disease, thereby creating such counteraction and distress in the organism, as to deprive the patient of much strength, and even to endanger life.* But if the medicine is given just after the termination of the attack, when the fever has entirely subsided, and before the premonitory symptoms of the next paroxysm have time to appear, the vital force of the organism is in the most favorable condition to be gently modified by the medicine, and restored to healthy action."

§ 237: "If the feverless interval is very brief, as in some severe fevers, or if it is disturbed by the after-effects of the preceding paroxysm, the dose of homœopathic medicine should be administered when the perspiration diminishes, or when the subsequent stages of the paroxysm decline."

§ 238: "One dose of the appropriate remedy may prevent several attacks, and may actually have restored health; nevertheless, we may perceive threatening indications of a new attack, and in this case only, the same medicine should be repeated, provided the complex of symptoms continues to be the same."

If, after the exhibition of the proper remedy, the next paroxysm be *earlier* and *more severe,* or *later* and *milder* than preceding one, the action of the remedy should not be interfered with; wait for succeeding paroxysm, which may be lighter still or not return at all.

§ 245. "Perceptible and continued progress of improvement in an acute or chronic disease, is a condition which, as long as it lasts, invariably counter indicates the repetition of any medicine whatever, because the beneficial effects which the medicine continues to

---

* There are proofs of this, unfortunately, in the too frequent cases of where a moderate allopathic dose of Opium, administered to the patient during the cold stage of the fever, has quickly deprived him of life.—Note to Organon, p. 195.

exert is rapidly approaching its perfection. Under these circumstances every new dose of any medicine, even of the last one that proved beneficial, would disturb the process of recovery."

To many, as it was to Hahnemann for years, this is one of the most perplexing problems in practice. Those who have given it a trial are convinced not only of the soundness of Hahnemann's teaching, but of its superior success in practice. Those who have never tried it can never know.

## THE SIMILLIMUM.

The selection of the remedy is the question of questions—the one of vital import to the physician as well as his patient. Once unmistakably found, a cure will as certainly result. The potency question, in comparison, sinks into insignificance. The more perfect the simillimum, the quicker and surer the cure. On the other hand, if the remedy be not the proper one, no matter how high or how low the potency, how crude the drug, or how massive the dose, we will utterly fail; or, at most, only partially cure by suppressing the attack. We are slow to learn the great lesson inculcated by Hahnemann from the first to the last page of the Organon: **that it is quality, not quantity, that cures**; that the proper selection of the remedy is of much greater moment than the quantity to be given; that *disease is not an entity, and cannot be expelled from the system by* **quantity**; *nor can quantity ever take the place of, or atone for, an improper or imperfect selection of the remedy.*

Dunham says: "The selection of the remedy for a case of sickness, is a process of comparison. We compare the symptoms of the case with the symptoms which drugs have produced in the healthy; and we select the drug of which the symptoms are most similar to those of the patient. We seek a parallelism between drug symptoms and those of the patient. The symptoms of a case of sickness, like the physiological phenomena of healthy persons, are not always and during all time the same; they vary from day to day, from hour to hour or from minute to minute. Indeed it might properly be said that life is, in so far as every physiological process is concerned, a series of oscillations within physiological limits; now action is vehement, now mild; waste is now in excess, now in deficit.

"Just so it is with morbid phenomena or symptoms, whether they be of natural, or of artificial or drug, disease. We are then instituting comparisons between, as to speak, oscillating and continually shifting series of phenomena.

"Now, the point of importance here is that this oscillation and shifting require time, and that therefore our summary of the symptoms must cover not merely the moment of time at which we observe the patient, but also some previous time during which the symptoms may have been different from those of the present time. This remark applies both to the drug and the case. It is necessary not simply for the purpose of getting a full picture of the case, but also to make certain that there is a complete parallelism between the case and the drug we think of giving the patient.

"Two lines, each an inch long, may appear to be parallel. If we would be certain whether or not they are so, let us project each line until it is a foot long. We shall then more easily see the divergence or convergence if there be any. Just so, at some particular moment, the symptoms of a case and of a drug may appear to be very similar; but if we compare the succession and order of the symptoms, for the space of a day or two, with the succession and order of the drug symptoms, we may notice a marked difference.

"This is illustrated by comparing the symptoms produced by two drugs in the healthy prover. There is a period in the action of each, when, to my mind the symptoms of Aconite and Carbo vegetabilis are very similar, and yet, taking a broader view of these drugs, we can scarcely find any more unlike.

"Shall I shock any of my hearers by stating this necessity for taking into consideration the course and succession of symptoms in selecting a remedy and shall I be told that strict homœopathy requires that a prescription shall be made for the symptoms that are present, the remedy to be changed when the symptoms change? I believe that some consciencious physicians too closely follow this method—too closely for the best success. Let us take a practical instance; a case of intermittent fever. The patient has certain symptoms which precede and usher in the chill. Then, for two hours or more, he has the symptoms which constitute the chill; then, after an interval, those which constitute the hot stage; then those of the sweating stage; after which comes a period of from ten to forty hours, constituting the apyrexia, during which the patient probably may have some symptoms which serve to characterize his case, and individualize it. We may see the patient during one or all of these periods. His symptoms at the different times are certainly very different. Is it our custom, is it good practice, to give the patient a different remedy, corresponding to each of these stages; or, would the nicest faculty of selection lead us to select for each stage the same remedy, to which a survey of the whole case would bring us? The former is not our custom. It would not be good practice. We could not so select. On the contrary, we extend our lines of symptoms—unless they correspond with the complete paroxysm and apyrexia—and then we can judge of their parallelism. We seek a remedy which produces just such cold, hot and sweating stages, in just such order and with just such concomitant symptoms, and that likewise produces such symptoms in the apyrexia. Do you point me to cases in which no such parallelism is found, and yet a successful prescription is made? I reply that, as I said at first, we are like the Israelites, and must make bricks whether we have straw or not. We must prescribe from our Materia Medica as it is. Where we can do no better, we must prescribe on a few symptoms. on an inference or an analogy, rather than refuse to prescribe at all, Yet nobody will deny the greater certainty of the prescription where such a parallelism can be established. In such a case then we follow the patient along a series of violent oscillations, between cold, heat, sweat, and the normal state again, and this we do, to a greater or less extent, in very many illnesses in which the oscillations are not so violent. I believe that a broad enough consideration of this subject would lead physicians to abstain from alternation of remedies even in the few instances in which Hahnemann sanctioned it, and would deter them from the error, as I deem it, of leaving a patient several remedies to be taken, variously, as different phases of sensation or objective phenomena succeed each other. But to be able to prescribe in this large-viewed way for your patient, you must have studied the Materia Medica in the same comprehensive way; you must have studied the connection and succession of the symptoms. A mere repertory study for the case in hand will not suffice. \* \* \* \* \* Seeking the means to cure the patient then, we look among drug provings for a similar series of phenomena. Let us suppose that we find one, which corresponds pretty well. Not exactly, however, for here are certain symptoms characteristic of that drug of which the patient has not complained. We examine the patient as regards those symptoms. No! his symptoms in that line are quite different. We try another similar drug, comparing its symptoms with the patients, and questioning the patient still further; and thus the comparing and trying proceed until we find a fit. This is a mental process, so expeditious sometimes that we are hardly aware how we engage in it. But it shows how difficult it is to take a case unless we have some knowledge of the Materia Medica, and how much an extensive knowledge of the Materia Medica aids us in taking the case; and this explains why the masters in our art have given us such model cases.

"To cure an intermittent fever we must: 1. Study the patient during the apyrexia, to form an exact idea of the functional action, regular or otherwise, of all the organs. 2. Observe all the symptoms of the pyrexia in its three stages of cold, heat and sweat. 3. Particularly note if a stage is absent, and which among them is the most marked. 4. Expressly depend upon the bizarre, singular, exceptional, phenomena, because they, above all, are characteristic, and figure in the first rank of the symptoms to which the drug must correspond in order to cure."—A. CHARGE, M.D. The following:

## ANALYSIS

Case VI (Ignatia) is an example of the comparative or cancellation method of selecting the remedy:

| | |
|---|---|
| **Time.**—Paroxysm every other day, in the afternoon. | Common to many remedies. |
| **Prodrome.**—Violent yawning and stretching. | Ant. t. Arn. **Ign.** Ipec. Quinine. Rhus. |
| **Chill.**—Especially along the back and arms, for an hour, *with thirst*, followed by | Arn. Caps. Carbo v. **Ign.** |
| **Heat.**—(Without thirst) over whole body, with cold feet; accompanied with internal shuddering, not disappearing until the | Caps. Cinchona. **Ign.** Led. |
| **Sweat** has broken out, the sweat lasting several hours (without thirst). | **Ign.** Ipec. Puls. |
| Dull, aching pain in the pit of the stomach; heaviness in the limbs, with pain in the joints. | Bry. **Ign.** Rhus. |
| During apyrexia, great weariness and bending of the knees. | **Ign.** |
| Sleep sound, with snoring breathing. | **Ign.** Nux m. Op. |
| Tongue coated white; lips chapped and dry. Taciturn, indifferent, starting. | Ars. **Ign.** Nat. m. |
| Countenance pale. | Fer. **Ign.** Sec. |

## THE POTENCY.

The greatest calamity that in practice can befall a homœopathic physician, is to acquire a routine habit of thinking that a remedy can cure only certain conditions or diseases, and no others. This usually is the first step in a routine habit of prescribing, and keeps time and pace with that other habit of thinking that, "the potency I use is the only successful one." The objections that "there is no power in potentized drugs, hence I have never used them;" or, "I do not believe they can possibly cure, or I would use them;" or, "I cannot understand how they are made," are offered as objections daily by the allopath to our low dilutions and even drop doses of the tincture. Truth is truth, whether we believe it or not. The potency, whether high or low, will never be affected in the slightest degree by such objections. Faith can have no place in science, where a fact can be demonstrated by experiment. The question of potency can only be settled by the test of experience; and each individual member must make the experiment for himself. Those who never use but one potency can never have any experimental knowledge of any other. Hahnemann asked to have his great discovery, under the rules he laid down, subjected to the test of practice, and the failures published to the world. Submit the potency question to the same test, write out the case, *in extenso*, with the remedy and potency, and publish the failures; the profession can then decide whether it was in the selection of the remedy used, or in the potency. Columbus had no difficulty in making the egg stand. The calling of hard names can neither decide the question, nor reconcile the conflicting views. In the interests of science, published facts, which bear on their face the stamp of reliability, should, both in justice to ourselves and others, be accepted as such, irrespective of potency, instead of being met with the weapons used by the cotemporaries of Hahnemann and Jenner. **Hahnemann decreased the dose as he increased his knowledge of Materia Medica. Can we adopt a better rule?**

"Boastful homœopathic physicians often claim that they can cure *any* case of ague with the high potencies. But those who have practiced many years in malarious districts know that such assertions are false. I need only refer

"Every case of intermittent fever, *can, has and must be cured*, with the potentized remedies, under the law of the similars *homœopathically.*"—*Lippe.*

This statement is endorsed by the writings and experience of such men

you to the writings and experience of such men as Holcombe, Ellis, Douglas, Marcy, Pulte, and hundreds of others in this country; also Hughes, Baehr, Roth, Kafka, and others, in England and on the continent."—*Hale's Therap.*, p. 610.

as Hering, Raue, Guernsey, Wells, Dunham, Bayard, Joslin, Bell, Gallupe, H. V. Miller, Baer, Wilson, and many others in this country; also Hahnemann, Berridge, Bœnninghausen, Müller, Meyhofer, and others, in England and on the continent.

Dunham says: "Nothing will gain the confidence of a patient so surely as *success*. His confidence, once gained by *success*, cannot be shaken by the form of your dose! Yes; it may though! If he sees that while your doctrines require you to give small doses, you yet dissemble and juggle, and, by using large pills and lozenges and mixtures, try to make it appear that you are giving as large doses as your Old-School neighbor, he will suspect that your faith in the system you profess is not really strong, and he will have doubts of both you and your system. The sick man who feels that you are *curing* him, cares not a straw for the logical improbabilities of your doctrines, nor for the scientific difficulties attending the explanation of the action of your little dose. Large or small — much or nothing — if under your auspices, his health return, he will have faith equally in yourself and in your methods."

"Patients are like soldiers; they believe in a man who believes in himself. We say this with all humility, for, in a matter of science, belief in one's self is faith in the laws one has undertaken to carry out in practice. And if the physician show confidence in his methods, his patients will yield themselves implicitly to his guidance. The prejudice in favor of large and many doses is a relic of past ages, when the practitioner was paid, not for his skill and personal services, but for the medicines he furnished."

A homœopathic cure is as beneficial to our patients as an allopathic one; and if it be quicker, surer, safer, and more pleasant, why not cure him homœopathically.

## CHARACTERISTIC.

I am convinced that in the treatment of intermittent fever, as well as of many other affections, we pay too much attention to the local manifestations of diseases—to the local symptoms of the drug—and too little to the general symptoms of the patient and the constitutional action of the remedy. For this reason we fail to get a true picture of the disease — the totality of the symptoms, objective and subjective — and are apt to fall into the routine practice of treating the disease instead of the patient. This is especially true in that large class of chronic intermittents, in which the *psora* of Hahnemann—the constitutional dyscrasiæ of the German pathologists—becomes such an important factor.

In "masked intermittents," also, where the character of the disease is not marked by the usual chill, heat, and sweat, our only guide is the constitutional symptoms of the patient. In this way we may relieve a multitude of ailments, as well as intermittents, for whose local symptoms and tissue lesions we have as yet been unable to find an analogy in our drug provings. For this reason, and to make the book a more complete work of reference, I have added some of the leading peculiarities of each remedy under

### CHARACTERISTIC.

Dunham says: "The fact cannot be too often called to mind, nor too strongly insisted upon, that our most characteristic indications for the use of a drug, which presents well-defined general symptoms, as Arsenic does, and indeed as every well proved drug does, are derived not from its local action upon any organ or system, not from a knowledge of the particular tissues it may affect, and how it affects them, but upon the general constitutional symptoms and their conditions and concomitants. If this were not so, in the presence of how many maladies, of the intimate nature of which we are wholly ignorant and which nevertheless we cure, should we be utterly powerless for good.

"A case will serve to illustrate not merely this point but also another, viz: the detection and treatment of what is sometimes called 'masked intermittents,' by which is meant a disease clearly resulting from marsh-malaria, but which nevertheless does not manifest itself by the customary paroxysm of chill, heat and perspiration, which constitute intermittent fever.

"A precocious child in Dutchess Co., twelve years old, had complained for more than eighteen months of a severe pain in left ear. She was brought to my office for treatment, with the statement that for this affection she had been treated, both locally and constitutionally for an inflammation of the middle ear, by some of the most distinguished surgeons of the city of New York but with no good result. I could discover no distinct signs of local lesion, but nevertheless supposed it to be a case of otalgia, and from a very close correspondence of the case, as described to me, with the symptoms of Chamomilla, gave that drug. She got no better. I then learned, that she had been under the care of a good homœopathic physician, who, if it had been simple otalgia, would surely have cured her. This fact induced me to scrutinize the case very carefully before I prescribed again. Visiting the patient repeatedly at her residence, at different times in the day, I found that the attacks of pain were regularly and distinctly paroxysmal; that they were attended by the peculiar thirst so characteristic of Arsenic, by the restlessness and anguish, and followed by the prostration, equally characteristic. Furthermore, concomitant symptoms of an Arsenic gastralgia and diarrhœa were also present. It then occurred to me that this was probably a case of masked intermittent. The situation of the house and the topography of the neighborhood favored the idea. On the strength of the symptoms recited, I gave Arsenic $^{200}$. Within five days the pains had ceased to appear, but in their stead came a regular paroxysm of chill, fever and sweat, indicating the existence of quotidian intermittent fever. These paroxysms recurred for four days, gradually diminishing in intensity. They then ceased, leaving the patient well.

"Whatever, then, may be the local name of the disease, whatever pathological name it may bear, if the general symptoms correspond to those of Arsenic, in the way that I have pointed out, do not hesitate a moment to give that drug."

## THE CLINICAL CASES

Are taken from the periodical literature of our school, wherever found, or have been kindly furnished by professional colleagues to whom the author is under many obligations. They are intended to illustrate the sphere of action, as well as the selection of the remedy, and at the same time dispel the delusion honestly entertained by many, "That patients will not *wait* for the homœopathic remedy to act, hence, must resort to Quinine." Patients *wait* for the prompt action of the homœopathic remedy in croup, cholera, diphtheria, dysentery, pneumonia and yellow fever! The *remedy* is not at fault; **it acts just as promptly in intermittent fever as in any other disease.**

# THE THERAPEUTICS OF INTERMITTENT FEVER.

## ACONITUM NAPELLUS.

**Characteristic.**—Aconite is most frequently indicated in recent cases occurring in young persons, especially girls of a full plethoric habit, who lead a sedentary life; persons easily affected by atmospheric changes.

On rising from a recumbent posture, the red face becomes deathly pale, or he becomes faint or giddy and falls over; he fears to rise again; often accompanied by vanishing of sight and unconsciousness.

Great fear and anxiety of mind, with great nervous excitability; afraid to go out, to go into a crowd where there is any excitement or many people, to cross a street. His countenance is expressive of fear; his life is rendered miserable by it.

Hahnemann says: "Whenever Aconite is chosen homœopathically, you must, above all, observe the moral symptoms, and be careful that it closely resembles them: the anguish of mind and body; the restlessness; the disquiet not to be allayed."

**Aggravation.**—In the evening and night the pains are insupportable; in a warm room; when rising in bed.

**Amelioration.**—During the day; in the open air; while at rest (except at night in bed); after perspiration; from wine.

**Type.**—Quotidian; quartan. No regularity; periodicity not marked. Apt to become synochal, or inflammatory symptoms with congestion of local organs, as head and chest, may form a complication.

**Time.**—Usually in the evening.

**Cause.**—Dry, cold winds; hot days and cool nights; getting wet (**Dulc.**, **Rhus**); suppressed perspiration by uncovering or sitting in a draught; *by fright;* rheumatic exposure.

**Chill.**—*Ascends from feet to chest,* with internal heat and sensation of hot water in the head; chilly *when uncovered or even touched;* chilliness on *the slightest movement, even by lifting of bed clothes* (**Nux v.**). *Coldness,* with **redness and heat of one, coldness and paleness of the other cheek** (**Cham., Ipec.**). Chill with *one hot cheek;* contracted pupils; anxiety; or *body chilly,* with *red face, hot cheeks, hot forehead* and *ear lobules;* face hot, hands and feet cold. *Chill from extremities to head and face; heat, vice versa.*

**Heat.**—With thirst. *Towards evening, dry heat in the face, with anxiety; high fever; dry burning heat,* which extends from head and face; burning heat, with chilly shiverings running up the back. *Great fear; nervous excitability; restlessness* and *anxious tossing about. Cough during heat,* with palpitation and pleuritic stitches in the chest (cough during chill and heat, **Bry.**—cough before and during the chill, **Rhus**). *Red face while lying,* and *pale face and fainting when rising up. Great thirst for large quantities of water; everything else tastes bitter* (thirst for large quantities in every stage, **Bry., Natr. m.**—only during heat, **Ipec.**). Can not bear to be covered, yet fears to be uncovered (**Camph., Sec.**).

**Sweat.**—*Must be covered as soon as sweat begins; covered* or *affected parts sweat most profusely,* (**Ant. t.**) or *perspiration only on side on which he lies* (**Cinch., Nitr. ac.**)—sweat on single parts only (**Bry.**). Profuse warm perspiration over whole body, by which nervous excitability, restlessness and anxiety are relieved (sweat brings relief of all suffering, **Natr. m.**). General warm steaming sweat.

**Tongue.**—Coated white; papillæ red and elevated. "Strawberry tongue."

**Pulse.**—During chill, intermittent, thread-like; during heat, quick, full, hard, bounding.

**Apyrexia.**—*Never clear.* Loss of appetite; sleep restless and disturbed by dreams; *very anxious* about recovery; weak and exhausted by slightest exertion, either mental or physical.

Is rarely indicated, *per se*, as the remedy to cure (but frequently used during paroxysm when not indicated). Cause, often the characteristic indication; then it acts promptly and cures permanently.

"Aconite is never to be given first to subdue the fever, and then some other remedy to meet the case; never to be alternated with other drugs for the purpose of controlling the fever. If the fever be such as to require Aconite, no other drug is needed. If other drugs seem indicated, one should be sought which meets the fever as well; for many drugs beside Aconite produce fever, each after his kind."— *Dunham*, I, p. 87.

## CLINICAL.

CASE I.—Mrs. H., æt. 49, after a fatiguing walk, sought a cool retreat to rest; she soon began to feel rigors passing down her back, followed by shuddering and indescribable aching from the head to the lower extremities; could scarcely endure contact with bed-clothing, and this sensitive and sore feeling was all over the body; great thirst; thick, white coating on the tongue; tumefied countenance, expressive of much pain. Pulse not much accelerated; chilliness and heat in rapid alternation; intolerable aching; thirst and dry skin continued all night. In the P.M., frightful pains tending to the head. Acon.$^3$ in water. First dose had a quieting effect; pains less; skin moist; sensitiveness to contact removed; slept till morning. Made a good recovery.—A. E. SMALL, *U. S. Med. and Surg. Journ.*, 1871.

CASE II.—Aconite given during the apyrexia, four doses, removed intermittent fever in a plethoric individual, the chilliness being very violent, and succeeded by *dry, glowing heat, excessive anguish and oppression.*—*A. H. Z.*, I, p. 146.

CASE III.—Acon.$^3$, two doses, freed a child of two years, of a quartan fever, which had lasted upwards of a year, commencing with *a chilliness in the evening*, and succeeded by *a ten hours heat.*—*Hygea*, I, p. 79.

## ÆSCULUS HIPPOCASTANUM.

**Characteristic.**—Most suitable to persons with hemorrhoidal tendencies, who suffer from gastric, bilious or catarrhal troubles.

Constant backache—severe, dull, aching pain—affecting the sacrum and hips, sacro-iliac articulations, worse when walking or stooping forward.

Back gives out at that point when walking, must sit or lie down.

Venous congestion (portal and hemorrhoidal), as if parts contained too much blood; heart, lungs, stomach, brain (Aloe, Sulf.).

Mucous membranes dry, swollen; burn and feel raw; mouth, throat rectum.

Constipation; stool large, hard, dry; passed with difficulty, with dryness, heat and constriction of rectum which feels as if full of small sticks; knife-like pains shoot up the rectum after stool (Ign., Nitr. ac.).

Hemorrhoids; blind and painful, rarely bleeding; small, like ground-nuts, of a purple color, with severe lumbo-sacral backache.

**Type.**—Quotidian; tertian; double tertian. Periodicity marked. Autumnal fevers.

**Time.**—4 P. M. (**Lyc., Puls.**). Evening. Fever without chill from 7 to 12 P.M.

**Prodrome.**—Yawning, stretching and bursting headache. Without thirst.

**Chill.**—At 4 P.M., with goose-flesh, relieved by heat of fire (**Ign.**); along the spine; runs up the back or creeping up and down the back (**Gels.**), with heat and burning in the rectum and anus. Severe chilliness, with rigor; cannot get warm.

**Heat.**—Flushes of heat over the face, occiput, neck, and shoulders or over whole body. In evening fever from 7 to 12 P.M., skin hot and dry, palms and soles burn, disposed to yawn and stretch; head aches as if it would burst. Lungs feel engorged; heart beats violently.

Burning in the mouth and profuse salivation. Burning dryness and constriction of the throat, constant inclination to swallow, and frequent spitting of mucus from the mouth.

**Sweat.**—Profuse, hot, and comes with the heat, not after it: on head and face. The congestions of head, face, and chest decline and abdominal symptoms disappear during sweating stage.

**Pulse.**—Soft, slow, and feeble. Functional disturbances of heart from hemorrhoidal complications; heartbeat full and rapid; can feel pulsations over whole body (Natr. m.).

**Tongue.**—Coated white or yellow; tip sore as if ulcerated; feels scalded. Taste sweet with ropy mucus; metallic, coppery, with salivation.

In France during the continental wars of the Empire, the blockade of the European ports by the English navy was so rigid, that Peruvian bark—the recognized specific for intermittent fever—was effectually excluded.

It was during this time that a vigorous search by the faculty for a substitute for bark, brought into experimental use many remedies, and among others Arsenic and Æsculus.

The *Bulletin des Science Médicales*, in 1808, Vol. II., p. 560, published a large number of cures obtained by the bark of the horse-chestnut. Dr. Ranque reports 43 cases; Dr. Cazin 2 cases of tertian and one of double tertian; and Dr. Lacroix in an epidemic of intermittent fever in the department of Loire et Cher, successfully treated over 200 cases with Æsculus alone.

## CLINICAL.

CASE.—A woman of 44 years presented herself at my office in the following condition: For fourteen months, every day at 4 P.M., paroxysm of cold without shivering, followed by heat and sweat; the paroxysm lasted altogether from four to five hours. During the paroxysm she suffered cruelly in the throat and could swallow nothing; it seemed to her as if the inside of her throat were rubbed with a live coal; she was thirsty and the difficulty of swallowing was so great that she could not drink; moreover, saliva flowed abundantly and her whole mouth was lined with mucus. Being interrogated, she told me that, in the interval of the paroxysms, her throat always hurt her, but in a less degree; she was constipated and sometimes suffered from hemorrhoids. The numerous physicians previously consulted were unaminous in attacking the intermittent with the antiperiodic, *par excellence*, Quinine, and always without effect. In consideration of the periodicity of the symptoms, the sore throat, the constipation, the hemorrhoidal affection, all pathogenetic effects of Æsculus, I gave this remedy 30th, and two doses of three globules each, sufficed to relieve the patient of all her sufferings.—A. CHARGE.

## ALUMINA.

**Characteristic.**—Adapted to spare, dry, thin subjects of scrofulous habit, who suffer from chronic diseases; dark complexion; anxious, mild, tearful disposition; constitutions with lack of vital heat; old people; hypochondriacs.

Dry, tettery, itching eruption, worse in winter (Petr.); intolerable itching of whole body when getting warm in bed (Sulf.); scratches until bleeds, which then becomes painful.

## ALUMINA.

Constipation; no desire for, and no ability to pass stool until there is a large accumulation; with great straining, must grasp the seat of closet tightly; stools hard, knotty, covered with mucus; or soft clayey, adhering to parts (Plat.); of nursing infants, from artificial food; inactive rectum.

Urine voided while straining at stool, or cannot pass it without such straining.

After menses; exhausted mentally and physically (Carb. an., Cocc.).

Leucorrhœa; acrid, profuse, running down to heels in large quantities, relieved by cold bathing.

**Aggravation.**—Generally in cold air; out-doors; on alternate days, while sitting.

**Amelioration.**—Generally in warmth; in mild weather; walking. *Alumina* and *Bryonia* are complementary.

**Type.**—Tertian.

**Time.**—Chilliness at 4 A.M., lasting till evening. Evening paroxysm from 5 to 8 P.M.

**Chill.**—*With great thirst; with nausea* (**Arn., Caps., Ign.**). Internally cold and chilly, with desire for warmth of stove without relief from heat (**Lach.**—relieved by heat of stove, **Ign.**), and stretching and bending of the limbs; *worse after warm drinks*, and *after eating warm soup* (after cold drinks, **Ars., Caps., Eup. perf.**). Chilliness of whole body, feet cold as ice the whole day, with heat of head, *external chilliness* and *external heat*, especially *dark redness of the cheeks*. Frequent repetition of *chills in the evening*, every other day. Chills near the warm stove. Violent chilliness in evening, especially feet and back, that could not get warm near stove. Chilly during the day, heat all night (chill lasting 12 hours, **Canth.**). Chill increased by slightest motion (**Acon., Bry.**—increased by uncovering, **Amm. m., Nux v., Sep.**).

**Heat.**—*Without thirst; heat, with anxiety at night, and sweat.* Heat in evening beginning in and spreading from face and head, frequently *only of right side of body*. Heat aggravated by motion (**Bry.**—lessened by motion, **Caps.**).

**Sweat.**—*At night, in bed, toward morning;* most profuse in face, *often only on right side of face* (**Nux v., Puls.**). Sweat upon every motion (**Bry., Sep.**), followed by cold shivers as if taking cold. Sometimes entire inability to sweat (**Hep.**).

**Tongue.**—Clean. Appetite good. Longing for fruit and vegetables. Longing for indigestible things, acids, chalk, charcoal, clean rags, coffee or tea grounds; always worse from eating potatoes, which disagree, cause colic. All irritating things: salt, vinegar, pepper, bread crumbs, immediately start cough. Aversion to meat (**Arn.**).

**Apyrexia.**—*Continual empty eructations which afford relief.* Great *lassitude of the whole body;* great exhaustion and inclination to lie down; unconquerable disposition to lie down.

If patient has had frequent attacks of painter's colic. Rarely indicated, but when required, chronic constitutional ailments will almost always be present. Often completes a cure begun by Bryonia, and should always be thought of as the next remedy if symptoms correspond.

## AMBRA GRISEA.

**Characteristic.**—Adapted to bilious or nervous-bilious temperaments; lean persons; children, especially young girls who are nervous, exitable, weak.

Ranula, with fetid breath.

Sleepnessness; after business embarrassment, must get up (**Act. rac.**).

Frequent ineffectual desire for stool which causes anxiety; at this time the presence of other persons becomes unbearable (while urinating, **Natr. m.**).

Metrorrhagia between menstrual periods at every little accident, as a longer walk than usual, or every hard stool.

Violent cough in spasmodic paroxysms, with eructations and hoarseness.

**Aggravation.**—Warm drinks; warm room; lying down; at night; too little sleep.

**Amelioration.**—After eating; cold air; cold food and drinks.

**Type.**—No periodicity.

**Time.**—In the forenoon. Fever, without chill, 7 to 8 P.M.

**Chill.**—Of *single parts of body*, with heat of face. Chill, with lassitude and sleepiness, relieved by eating (sweat lessened by eating, **Anac.**); chills before dinner. Skin of whole body, except face, neck and genitals, cold (ice cold genitals, **Sulf.**).

**Heat.**—In face and over the whole body every quarter of an hour, most violent from 7 to 8 o'clock in the evening.

**Sweat.**—Profuse night-sweat, worse after midnight, the body being warm. Sweat every morning, **worse on affected side** (**Ant. t.**). Profuse sweat of abdomen and thighs (during exercise).

Should not be given in the evening, apt to produce nightly aggravation.

## AMMONIUM MURIATICUM.

**Characteristic.**—Suitable to those who are fat and sluggish; or body fat but legs thin (see Lyc.).

Watery, acrid coryza, excoriating the lip; mouth and lips sore and excoriated (Natr. m.).

Constipation extremely obstinate; stools hard, crumbling, requiring great effort for expulsion (Magn. m.), with much flatulence.

During menses; bloody discharge from the bowels (Phos.); diarrhœa and vomiting (Amm. c.); neuralgic pains in the feet.

Blood seems in constant ebulition. Chills alternating with heat every half hour.

**Aggravation.**—From uncovering during fever paroxysm (**Nux v.**).

**Type.**—No periodicity.

**Time.**—3 till 4 A.M.—5, 6 and 7 P.M.

**Septimani.**—Chill and fever followed by profuse sweat every seventh day (**Cinch.**).

**Prodrome.**—Thirst; sleeplessness.

**Chill.**—Without thirst. Chilliness evenings after lying down, and *as often as she awakes*, lasting entire night. Violent shivering, without subsequent heat (without subsequent heat or sweat, **Bov.**). Chill running up the back; warm covering does not relieve the coldness. Chill with external coldness day, evenings and nights; *worse from uncovering, dares not uncover on account of chilliness* (**Nux v.**). *Chill alternating* **every half hour**, *with heat and bloated red face* (yellowish, mahogany-red, **Eup. perf.**). Severe pain in lumbo-sacral region.

**Heat.**—With thirst; over the whole body, with redness of face and a kind of stinging heat in skin, especially over whole chest (**Apis, Nitr. ac.**—itching over whole body, **Led., Petr.**).

Flushes of heat frequently coming on, always ending in sweat, which is most profuse in face, palms of hands and soles of feet.

**Sweat.**—Without thirst; day and night; following heat. Increased transpiration; every movement makes him sweat (**Bry., Sulf., Verat.** —when sitting quietly, **Staph.**). Sweat on the lower part of the body. Night-sweat, most copious after midnight and towards morning, in bed. Fever paroxysms begin with chilliness, then heat, and end with sweat.

# ANACARDIUM ORIENTALE.

**Characteristic.**—Adapted to ill-natured, nervous, hysterical persons, in whose diseases mental symptoms predominate.

Sudden loss of memory; everything appears as in a dream; patient much troubled about his forgetfulness. Hypochondriasis.

Disposed to be malicious, seems bent on wickedness; irresistible desire to curse and swear.

Suspects every one and everything around him; when walking he felt anxious as if some one were pursuing him; lack of confidence in himself and others; weakness of all the senses.

Strange temper; laughs at serious matters, and is serious over laughable things; thinks herself a demon; swears.

Sensation as of a hoop or band around the part (**Sulf.**).

**Type.**—Quotidian; tertian; quartan.

**Time.**—4 P.M. Afternoon. *Every P.M., at four o'clock, fever without chill* (**Lyc.**).

**Chill.**—Especially in the open air, relieved in the sunshine (**Con., Sec.**). Shivering over the back and whole body, as from cold water being thrown upon the person, with heat of face (**Rhus, Ant. t., Arn.**). Repeated icy cold creeping; feeling of chilliness of limbs, hands and feet, which causes trembling; internal chill even in a warm room; worse in open air. Shaking chill, with ill-humor and restlessness. Forehead cold and cheeks red. External heat with internal chill. Internal heat with cold sweat. Heat of left side only.

**Heat.**—From 4 P.M. till evening, daily *relieved by eating;* heat of upper part of the body; with hot breath, cold feet with internal shiverings; external heat, especially of face and palms; abdomen and knees weak; heat over whole body, but complains of being cold. If any thirst, between heat and sweat (between cold and hot stage, **Sabad.**).

**Sweat.**—Night-sweats; frequently waking up from sleep, with general sweat. At night he sweats on the *chest* and *abdomen*. Clammy sweat in the palms, especially the left. Sweat better by eating. *Sweats when sitting.* Dyspnœa and distressing shortness of breath (during chill, **Apis**).

**Tongue.**—Is white and rough; taste, like herring brine; *bitter taste after smoking.* Flat, offensive taste in the mouth. Apt to choke when eating or drinking.

In fevers of nursing children, which return every afternoon at four o'clock, Anacardium vies with Lycopodium; but the fever is not so severe in character, all stages being of a milder grade. *Child is very irritable, a slight offence or contradiction makes him excessively angry* (**Bry., Cham.**).

## ANGUSTURA.

**Characteristic.**—Very much fatigued, feels it most in the thighs.

Caries and very painful ulcers, which affect the bones and pierce them to the marrow, particularly if the patient has longing for coffee and a very touchy, sensitive mind; very susceptible, will not bear the slightest joke. Timid; dyspeptic.

Traumatic tetanus (**Hyper.**).

**Aggravation.**—From touching the affected part; 3 P.M., in afternoon.

**Type.**—Periodicity not marked.

**Time.**—3 P. M.—(**Apis, Ars., Chin. s.**)

**Cause.**—Fevers occurring in tropical countries; after travelling through swamps in a hot climate (**Ced.**).

**Chill.**—Violent chill every afternoon at 3 P.M. *Shivering with goose-flesh, without thirst,* for several days in succession. Severe cold sensation over back; cold hands, fingers and feet; drawing pain in elbows, knees and toes (pains in ankles and wrists, **Pod.**). Chill lasts half an hour. Creepings up the back, with restlessness extending to inner parts, causing trembling with warm lips without thirst. Coldness, followed by heat the same day; recurring now in the evening, then at noon, then in the morning, with thirst in the beginning of the fever, and vomiting of bile.

**Heat.**—Warmth of the whole body, except head, towards evening, so that she is unable to sleep again after 3 A.M. (worse at 3 A.M. and 3 P.M., **Thuya**). Cold cheeks. The heat ascends (**Sep.**). Flushes of heat with anxiety.

**Sweat.**—Perspiration at night in bed. Sweat in the morning; on the forehead.

## ANTIMONIUM CRUDUM.

**Characteristic.**—Gastric complaints from over-eating; stomach weak, digestion easily disturbed; thick milky-white coating on the tongue.

Young people disposed to obesity (Calc.). Old people with diarrhœa suddenly get costive; alternate diarrhœa and constipation (see Nux v.).

Child is fretful, peevish, cannot bear to be touched or looked at; sulky, does not wish to speak (Ant. t., Iod., Sil.).

Anxious, lachrymose mood, the slightest thing affects her (see Puls.). Irresistible desire to talk in rhymes or repeat verses.—Hering.

Disposition to abnormal growths of skin; finger nails do not grow as rapidly; crushed nails grow in splits, like warts, and with horny spots.

Large horny places (corns) on soles, which are very sensitive when walking, especially on stone pavements. When symptoms re-appear, they change locality, or go from one side of body to the other.

**Aggravation.**—After eating; cold bathing; sour wine or acids.

**Amelioration.**—During rest; in the open air.

**Type.**—Quotidian; double quotidian; tertian. Remittent of children.

**Time.**—12 M. or afternoon. *Sweat at same hour every other day.*

**Prodrome.**—Ushered in by gastric disturbances; with **great melancholy, sadness, and a woeful mood.**

**Chill.**—*Without thirst* (**Apis, Puls., Cinch.**). Violent shaking at noon; or chill in the afternoon with shivering in the back; chill with sweat at same time; chill and shivering over the back, feet cold as ice, with sweat on rest of body; **chilliness predominates (Meny.)**; even in a warm room, cold and chilly during the day (chill worse in warm room or near a stove, **Apis**—chill increased by external heat, **Ipec.**). Painful coldness of nose during inspiration, as if inhaling cold air. Great desire to sleep (wants to sleep during hot stage, **Apis**). Drawing pain in sacrum.

**Heat.**—When sweat sets in with the heat; great heat for an hour, then sweat ceases suddenly, followed by dry heat for two hours, or even all night. *Heat with sweat.* Great heat from the least exercise, especially in the sun. Heat at night, before midnight, with cold feet. During heat, pain in chest. Vomiting during the heat—(Natr. m.).

**Sweat.**—Sets in simultaneously with or immediately after the chill. (See **Pod**.) Sweat in the morning when awaking which causes shrivelling of tips of fingers (**Canch., Verat.**). Sweat which returns at precisely the same hour every other morning. Sweat alternating with chilliness, or vice versa. Sweat soon disappears, dry heat remaining.

**Tongue.**—Thickly coated; milky white; characteristic of Ant. crud. Taste bitter. *Great desire for pickles.* Saliva saltish. Hunger, which eating does not relieve.

**Pulse.**—Irregular; rapid, then slow; changing every few beats.

**Apyrexia.**—*Predominance of gastric symptoms* (**Ipec., Puls., Nux v.**). Want of appetite, nausea, vomiting, and bitter taste in mouth (**Ipec.**); tension and pressure in region of the stomach; belching with taste of ingesta, pain in bowels, with diarrhœa, or constipation; *aversion to food; longing for acids, particularly pickles;* (longing for salt, **Natr. m.**); *disgust for drink and food; increasing sweat.*

## Antimonium crud.

**Prodrome.**—Great sadness, and a woeful mood.

**Chill.**—Predominant, followed by sweat, then *heat;* or chill and sweat simultaneous; or chill and sweat, or sweat and heat, alternating.

**Tongue.**—*Thickly coated; milky white.* Diarrhœa or constipation. No thirst in any stage.

## Pulsatilla.

**Prodrome.**—Thirst and *diarrhœa at night.*

**Chill.**—*Heat* and *sweat* in usual order, but apt to run into each other. One-sided coldness. No two chills alike.

**Tongue.**—Coated with yellow mucus; feels sore, as if scalded. Diarrhœa. Thirst before chill.

Antimonium crudum will often relieve, where Pulsatilla or Ipecacuanha seem indicated and fail. One of the few remedies where sweat follows chill and is followed by heat. Gastric symptoms usually present; acts promptly and cures completely.

Relapses often occur from derangement of stomach. Quotidian or tertian fever with *loathing, nausea, vomiting, cutting in bowels and diarrhœa* or constipation (Puls., but no constipation.)

## CLINICAL.

In the spring of 1876, Ant. crud. did me good service in two cases of double quotidian, where there was much nausea and vomiting, with *tongue thickly coated white;* the algid stage being followed *by sweat with great heat for an hour,* when the sweating ceased, *dry heat remaining for two hours.* Puls. previously had failed to make any impression on the cases, while convalescence was established in twelve hours after the Ant. crud. was commenced.—A. L. FISHER, *N. A. J.*

I have found Ant. crud. an excellent remedy in remittent fever of children, with following symptoms: Child delirious: *drowsy, with nausea; hot and red face, tongue very white, and great thirst,* especially at night; does not like to be bathed; is fretful and peevish; *does not want to be looked at.*—E. B. NASH, *Am. Homœop. III.*, p. 161.

## ANTIMONIUM TARTARICUM.

**Characteristic.**—Adapted to torpid, phlegmatic constitutions: hydrogenoid (of Grauvogl). Intermittents from exposure in damp cellars or basements (Ars., Tereb.).

Child: clings to those around; wants to be carried; cries and whines if any one touches it; will not let you feel the pulse.

When patient coughs there appears to be a large collection of mucus in the bronchi, and it seems as if much would be expectorated but nothing comes up.

Nausea, vomiting and want of appetite in intermittents.

Nausea, vomiting and constipation, in remittents (Ant. c.).

Great sleepiness, or irresistible inclination to sleep, with nearly all complaints.

**Aggravation.**—In damp cold weather; in evening; lying down at night; motion; warmth.

**Amelioration.**—Cold open air; sitting upright; eructations; expectoration.

**Type.**—Quotidian; tertian; quartan. Apt to become remittent or typhoid. Epidemics of winter or early spring. *In tertian fever attacks anticipate several hours.*

**Time.**—9 A.M., severe rigor without shaking. **3 P.M.**, or evening at 6 P.M. *All periods;* no regularity.

## ANTIMONIUM TARTARICUM.

**Prodrome.**—Yawning and stretching (Cinch., Eup. perf.). When gaping, mouth remains open for a while, could not shut it.

**Chill** and **Heat,** *without thirst,* alternating during the day. (**Ars.** —chill and sweat, or sweat and heat alternating, **Ant. c.**) Chill as if cold water were dashed over one (**Rhus,** Opium), with goose-flesh, gaping, want of thirst; drowsiness following heat with dullness in head. Chill with trembling and shaking over whole body. Backache with the chill. He looks pale, and is so chilly on going into the open air that he trembles (chilly when going from open air into a room, **Ars.**—See **Rhus**). *Cold skin. Trembling and chilliness always from within outward. Short chill and long lasting heat, with somnolency and profuse sweat on forehead.* Chill, with external coldness, coming on at all times of the day, with somnolency; mostly with trembling and shaking. Chill lasting 45 minutes followed by vomiting, headache, heat, and thirst; after drinking, retching.

**Heat.**—*Violent short heat succeeding a long chill, aggravated by every motion* (feels chilly if he moves, **Nux v., Apis**). Thirst not constant during the hot stage, but marked between heat and sweat. Heat long and severe with much sweat, intense thirst and delirium, sometimes occurs in tertian type.

**Sweat.**—*Profuse all over;* may last all night; follows long after, in the afternoon during the sleep, or profuse sweat the following night, with increased secretion of urine. **Affected parts sweat profusely** (**Amb. g.**). Sweat often, *cold, clammy, sticky.* Worse while sweating, but rather better after (**Ipec.**).

**Tongue.**—**Characteristic,** *red edges,* or *red* and white in alternate streaks; papillæ red and *raised as in scarlatina;* tongue bright red and dry in the centre, covered with a thick, white, pasty fur. Food tasteless; tobacco has no taste. Desire for apples; acids (desire for juicy fruit, **Verat.**).

**Pulse.**—Much accelerated by slightest motion; strong and full during chill; feeble, slow and very weak as the heat passes off.

*During paroxysm, cannot keep his eyes open; irresistible sleepiness and deep stupefied sleep; when awake, hopelessness and despair.*

*Violent but not long-lasting heat succeeding a long chill, aggravated by every motion.*

*Long-lasting heat, after a short chill, with somnolency and sweat on the forehead.*—HERING.

**Apyrexia.**—The *gastric, rheumatic, soporous* character of the intermittents of Antimonium tart. will not fail to call our attention to this polychrest. In spring and autumn, especially with children, they are prone to take on a remitting type of fever, attended with nausea, vomiting, and drowsiness. Gastric symptoms are very pronounced, as in Antimonium crud. Nausea and vomiting may be present; if so, it is very prostrating. Weakness and exhaustion, with great depression of spirits. Weariness and lassitude with no appetite.

In some epidemics occurring in winter and early spring it often amounts to the *genus epidemicus;* especially when gastric and typhoid fevers predominate, or when every fever is inclined to become remittent or typhoid.

## APIUM VIRUS.

**Characteristic.**—Adapted to strumous constitution. Bilious, nervous temperament; women, especially widows; children and girls who though generally careful, become awkward and let things fall while handling them (Bov.).

Lachrymose disposition; cannot help crying; discouraged; despondent. Bag-like swelling under the eyes (over the eyes, Kali c.).

Great sensitiveness to touch (Bell., Lach.).

Pain: burning, stinging, sore; periodical, in sudden sharp paroxysms, suddenly migrating from one part to another (Kali b., Puls.).

Sudden, shrill, piercing screams while wakening or sleeping (Hellebore.).

Thirstlessness: Anasarca; ascites. Incontinence of urine with great irritation of the parts; can scarcely retain the urine a moment, and when passed, scalds severely. Frequent, painful, scanty, bloody urination.

**Aggravation.**—After sleeping (**Lach.**); closed, especially warm or heated rooms are intolerable. Worse from getting wet through (**Rhus**), but better from washing or moistening the part in cold water.

**Amelioration.**—Open air; cold water or cold bathing; uncovering.

**Apis** and **Natr. m.** are complementary.

**Type.**—Quotidian or double quotidian. Tertian most common. Congestive.

**Time.**—3 P.M. and 3 to 4 P.M. (4 P.M., **Lyc.**); 4 P.M., fever, *without chill;* 5 P.M., rarely, *then night and morning paroxysms.*

**Prodrome.**—Sudden vomiting.

**Chill, with thirst,** *always* (**Ign., Carb. v., Caps.**). Chill sudden, begins *in front of chest, abdomen, knees,* and runs down the back (reverse of **Eup. purp.**); chill **worse in a warm room**; from external heat (**Ipec.**). **Cannot bear heat of stove** (relieved by heat of stove, **Ign.**—relieved by external heat, **Ars.**); chilliness *renewed from the slightest motion* (chill increased by motion, **Caps.**—*cannot bear to move or be uncovered in any stage,* **Nux v.**). Chill, with *cold feet* and *fingers, heat of face* and *hands,* and *oppressed breathing* (during sweat, **Anac.**). **Oppression of chest as though patient would smother.** Falls into a *deep sleep* as the severity of the chill passes off, and breaks out with urticaria (urticaria before and during chill, **Hepar**—during heat and sweat, **Rhus**—during heat only, **Ign.**). Sensation of cold without external coldness of the skin; cold limbs and feet, with burning toes and burning cheeks.

**Heat.**—*Rarely with thirst;* heat, with inclination to uncover (**Acon., Sec.**); more or less violent headache and generally a continuous deep sleep (**Op.**); chilliness on moving or uncovering *during heat* (**Arn., Nux v.**). *Burning, hot, dry skin all over,* particularly felt in *abdomen, epigastrium* and *chest* and *hands; alternate dry and hot skin,* or cool in some places and *hot in others, with occasional spells of sweating.* **Great oppression and burning in the chest, with sensation of smothering.** Itching, burning nettle-rash, in this stage (**Ign., Hepar**). *The heat of the room is intolerable.* Sensation of heat through whole body, especially on chest and region of stomach, without heat of skin.

**Sweat.**—*No thirst in sweating stage. Sweat after trembling and fainting, then nettle-rash. Perspiration may alternate with dryness of the skin.* Sweating stage often absent, or of a light grade. Weak and trembling. Sleep, or sleepy.

"This stage is usually wanting, and is characteristic of Apis fever in old protracted cases."—CARROLL DUNHAM.

**Tongue.**—Clean in old cases. In acute attacks, dry, red, with a raw, sore, painful tenderness; does not care to talk or protrude it. *Swelling and burning of lips during entire paroxysm.* No appetite, nor desire for food; craves milk, which relieves.

**Apyrexia.**—Soreness and pain under ribs of left side, in region of spleen; great soreness of all the limbs and joints; feet swollen; urine scanty; restless; sleepless; urticaria and great debility. In old cases, badly treated by domestic and patent medicines. Natrum mur. often indicated if Apis fails to permanently cure. In either acute or chronic cases occurring as sequellæ of eruptive diseases.

In ascites: "*sensation in abdomen as if something would break, if much effort were made to void a stool.*"—GUERNSEY.

Chills and fever in seasons when the flies sting with unusual vigor. —HERING.

A very important anti-pyretic (in one of the most malarial countries) given according to Wolf in the third centesimal; but for two years in the one hundredth centesimal potency, they have seen results, such as they had not many years witnessed from any other homœopathic remedy against intermittent fever—at least as regards the rapidity of the result.—DRS. STERN AND MISKOLEZ.

Since a year 65 intermittent cases of various age and sex; 19 among these had been suppressed by large doses of Quinine, etc. No relapse ever occurred.—*Guiding Symptoms.*

## Apis.

**Time.**—3 P.M.; 3 to 4 P.M.
**Prodrome.**—Free from pain.

**Chill.**—*With thirst* always, in chill, absent in heat and sweat. Begins in *front of chest, abdomen, knees.* Oppression of chest as though he would smother. *Sleep* and *uticaria* as chill passes off.

**Heat.**—Oppression of chest, with burning, smothering. Heat worse in the chest, abdomen, epigastrium. Urticaria. Sleep.

**Sweat.**—This stage is usually wanting. Sleepy. Urticaria.

**Apyrexia.**—Soreness in spleen—in all limbs and joints; feet swollen; urine scanty; urticaria.

## Bryonia.

**Time.**—All periods.
**Prodrome.**—Stretching and drawing in the limbs; headache, vertigo, and *great thirst.*

**Chill.**—With *great thirst* in all stages. Begins in *tips of fingers, toes* and *on the lips.* Violent, dry, racking cough, with plueritic stitches in chest; stitching pain in right hypochondrium.

**Heat.**—Cough, with pleuritic stitches. Heat as if blood in the veins was burning; headache and vertigo.

**Sweat.**—Profuse, sour, easily excited by exercise. Thirsty. Irritable.

**Apyrexia.**—Constipation of dry, hard, lumpy stools. *Exceedingly irritable;* everything makes him angry.

## CLINICAL.

Apis cured a case of intermittent fever; the patient *sleeping during the fever;* thirst only in chill, wanting during *heat* and *sweat.* Chill aggravated by external heat.—C. PRESTON, in *H. M.*, p. 296.

Mr. H., aged 28, from cold, exposure, and sleeping in a wagon in Missouri, was taken September 28th, 1865, with a violent congestive chill at 8 A. M., which lasted one hour. He was very pale and faint, with much inward fever; pulse weak, 130; little thirst; inclined to diarrhœa; severe pain in small of back; complained most of *pressure* or a *stricture across the chest, exciting a cough;* tongue furred, but not heavily coated. The chill began by a violent fit of coughing, with *feeling of suffocation;* heat lasted some hours; *perspiration slight.* September 29th, was free from fever, but was restless, wakeful, and had some pain in the back.

Next A.M., 30th.—Severe chill at 7 A.M.; thought he was dying. His extremities were cold; nails purple; veins resembling dark lines; nose cold and pointed; features contracted; pulse fluttering and scarcely perceptible, and general appearance that of collapsed state of cholera. *Had great anguish from a smothering sensation; desired to be raised up to get breath,* but on raising was seized with paroxysm of coughing and retching, with faintness amounting to insensibility. Gave Verat.$^4$ in water, two teaspoonfuls every fifteen minutes, until chill subsided. In about an hour fever severe and continued all day, terminating with slight perspiration as before. Sac. lac. until 9 P.M., when I gave him Apis$^{100}$, and left another to be taken next A. M.

Oct. 1.—Here was a bad case of congestive chills, such as I think we seldom meet in practice. Two paroxysms had already occurred. We are told the patient never survives the third. It is folly, the allopaths say, to trust to anything but Quinine— give 10, 20, or even 30 grs.—prevent the next chill or your patient will certainly die. But the chest symptoms pointed clearly to Apis (there was not enough cold perspiration for Verat.—H. C. A.), and giving Sac. lac. during the day, I left another powder of Apis$^{100}$ to be taken at night; preferring to rely on *Homœopathy* and *my own judgment.* Next morning I saw him early. He had only a slight chill. A powder was given at night for five or six days. No return.—C. PEARSON, *U. S. M.* and *S. J.*, 1–208.

## ARANEA DIADEMA.

**Characteristic.**—Headache and confusion of the head, relieved by smoking, and ceases entirely in the open air.

Sudden violent pains in the teeth of the whole upper and lower jaws, at night, immediately after lying down.

**Aggravation.**—In cold rainy weather; damp dwellings; cold bathing.

**Amelioration.**—From tobacco smoke; in the open air.

**Type.**—Quotidian, tertian. Remarkable periodicity in every type.

**Time.**—At precisely same hour, *every day, or every other day* (Ced , Sab.). Great regularity of paroxysm.

**Cause.**—Rheumatic exposure: getting wet; working in the rain; working while standing in water (**Calc., Led., Rhus**).

**Chill.**—*Long-lasting,* often 24 hours; chill predominates. Constant chilly feeling, *worse on rainy, cold days; from bathing with cold water; from damp dwellings.* Chilly all the time, day and night, in midsummer. Bone pains for four weaks; fever attacks, consisting almost wholly of coldness. Chill without *heat, sweat* or *thirst. Headache, which ceases entirely in the open air.* Great exhaustion; lassitude. Painful feeling of coldness in lower incisors every day at same hour.

**Heat.**—Slight, preceded by chill. Evening heat, with fullness and heaviness in epigastrium as from a stone; qualmishness in pit of stomach, and heaviness of the thighs so that she is scarcely able to drag her limbs along. Forearms and hands so heavy that he imagines he cannot lift them. *This stage often wanting.*

**Sweat.**—Wanting.

**Tongue.**—Slightly coated, nauseous, bitter, relieved by smoking.

**Apyrexia.**—Clear. Spleen enlarged. Menses eight days too early, too strong and too copious.

The paroxysm of Aranea is often unattended by either heat or sweat, consisting only of coldness, which is persistent and severe, and *not relieved by anything.* It is usually without thirst in any stage; if any thirst, usually during the heat.

## CLINICAL.

A lady, 40 years old, slender, of erethic nature, hydræmic constitution, was attacked, in consequence of taking cold, with *a violent shaking chill, lasting uninterruptedly for twenty-four hours, without being followed by heat or sweat,* or any other affection. Internal application of warm things gave no relief. Diad.⁴″, a few globules in water, relieved the chill within half an hour. Perfectly well next day.—C. HEINIGKE, *H. Kl.,* 1870, p. 44.

A teamster, 43 years old, 6 feet, 2 inches in height, and well developed, never been sick before, slept on some straw on the bar-room floor in Frankfurt, on a winter night. In the morning *felt stiff in his limbs, tired and sick.* Chill began at 7 P.M., *and lasted till precisely* 8 *in the morning, every day at same hour, without heat or sweat*, with cough, loss of appetite, sleeplessness, and great exhaustion, which distressed him most because it interfered with his occupation. Being yet unskilled in Homœopathy, and not having the least confidence in it in fever and ague, I gave him two grain doses of Quinine every two hours at first, then every hour during the day, until he had taken forty powders without the least improvement; on the contrary, his general weakness had increased. I now consulted the original provings, and found that according to the law of similarity, *Aranea diadema* must be the remedy. He received five drops of second dec. attenuation every hour. Next day the patient exclaimed, "Now you have hit the right medicine; after the second hour I felt warmth again in my whole body, and the first time for three weeks I slept some hours at night again, without any chill." The cure was complete in six days, and for seventeen years he had no relapse.—GRAUVOGL, p. 204.

Like many of our colleagues of the present day, Grauvogl's lack of confidence in Homœopathic treatment of fever and ague (in his early investigations) was only equaled by his imperfect knowledge (at that time) of the true curative sphere of Quinine in the same disease. Here was a fever with *chill prolonged* and *predominant; heat and sweat absent.* It could never be cured by Quinine, which has all three stages, but *particularly heat and sweat*, prominently developed. Possibly, owing to its rheumatic character, Quinine would not seem even to suppress it and there certainly was enough given (80 grs.) to fairly test its curative power.

## ARNICA MONTANA.

**Characteristic.**—Hydrogenoid constitution. Dark hair; rigid muscles. Plethoric; red face. Especially adapted to those who remain long impressed by even slight mechanical injuries.

Nervous, cannot stand pain; whole body over-sensitive (Cham., Coff., Ign.); sore bruised feeling all through the body, as if beaten.

Everything on which he lies, seems too hard; complains constantly of it and keeps moving from place to place, in search of a soft spot (must move continually to obtain relief from the pain, Rhus.—See Bapt.).

Heat of upper part of body; coldness of lower.

The face, or head and face alone is hot, while the body is cool.

## ARNICA MONTANA.

Diseases of traumatic origin, the muscular fibre being chiefly involved.

Unconscious; when spoken to answers correctly but unconsciousness and delirium at once return (falls asleep in the midst of a sentence, **Bapt.**).

Fears being touched or struck by persons coming near him.

Cannot walk erect on account of a bruised sore feeling in pelvic region.

Tendency to small painful boils, one after another; extremely sore (small boils in crops, **Sulph.**).

**Aggravation.**—At rest, when lying down; from wine.

**Amelioration.**—From contact, motion.

**Type.**—Tertian; quartan. CONGESTIVE. Malaria intermittens.

**Time.**—Not characteristic; usually 4 A.M.; *afternoon or evening.*

**Prodrome.**—Thirst for large quantities of cold water (**Eup. perf.**). Much yawning and stretching; drawing pain as if in the periosteum; drinking refreshes (**Natr. m.**).

**Chill.**—With thirst, and, if he drinks a great deal, vomits afterwards (**Ars.**). Chill, as if cold water were poured over him. (**Rhus**—as if cold water were dashed over him, **Ant. t.**). Chill with **pain in muscles of back and extremities as if bruised; aching in bones** (**Natr. m., Rhus**); *soreness of the whole body* (whole body feels sore, **Bapt.**). Chill *felt most severely in* PIT OF STOMACH. *Chill after every sleep; with heat and redness of one cheek;* with burning of head alone, or *face alone, rest of body being cold.* Internal chill with external heat (**Ars., Thuya**). Chilliness on one (right) side; on side on which he lies. **Chilly, with heat and redness of one cheek. Shivering over the whole body and the head, at same time heat in the head and redness and heat in the face,** *accompanied by a coolness of the hands, and a feeling as of the hips, the back and anterior surface of the arms being bruised. Morning, chill while in bed;* begins before she rises and lasts four hours. Chilly from the slightest movement of the bed-clothes (**Acon., Rhus**—constant desire to be covered up, **Nux v.**).

**Heat.**—*Thirst* continued, but less than during chill, except early in the morning, when it is violent. Dry, general heat, with *indifference, stupor* and such *weakness,* that when he attempts to sit up he faints

ARNICA MONTANA.

(**Acon.**). During heat, *slightest lifting of bed-clothes, or even moving in bed, makes him chilly* (**Apis, Nux v., Rhus,** same in all stages of paroxysm). *Great internal heat, with coldness of hands and feet.* **The heat becomes intolerable to him** (**Apis, Puls.**), *and he tries to uncover himself, but upon uncovering he feels chilly.* Dry heat over the whole body after waking early in the morning. Burning heat in one spot, which is cold to the touch; alternate heat or coldness here and there over the entire body.

**Sweat.**—*Sour, fetid, offensive,* like *mouldy earth;* in old cases, sometimes cold and clammy. The exhalations smell sour; the night-sweat is sour. Worse when sweating (**Ant. c., Ipec.**). Partial sweat on front of body; on plantar surface of hands and forearms. Headache (which begins in hot stage) and soreness continue, but pain and drawing in the periosteum, which occurs before the chill, disappear gradually (*all pains disappear with sweat,* **Natr. m.**).

**Tongue.**—*Never clean.* Dry, yellow, or dirty white coating, and often, in acute cases, with a brown streak down the middle. **Breath sour, fetid.** Taste *bitter,* **putrid, of rotten eggs.** Longing for alcoholic drinks; acids. Repugnance to food.

**Apyrexia.**—Headache, *soreness and bruised feeling of muscles* continue; **eructations tasting like rotten eggs.** *Yellow face; bitter taste; aversion to meat;* and, especially in chronic cases, debility and aversion to exercise. The apyrexia is not marked in recent attacks, but is always a characteristic in chronic cases where large quantities of Quinine have been taken, then the soreness and bruised feeling are always indicative.

All three stages, chill, heat and sweat are well marked; and in each stage the same characteristic of the remedy is usually found.

### Arnica.

**Prodrome.**—Drawing pains as if in the periosteum.

**Thirst.**—For large quantities of cold water, which refreshes him.

**Chill.**—*With thirst,* pain in muscles of back and extremities, as if *bruised;* great soreness of whole body.

**Heat.**—*Less thirst,* but increased

### Eup. perf.

**Prodrome.**—Pain in back and bones of extremities, as if broken.

**Thirst.**—He cannot drink enough, but drinking hastens chill, and produces nausea.

**Chill.**—*With thirst,* but drinking causes nausea. Headache, with intense pain in back and bones, *as if broken.*

**Heat.**—*Less thirst,* but increased

soreness of flesh; must lie down, yet bed feels too hard; he cannot find a soft place and keeps constantly changing position in search of one.

**Sweat.**—Generally absent in recent attacks. In old cases, sour, and offensive.

**Apyrexia.**—Bruised feeling and soreness continue through every stage, and persist during apyrexia.

cephalalgia and bone pains. *Vomiting of bile before heat begins* (Lyc., is sour).

**Sweat.**—Generally absent, scanty if any. Headache continues for several hours after fever is gone; sweat relieves all pains except cephalalgia (all pains, Natr. m.).

**Apyrexia.**—Bone pains begin before the chill, but disappear with disappearance of sweat. None in apyrexia. Loose cough; night-sweats.

The "key note" of Arnica is the same in intermittent fever as in all other diseases (Quinine druging always on additional indication), viz.: **Bruised, sore, weary; great weakness, and must lie down in consequence, yet bed feels too hard; hence frequent change of position in search of a soft place, which may cause pain.** In old cases, where Arnica is indicated, the symptoms of apyrexia should be carefully studied.

In the Materia Medica Pura, Hahnemann recommends Arnica as a remedy, that in its pathogenesis corresponds with the Quinia cachexia; and clinical experience for many years has confirmed his observation. Arnica is probably more frequently indicated in cases maltreated with Quinine than any other remedy; and here lies its chief value in the treatment of intermittent fever. It is also a fact, that in acute cases, where Arnica is indicated, relapses are more frequent perhaps than with any other indicated remedy. It apparently antidotes the previous mal-treatment, but some other remedy is required to complete the cure. The patient does not feel well, but can scarcely tell why, and in four or five days has another paroxysm. This paroxysm, however, will differ materially from the preceding ones, Arnica having apparently paved the way for Apis, Arsenicum or Natrum muriaticum (which follow Arnica well) to complete the cure. Has been recommended for "congestive chills," but I can find no case in our literature treated with it.

## CLINICAL.

A youth of 18, tall and well formed, had chills, and had been under allopathic treatment for several months. Carefully selected remedies failing, inquiry was made for hidden cause, when it was found that six months before, he had received an injury in the back (dorsum) by a fall from a wagon. In every access of fever *the seat of the injury became painful.* Arn. ³⁰ in water, every six hours, relieved the chills at once. —C. P. JENNINGS, *Med. Ind.*, VII.—257.

Patient, a lady, suffered for many months with tertian ague, temporarily suppressed by Quinine. Appetite failed and grew continually weaker. She complained of *soreness of the scalp and of the muscles generally*, and a cough that occasioned much distress on account of *soreness of the chest and pectoral muscles*. Arnica in drop doses, for two days, at intervals of two hours. Fully recovered in ten days.—A. E. SMALL, *U. M.* and *S. J.*

Mathias Novak, aged 23 years, had a daily fever for nine days, which began in the morning by hard chill, followed by a violent heat and abundant sweat. Mediocre thirst during chill, but great during heat. First attack, vomited during chill and complained of pains in epigastrium; had no appetite, *dislike and horror for meat*, which he said would increase his fever. Arnica⁶, two doses, cured in three days.— "M. K.," *Gazette Homœop.*, VIII, 234, 1836.

Arnica⁶ *cured* a quartan fever. Paroxysm every four days, generally in the afternoon or evening. *Violent thirst before the chilliness*, and until the heat set in, when the thirst abated. Aching pain in the anterior part of the vertex. Headache during the apyrexia, yellowish complexion, bitter taste in the mouth.—*Clinique Homœop., Pr. Com.* 1, p. 179.

## ARSENICUM ALBUM.

**Characteristic.**—Great prostration, with rapid sinking of the vital forces. Fainting.

The disposition is:

*a.* Depressed, melancholic, despairing, indifferent.

*b.* Fearful, restless, anxious, full of anguish.

*c.* Irritable, sensitive, peevish, easily vexed.—Dunham.

Burning pains, the parts burn like fire. Excessive anxiety; great anguish; extreme restlessness; fear of death. Burning thirst, without special desire to drink; the stomach does not seem to tolerate, because it cannot assimilate cold water; it is wanted but he cannot drink it.

Great thirst for cold water; drinks often but little at a time; eats seldom but much. Teething children are pale, weak, fretful and want to be carried rapidly.

## ARSENICUM ALBUM.

Diarrhœa after eating or drinking; stool scanty, dark color, offensive odor, followed by great prostration.

Cannot rest in any place; changing his position continually; wants to go from one bed to another, and lies now here, now there.

Rapid emaciation, with cold sweat and great debility (see Verat.). Excessive exhaustion from least exertion.

**Aggravation.**—After midnight (1 to 2 A.M.); from cold; cold drinks or food; when lying on the affected side or with the head low.

**Amelioration.**—From heat in general.

**Type.**—Quotidian; tertian; quartan; double tertian and quartan. Anticipating (Bry., Cinch., Nux v.). Every fourteen days. Yearly (Lach., Natr. m.). Irregular, both in type and stage (Nux v.). Remitting and relapsing both tend to typhoid and typhus, especially after abuse of Quinine.

**Time.**—All periods—*mostly afternoon paroxysms*, 1 to 2 P.M.; 12 to 2 A.M.; 3 to 6 P.M.; 5 P.M.; 12 M. *Every fourteen days* (Calc. c., Cinch., Puls.). *Anticipates,* one hour every other day.

Yearly return of complaints (Carb. v., Sulf., Thuya).

Fever without chill—2 A.M.; 4 P.M.; 10 P.M.

Afternoon intermittents of nursing children, *without chill, must be covered,* and *very thirsty; fever lasting all night.*

**Prodrome.**—"Sleepiness night before paroxysm."—H. V. MILLER.

*Yawning and stretching; malaise; debility; weakness;* headache; vertigo; *great weariness and inclination to lie down;* slight creepings over the back after drinking; cutting pain in chest and bowels like knives, and watery diarrhœa; shuddering. Every morning stretching of limbs, gaping, emptiness in head, anxiety, thirst, and immediately after drinking, chilliness and crawling.

**Chill.**—*Without thirst; irregularly developed; never clearly defined; simultaneously, or alternating with heat; mingling of heat and chilliness;* all ameliorated by external warmth (Ign.—*aggravated* by external heat, **Apis, Ipec.**). Irregular chills at any time of day. *Shuddering when walking in the open air.* Generally little if any thirst during chill; if thirsty, *frequent drinking but little at a time,* but drinking increases the chilliness and causes shuddering, nausea and vomiting (drinking hastens and aggravates chill and causes nausea, **Eup. perf.**

—causes headache, **Cimex**—every drink causes shivering and chill, **Caps.**); oppression of the chest (**Apis**); coldness of abdomen (**Men.** blue nails and lips (**Nux v.**); tastelessness of food; shuddering without thirst, worse in the open air. *Internal chill, with external heat and red cheeks;* coldness of body and dryness of the skin; burning heat of skin, cold to the touch; headache.

Coldness of the whole body; pale, sunken face; very sickly appearance; lips pale, rigor, pains in limbs, back and chest; breathing impeded, restless, trembling.

*Crawling in the evening, with stretching of limbs and anxious restlessness. Chill gradually increasing to shaking rigor.*

Concomitants of chill: colic and nausea, diarrhœa, unconsciousness, drawing, tearing in limbs, thighs feel as if beaten, cramps and contraction in chest, difficult breathing, desire to urinate and frequent urination; hunger.

With the shivering and coldness, aggravation of other complaints. Coldness and chilliness renewed after drinking and after eating.

"Chill in forenoon not relieved by anything; external coldness, with cold, clammy sweat."—HERING.

Chill or chilliness without thirst; if there be thirst during chill except for hot drinks, do not give Arsenic.—H. N. GUERNSEY.

**Heat.**—The hot stage of the fever is *intense, long lasting, dry, burning* and *pungent to the touch,* with *inclination to uncover* (**Apis, Sec.**) and **insatiable thirst for cold water;** *drinks little and often, with vomiting after drinking several times.* Internal, burning, dry heat at night, must be uncovered. Burning heat as if *hot water were poured over one,* or as if *hot water were coursing through the blood-vessels* (**Bry., Rhus**). Oppressed breathing (**Apis**); **great restlessness,** and pressing, burning pain in region of the spleen. Burning pain in stomach and bowels. **During chill and heat, aggravation of previously existing symptoms.** Heat following the chill is *dry, burning, unbearable,* lasts three or four hours, with painful pressure and tension in both hypochondria; fulness in epigastrium; pressing pain in forehead; *restlessness, anxiety and unquenchable thirst;* sometimes a great desire for acids and acid drinks.

**Sweat.**—This stage is as variable as that of chill—*with* **unquenchable thirst for large quantities of cold water** (**Cinch.**), *which causes vomiting.* Sweat, with cessation of all the previous symptoms (**Natr. m.**—of all except headache, which is increased, **Eup. perf.**).

Sweat; sometimes *offensive and sour smelling.* Sweat during first sleep. or during entire night; **cold, clammy sweat.** *Sweat with excessive thirst.* Sweat with thirst, coming on *several hours after the heat,* or *what is oftener the case, there is no sweat at all, the dry heat continuing all night.* **After the paroxysm**—*with or without sweat*—**great weakness and prostration** *and a desire for stimulants, wine or coffee.* There is more headache than in the hot stage, unless there be copious sweat (most intense in hot stage, **Natr. m.**). **Drinks large quantities in sweat; little and often in chill and sweat.**

With the various stages of the fever always appear other symptoms.

**Tongue.**—Sides furred with red streak down the middle (**Ant. t.**) and red tip; yellowish-white; brown; bluish. Water tastes bitter; desire for acids; brandy. Aversion to food (aversion to meat, **Arn.**).

**Pulse.**—Weak, small, easily compressible. Very frequent in morning, slower at night. Pulsations through whole body (**Natr. m.**).

**Apyrexia.**—*Never clear of symptoms. Great debility;* lassitude; weakness of all the limbs and constant inclination to lie down (**Arn.**). Face *pale, sunken, sallow, clay-colored, bloated;* dull aching in region of liver and spleen, painful on pressure, with sensation as if swollen. Abdomen bloated (**Apis**); *fœtid, watery, diarrhœic stools,* which are *very debilitating;* urine scanty and turbid. Constant desire for acids or something refreshing. The patient is constantly chilly and must be in a warm room. *General anæmic appearance* (**Eup., Cinch., Ferr.**). Skin pale, often covered with cold perspiration. *Icterus after the fever. Fevers contracted at sea-shore watering places,* coming on in the autumn, or " wintered over " and not coming on until spring (**Gels.**).

" The paroxysm is not complete. One (especially the cold) stage is generally wanting."—CARROLL DUNHAM.

The following admirable analysis of the indications for Arsenic in intermittent fever is by Dr. Wurmb in *Homœopathische Clinische Studien,* 1, p. 179.

" Arsenic is one of those few drugs whose action is distinguished not alone by its intensity, but equally by its extent; it involves the entire organism. Every system, every organ of the body, every nervous filament, is so subjected to its powerful influence that we are not able to say which of its symptoms are primary, which are secondary, and where the focus of its action chiefly lies. We see the entire nerve-life attacked in all directions, from the slightest excitement to the most violent irritation; from the mere sensation of weakness to actual paralysis, and then we see, likewise, another series of disturbances arise from its action, which advance in regular gradation from the most inconsiderable acceleration of the circulation to the most violent febrile storm; from the slightest irregularity in the vegetative sphere to a cachectic dyscrasia; yes, even to decomposition and destruction of the organic substance.

In addition, we remark the striking similarity between the symptoms of chronic arsenical poisoning and those of the intermittent cachexy, as well as the fact that Arsenic has the property of causing the periodical recurrence of symptoms in so high a degree as to surpass in this respect all other drugs; in a word, no other drug known to us has such a power of affecting so intimately and so variously those organs that are especially affected in intermittent fever, and none corresponds so well as Arsenic does to all the requirements of a remedy for intermittent.

"Arsenic is indicated in cases which are distinguished not only by weakness in the vital power and deterioration of the organic substance, but also and at the same time by symptoms of excitation of the circulation, or of the nervous system alone, or of both together. Again, it seems to be more especially indicated the more malignant the influence from which the disease has sprung. Marsh-miasm is the chief of these influences; in this originate the most serious and most dangerous cases of fever, and in these Arsenic is often the only remedy that will rescue the patient. Again, the longer the disease has lasted, the more is Arsenic generally indicated, because the more deeply have the organs and tissues been affected, the more nearly has the patients' condition approached that known as the intermittent cachexia, and which so nearly resembles the arsenical cachexia. Especially is this the case when the liver and the spleen have become swollen.

"The intermittents which find their homœopathic remedy in Arsenic present in their paroxysms the following peculiarities: The paroxysms are general, violent and of long duration; the stages are either distinctly developed and equally proportioned to each other, or else, as is most frequently the case, one of the stages is absent or is very feebly present; if the latter be the case, it is generally the cold stage which fails, and the hot is all the more violent. The more intense the heat, the longer it continues, the higher the degree of development of the accompanying excitement in the vascular system, and the more burning and insatiable the thirst, the better is Arsenic indicated. The sweating stage may be altogether wanting, or the perspiration may be very copious; it breaks out generally several hours after the hot stage and lasts a long time.

"With the paroxysms are associated many distressing accessory symptoms, which are connected, some with the disturbances in the nervous system, some with those of the vascular system, *e. g.*, spasms, pains, delirium, paralyses and the anguish and restlessness that are so characteristic of Arsenic.

"The apyrexia is not pure, but is disturbed by symptoms of the most various kinds; restlessness, sleeplessness, spasms, digestive disorders, feeling of weakness and general prostration, and it is especially characteristic for Arsenic that after every paroxysm there is a notable increase of prostration."

## Arsenicum.

**Time.**—Characteristic; 1 to 2 P.M.—12 to 2 A.M.

Anticipates.

"Sleepy, night before the paroxysm."—H. V. MILLER.

**Prodrome.**—*No thirst.* Headache, with vertigo and *pale face;* pain in bowels and watery diarrhœa.

**Chill.**—Irregular; mingling of heat and chilliness; chills alternating with heat; *ameliorated* by external heat. *Great thirst;* drinks little and often.

**Heat.**—*Dry, burning, intense, as if hot water were coursing through the blood vessels.* Great restlessness; uncovering brings relief. *Insatiable thirst;* drinks little and often.

**Sweat.**—*Rarely occurs,* light if any; but cold and clammy. *Unquenchable thirst* for *large quantities* of cold water, with vomiting after drinking.

**Tongue.**—Sides furred, with red streak down the middle. Tongue brown; blue; desire for acids; *aversion to food.*

## Cinchona.

**Time.**—Not characteristic. 5 A.M.—5 P.M.

Anticipates or postpones.

"Restless sleep, night before the paroxysm."—HAHNEMANN.

**Prodrome.**—*Great thirst.* Canine hunger, headache, with *flushed face* and palpitation of the heart.

**Chill.**—General, violent chill over whole body, with icy cold hands and feet; external heat *increases* chill. *No thirst during chill.*

**Heat.**—*With distended veins and congestive headache,* often *delirium.* Wants to uncover, *but chilly when uncovered. Rarely any thirst;* if any, at close of heat. Hunger instead of thirst.

**Sweat.**—*Debilitating; profuse.* On being covered, he sweats profusely all over. *Sweating during sleep. Thirst returns;* large quantities, or little and often.

**Tongue.**—White; yellow. Thick, dirty coating; taste too acute; food tastes bitter; too salt; *hungry.*

5

**Pulse.**—Weak, small and easily compressible. Frequent in morning; slower at night.

**Apyrexia.**—*Great weakness and prostration;* pale, sunken face; fetid, watery diarrhœa; abdomen bloated; great desire to lie down.

**Pulse.**—Hard; full; quick. Uncommon distension of blood-vessels.

**Apyrexia.**—*Sweats easily; exhausting night-sweats;* pain in both hypochondria; complete loss of appetite.

Arsenicum is often given (by some homœopaths) in alternation with Cinchona or some of its alkaloids in this disease; but with the above comparison, to those who differentiate, there ought to be little danger of confounding them. *Where one is indicated the other never is.* Fowler's solution, and massive doses of the lower triturations of Arsenicum, frequently repeated, are wholly unnecessary in the treatment of intermittent fever. If the remedy be indicated, the potentized drug will effect a more prompt and radical cure.

Arsenicum is probably more often indicated than any other remedy, in the so-called "dumb ague," "masked intermittent," so often met with after abuse of Quinine. Also, in the afternoon intermittents of nursing children—who never have chills, and from whom it is impossible to obtain many indications—it frequently suffices to complete a cure. The general constitutional symptoms are guiding.

## Clinical.

Chill without thirst; at 10 or 11 A.M., shaking chill, felt as though water was running down the back, *blue surface, shrunken skin.* Fever burning, great thirst, drinking little at a time, but often; marked prostration, dry parched tongue, little or no sweat, irritable and melancholy. Ars.$^{30}$, cured.—T. D. STOW, *N. Y. Trans.*, 304.

Mr. B., æt. 69, treated allopathically for six weeks. Has now slight chills or none at all, beginning *at midnight*, followed by heat or *chilliness and heat in rapid succession;* great thirst, drinks little at a time; *oppression of chest* and *short breathing;* some time after, heat and sweat, when thirst is increased and *drinks large quantities* of water. Ars.$^{3}$, cured in four days.—H. M. BROWN, *H. M.*, Aug., '72.

Quotidian fever. Afternoon; anticipates one hour each day; first chill, then heat, then perspiration with heat.

*Before chill*, pricking of the nose, grinding of the teeth, stretching, sour eructations and coryza. *During the chill*, hands, feet and nose cold; thirst, yawning, blueness under the eyes and pain in the stomach. *During heat and perspiration*, more of these symptoms were present. Stools slimy; urine of a dark red color. Ars.$^{200}$, cured.—B. F. JOSLIN, "*Homœopathic News*," 1855.

Tertian intermittent fever: first chill, then heat, then perspiration; thirst during the whole paroxysm; *drinks often, but little at a time;* during the cold stage, nausea; pain in the small of the back and lower limbs; *tongue blue; great debility after the paroxysm.* Ars. cured.—B. F. JOSLIN, "*Homœopathic News,*" 1854.

Mr. H., æt. 25, had intermittent fever, early in September, was checked by Chin. sulph. only to return and again be suppressed by same until December, when paroxysm presented following symptoms; *chill* returning every day two hours earlier; during the chill, pain in the small of the back and all the bones (Eup. perf.); much thirst, drinking very often and little at a time; vomiting of the injesta and bile; chill lasts two hours and is followed by *heat* with continued thirst; less pain in the back and bones. No vomiting, but violent headache in the whole head; heat lasts three hours, the *headache continuing four hours after heat has passed off.* During entire paroxysms, but more particularly during heat, *great restlessness.* During the night, he sleeps well, but perspires profusely—perspiration sour and offensive. During *apyrexia,* dullness in the head; great debility; urine diminished; but appetite good. Gave him Ars.$^{8m}$ after the fever. Next day, paroxysm one and a half hours earlier; no medicine. Next day, paroxysm one hour earlier; less severe, no vomiting, no headache. Following day, at same hour but very slightly; returned no more.—A. LIPPE, *A. J. H. M. M.,* 1–224.

Mr. D., laborer, living in marshy region, had two chills before I saw him; forenoon every other day; anticipating. Before chill, diarrhœa, stools thin, bloody, frequent, with burning in the stomach, aggravated by drinking water. Chill *not clearly developed; mixed with heat;* with *anguish, thirst, headache,* and *restlessness.* In heat, which was very great and long-lasting, there was *great prostration,* increase of thirst and headache, stools smaller, more frequent, and contain much blood. *Very restless,* with *fear of dying.* Sweat not very profuse; but great relief of pains and diarrhœa. In apyrexia, weak, nervous, cannot walk without help. Ars.$^{200}$ in water every three hours during apyrexia. No return of chills or diarrhœa. Well in four days.—A. L. FISHER, *A. J. H. M. M.,* Vol. V., p. 177.

N. J., æt. 30, hitherto strong and muscular, had been exposed, eight weeks before on the Isthmus of Panama; and three weeks after he left Panama, had chill, fever and vomiting, which was suppressed by Quinine to enable him to travel. Three days before I saw him, an unusually severe chill, followed by high fever, and alternations of chill and fever, with severe constitutional symptoms, which continued notwithstanding large and repeated doses of Quinine. He had lost thirty pounds in weight during last month. Face of a dusky, red hue, hot and dry, eyes injected, pupils contracted, with a very restless, anxious expression. Patient had constant thirst, only a single swallow at a time. Stomach excessively irritable—drink rejected as soon as taken;

a profound disgust for food of all kinds. Tongue covered with thick, brownish coat, and felt dry, though not actually so. When protruded, trembled and was moved involuntarily back and forth, in spite of efforts to keep it still; hands trembled excessively; indescribable weakness and prostration; uncontrollable restlessness, literally impossible to remain in one position—the recumbent posture was impossible; alternations of chill and heat, partial and fugitive in character, each lasting about fifteen minutes; heat yielding to partial, clammy sweat, again succeeded by chill. Dyspnœa, and short, dry cough. The spleen much enlarged. Last two nights, unable to sleep at all exeedingly restless and uncomfortable, tormented by thirst. Pulse 140, quick, small, wiry. Head confused, sensorium much clouded, it being difficult to get definite answers to my questions; had vague apprehensions of severe illness. Any one conversant with Panama fever could not fail to recognize the gravity of above, nor could there be any doubt of the remedy required. The indications being so clear, and the severity of the disease so undoubted, I deemed this a very fair case for the demonstration of the power of the high potencies. At 4 P.M. I gave him Arsenicum$^{200}$, to be taken dry, a powder every four hours.

The following day, better; had slept three hours the night before; stomach not irritable, tolerated beef tea and toast; chills and heat once in four hours, lasting for a few moments only. No cough or dyspnœa. Prostration still excessive, restlessness moderate, intelligence good, tongue and hands less tremulous.

Arsenicum$^{200}$ every six hours.

Third day: A better night, no chills or heat to day, strength increasing; no restlessness.

Arsenicum$^{200}$ every eight hours.

The fourth day: Slept well last night; feels like walking out; appetite good, tongue clean. Saccharum lactis.

Fifth day: Feels quite well and strong. Next day he resumed his journey. No relapse.—DUNHAM, *Science of Therap.*, p. 479.

"There are diversities in the form in which intermittent fever appears in different persons and in different epidemics; that these forms require different remedies, and that thus there is a form capable of being cured by Arsenic, and by nothing else; a form capable of being cured by Quinine, and by nothing else; and so of other drugs. In this view, when a case of intermittent fever presents itself, the question can never be: Is Arsenic a better remedy for this disease than Quinine is? Does it offer greater chances of a cure? There can be no better or worse. The question is between right or wrong; suitable and not suitable. Which remedy corresponds to this particular case, and is, therefore, indicated in it?—DUNHAM, *Lectures*, II., p. 201.

## BAPTISIA TINCTORIA.

**Characteristic.**—Lymphatic temperament.
Dysentery of old people; diarrhœa of children, especially when very offensive.
Great prostration, with disposition to decomposition of fluids.
Ulceration of mucous membranes; exhalations and discharges, offensive, fetid (Psor.)—breath, stools, urine, sweat.
Stupor; falls asleep while being spoken to, in the midst of his answer (when spoken to answers correctly, but delirium at once returns, Arn.).
Cannot go to sleep, because she cannot get herself together; feels scattered about, and tosses about to get the pieces together; thought she was three persons and could not keep them covered.
Face: flushed, dusky; dark red, with a stupid, besotted expression.
Can swallow liquids only; the least solid food gags (can swallow liquids only but has aversion to them, Sil.).
In whatever position the patient lies, the parts rested upon feel sore and bruised (Arn.).
**Type.**—Quotidian; double quotidian; intermittent or remittent; during epidemic typhoid; hot weather in autumn. Prone to become typhoid.
**Time.**—Every A.M. at 11. *Chill, fever and sweat every afternoon.*
**Prodrome.**—Great languor; wants to lie down. General malaise; feels weak, tremulous, as after severe illness; sore, bruised.
**Chill.**—*Chilly all day; whole body feels sore, bruised* (**Arn.**). Chills; up and down the back (**Gels.**); over the back, and limbs; over the back while sitting by the fire; on going into the open air; with severe aching in muscles of whole body.
**Heat.**—Whole surface hot and dry, with occasional chills, mostly up and down the back (**Ars.**). Flushes of heat; from small of back in all directions (**Gels.**); over the face; over the whole body; at 3 A.M. with feeling as if sweat would break out. Uncomfortable burning all over surface, especially face, as if sweat would break out; had to move to a cool part of the bed. Heat at night; burning in legs prevent sleep; limbs hot, but feel cold.
**Sweat.**—Fetid, frequent, but not profuse perspiration.

**Tongue.**—White, with red edges; brown streak down centre. Taste flat or bitter; cannot digest food.

**Apyrexia.**—Indescribable sick feeling all over. Generally weak, restless, uneasy; can confine himself to nothing; wants to be continually moving from place to place.

## BARYTA CARB.

**Characteristic.**—Especially adapted to complaints of first childhood; scrofulous, dwarfish children, who do not grow (children who grow too rapidly, **Calc.**); scrofulous ophthalmia, opaque cornea; attacks of colic; swollen abdomen; puffed face; general emaciation; mind and body weak.

Persons subject to quinsy; take cold easily, or with every, even least cold, have an attack of tonsillitis prone to suppuration.

Dwarfish hysterical women, with deficient vital heat, always cold and chilly.

Old cachectic people; scrofulous, especially when fat; or those who suffer from gouty complaints.

Diseases of old men; hypertrophied prostate or indurated testes.

Swelling and indurations, or incipient suppuration of glands.

Offensive foot-sweat; toes and soles get sore; throat affections after checked foot-sweat (see Silica).

Great sensitiveness to cold.

**Aggravation.**—While sitting; when thinking of his disease (Oxalic acid); lying on painful side.

**Amelioration.**—When walking in the open air.

**Type.**—Quotidian; tertian.

**Time.**—8 P.M. Afternoon or evening.

**Chill.**—Without thirst.

Constant coldness, *as if cold water were dashed over her* (**Ant. t., Rhus**), relieved by warmth of stove (**Ign.**), but aggravated by exercise or the least draught of air. Chill begins in face and descends over the body; or shivering, beginning in the feet, *with bristling of the hairs.* Chills in pit of stomach (**Calc.**) alternate with warmth of body; *cold feet*, then chilliness comes on again. Sudden chill, with goose-skin, external coldness and *the hair standing on end. Icy coldness of the feet* from afternoon till evening; after lying down, heat in the whole body. Alternate chilliness and heat the whole night. Chill generally one (left) sided. Chill alternating with heat; evening and night. *Horripilation.*

**Heat.**—Without thirst. Skin hot and dry; *heat at night and anxiety. She cannot lie upon the left side on account of violent palpitation,* with a feeling of *soreness* in the heart, and great anxiety. Dry heat the whole night, with sleeplessness; *if she puts her hands out from under the cover of the bed, she feels cold, chilly and thirsty* (feels cold, **Hepar**); *next day, violent thirst,* pours down whole glasses of water. Frequent flushes of heat during the day; night attacks, with great anxiety and restlessness. Heat and redness, frequently of one cheek, with coldness of the other. *Very sensitive to cold air,* or *to change of temperature* (**Calc., Hepar**).

**Sweat.**—Exhausting night-sweat; *anxious sweat. Sweat profuse, of the left side; offensive of one (the left) side;* returning *every other evening* (**Ant. c.**); increased by eating; increased in the presence of strangers. Sweat for several nights, after midnight. No thirst.

**Tongue.**—Very thick; white, fuzzy coating. Too weak to chew; too lazy to eat. Hungry, but cannot eat; sleepy, but cannot sleep. While at meals sudden disgust for food.

**Apyrexia.**—Excessive languor of all the limbs; prostration and inability to support one's self on the limbs. Constantly weak and weary, wishes to lean on something, to sit or lie down, and still feels weak and weary.

In fevers as sequellæ of scarlet fever or diphtheria; fevers occurring in young persons or old people of a psoric diathesis.

## CLINICAL.

The following case had been, for some months, treated without success by the usual Allopathic routine of Quinine, Iodine, Mercury, etc., in massive doses of the crude drugs:

Mrs. B., a large lady, dark hair, fair complexion, had spent some months in Florida the previous winter. Since her return, had some wandering rheumatic pains in left shoulder, left arm and left knee. Intermittent fever since first of June. *Chill* every afternoon; alternate chilliness and flushes of heat, *with ice-cold feet;* but it never amounts to a shake; lasts till evening. *Very sensitive to cold.*

*Heat*, with dry, burning skin, although she feels chilly and must be covered up. Great sensitiveness to cold air, or change of air, even going from one room to another makes her chilly. Chilly when undressing, and in bed must *wrap a woollen blanket around her* "to get warm," yet her skin is *burning hot to touch of others*. Soles of feet burn all night, yet *she cannot put either hands or feet from under clothes because it makes her chilly;* towards morning falls into an uneasy sleep with a light perspiration. No thirst in any stage. Tongue white; bitter taste; appetite capricious. Weak and tired for three days before the menses, which are two or three days too soon and too profuse. Baryta carb.$^{200}$ every morning, cured in a week.—H. C. A., *Counselor*, October, 1879.

## BELLADONNA.

**Characteristic.**—Adapted to bilious, lymphatic, plethoric constitutions; persons who are jovial and entertaining when well, but violent and often delirious when sick.

Women and children, with light hair, blue eyes, fine complexion, delicate skin; sensitive, nervous, threatened with convulsions.

Great liability to take cold, sensitive to draft of air, especially when uncovering the head; from having the hair cut (Hepar); tonsils swell after riding in a cold wind (Acon.).

Over-excitability of all the senses; convulsions during dentition; spasms of single muscles or the whole body; chorea, epilepsy.

Pains come on suddenly, last indefinitely, cease suddenly.

Pains usually in short attacks; cause redness of face and eyes; throbbing of carotids and head.

Head hot and painful, face flushed, eyes wild, staring, pupils dilated, pulse full and bounding, mucous membrane of mouth dry, stool tardy, urine suppressed.

Complementary—Calcarea ost.

**Aggravation.**—From touch, motion, noise, draught of air, looking at bright shining objects (**Stram.**); after 3 P.M. and midnight; while drinking; uncovering; hot sun.

**Amelioration.**—Rest; standing or sitting erect; warm room.

**Type.**—Quotidian, tertian. Sometimes the type is anticipating. Periodicity not marked.

**Time.**—6 P.M. In evening, or at night.

**Chill.**—*Without thirst.* Chill, beginning in *both arms* at once, thence spreads all over the body (**Hell.**—begins in extremities, **Gels.**); a violent chill seizes her *in scrobiculus cordis;* shivering running down the back, and terminating *in pit of stomach* (chill felt most severely in pit of stomach, **Arn.**—chill begins in pit of stomach with a *fixed, cold, agonizing weight,* **Calc.**). Chill, *alternating* with *dry, burning heat.* Chill, with *violent, bursting, frontal headache, dilated pupils, dread of light and noise;* restlessness; *pale face when lying down;* red face when sitting up (the reverse of **Acon.**). *Congestive chill,* with red face, delirium and bursting headache. Chill internal, with external burning heat. *Feet ice-cold; can scarcely be warmed, while face is red and bloated* (**Arn.**). Chill after eating (**Kali c.**—chill after eating and drinking, **Asar.**). Chilliness *in the arms,* with redness and heat of the ears and nose (with coldness of tip of nose during chill, **Cedr.**). Chilliness not relieved by heat of stove. *Rarely any thirst;* if any, it is during the alternate burning heat of the chill.

**Heat.**—INTENSE, *with great thirst* and desire for cold water, yet everything he drinks *feels as if too cold.* **Burning heat within and without;** *burning heat of the body, with extreme distension of the superficial blood-vessels,* the distended veins lie like cords on the skin (distension of veins and congestive headache, **Cinch.**). *Violent, bursting* headache, with strong pulsations of arteries, especially *throbbing of the carotids; dilated pupils; very red face;* delirium; restlessness. External coldness of the body, and internal burning heat. Head sometimes ice-cold, sometimes burning hot. Face hot, with extremities cold; forehead hot, with cold head and cold cheeks (**Rhus**). Heat the predominant stage of the paroxysm. *Averse to uncovering. Sensitive to light and noise.*

**Sweat.**—Beginning at the feet and rising up to head; during heat, or immediately after it, mostly on face and down the nose; on *covered parts only,* or *on covering parts ever so little* (**Cinch.**); sweat stains linen yellow or dark; empyreumatic, smoky odor; profuse sweat with diuresis; sweat of head, hands, face (which is very red) and feet, with burning heat; profuse sweat over whole body by the least exercise (**Bry., Camp.**); sudden, evanescent; during sleep, day or night, with gradual relief of pain (**Nat. m.**); *may be entirely wanting.*

**Tongue.**—*Red* and *dry,* with red edges and white coating in the middle; papillæ bright and prominent, like scarlatina (**Ant. t.**).

*Offensive, putrid taste in throat when eating or drinking, although food tastes natural.*

**Pulse.**—Strong, full, large and frequent, or small, wiry and hard; the former in chill and heat, the latter as paroxysm passes off.

## Aconite.

**Chill.**—Ascends from feet to chest.

One hot cheek; contracted pupils. Red face when lying down; pale face and fainting when sitting up.

Chilly from being touched, or even lifting bed clothes. Body chilly, forehead and ears hot.

**Heat.**—Redness and heat of one, coldness and paleness of the other cheek.

Sensation of coldness in the blood-vessels.

Likes to be uncovered.

**Sweat.**—Covered or affected parts sweat profusely.

Sour smelling sweat all over the body.

**Tongue.**—Coated white, "strawberry tongue." Everything but water tastes bitter; taste of rotten eggs.

## Belladonna.

**Chill.**—Begins in both arms at once, thence over body.

Hot face, dilated pupils. Pale face when lying down; red face when sitting up.

Chill after eating, with redness of the face. Chilliness, with redness and heat of ears and nose.

**Heat.**—Forehead hot, with cold face and cold cheeks.

Distended superficial blood-vessels, like whip-cords on the skin.

Averse to uncovering.

**Sweat.**—On covered parts only, or on covering parts ever so little.

Sweat stains the linen yellow.

Sweat of empyreumatic odor.

**Tongue.**—Red, dry, "scarlatina-like," mouth and fauces dry.

Food tastes salty: bread sour.

"Where there is a doubt whether Aconite or Belladonna should be given, I have always found that a disposition to perspire constitutes a valuable indication for Belladonna."—BAEHR.

It has been taught by some authors, and believed by many members of the homœopathic faith, that Aconite and Belladonna—except as incurrents during the congestive stage of heat—are useless in the treatment of intermittent fever. But the law of cure, as enunciated by Hahnemann, knows no such narrow restriction, and is not bound by the *ipse dixit* of individual opinion.

If Aconite or Belladonna cover the totality of the patient's symptoms, it will as certainly cure this fever, as any other remedy. They are comparatively rarely indicated, but will effectually do their work when called for. The characteristic symptoms of the remedy must always be the guide."—(See note to Arsenic by Dunham.)

## CLINICAL.

Case I.—Child had daily chill for three weeks. Chill at noon, *with marbled skin and blue lips*, with great weakness; then heat *with glowing red face and burning ears*. Soon after chill, or simultaneously with it, sweat, especially in drops on the head. One dose of Bell. cured.—Weber in *A. H. Z.*, 91, p. 146.

Case II.—Mr. T. had anticipating tertian ague. At 5 a.m. chill, with thirst and headache, lasts one hour. Hot stage was four to six hours long, there were increase of thirst and throbbing frontal headache, with delirium; talks of war and of being on the water; later he was stupid, hard to arouse; sick at stomach; eyes red, pupils dilated; throbbing of carotids and very red face, with constant desire for beer. *Not much sweat.*

During apyrexia, no appetite, but great and constant desire for beer, coffee and acids; is sleepless, though drowsy, some headache, and soreness across upper abdomen. Had taken Gels., Nux v. and Natr. m. in tincture or second dilution previously to my being called.

Gave Bell. $^{200}$ at once and every three hours during apyrexia. No return of paroxysm. Cured.—A. L. Fisher, *A. J. H. M.*, Vol. V., p. 177.

## BOVISTA.

**Characteristic.**—Sensation as if head were enlarging, or very much enlarged; dull, bruised pain, deep in brain.

Stool, first hard and difficult; then thin, watery, with much pain in abdomen (Pod.).

Diarrhœa before and during menses (cholera-like symptoms during the menses, Amm. c.).

Menses: flow, most profuse at night (Magn. c.) or early in the morning. During intermenstrual period, every few days a show.

Leucorrhœa: a few days before or a few days after the menses (before, Sep.; after, Kreos.; both before and after, Graph.); acrid, thick, tough, tenacious, yellow-green, leaving green spots on linen, causing soreness.

Adapted to old maids, subject to palpitation, leucorrhœa, tettery eruptions, urticaria.

Great weakness of all joints: as if the muscles of lower limbs were too short (Caust., Guai.). Drops things from the hands as from weakness (from awkwardness, Apis).

Unusually deep impression on finger from using blunt instruments (knives or scissors).

Stammering: in children. Intolerance of tight clothing around the waist (Lach.).

**Time.**—5 to 8 A.M., or 7 to 10 P.M. *Without heat or sweat* (Aran.).

**Chill.**—Generally with thirst. Chill predominates, even near a warm stove; constantly chilly on the uncovered parts, the neck and chest. Chilly the whole day, although she sat by a warm stove; must get near the stove as soon as chill begins (**Ign., Lach.**). *Severe chill every evening from 7 to 10 P.M.*, commencing with chilliness in the back, the first day with thirst, *without subsequent heat or sweat* (without heat or thirst, **Aran., Caust.**); with violent drawing pain in abdomen. *Chilliness the whole evening;* she could not get warm. Feet very cold at night; could not be warmed. Chill with the pains.

**Heat.**—In the evening, daily, at 7 P.M. Frequent heat and oppression of the chest, with thirst, anxiety, restlessness; relieved by uncovering. Flying heat, alternating with shuddering; thirst with the shuddering.

**Sweat.**—Especially upon the chest, every morning from 5 to 6 A.M. *Profuse sweat in axilla—smells like onions.*

**Tongue.**—Coated yellow. Taste putrid; bitter.

The characteristic of the Bovista fever is a well defined chill or shuddering; remaining stages of paroxysm being wanting, or if other stages occur, they are so light as not to produce inconvenience. Compare with **Aran., Camph., Dros.**

## BRYONIA ALBA.

**Characteristic.**—Suitable to the rheumatic diathesis; persons with bilious tendency, exceedingly irritable, inclined to be angry, black hair, dark complexion and firm muscular fibre.

Hering says: "Indicated in light complexions but more in dark."

The pains are stitching, tearing, worse at night, greatly aggravated by motion, relieved by rest. The parts which are the seat of subjective pain become subsequently sensitive to external pressure, and then swollen and red.

After anger: chilly; or head hot and face red.

In delirium: talks constantly about his business; desire to get out of bed and go home (Actea, Hyos.).

Headache: when stooping, as if brain would burst through forehead; from ironing; on coughing; in morning after rising, or when first opening the eyes; commencing in morning and gradually increasing till evening; from constipation; dull pain in forehead.

Headache: gastric, rheumatic, congestive, with vertigo, heaviness, pressure, and rush of blood to head.

Vicarious menstruation, epistaxis when menses should appear (Phos.).

Cannot sit up from nausea and faintness.

Pressure, as from a stone, at pit of stomach, relieved by eructation.

Constipation; no inclination; stool large, hard, dark, dry as if burnt.

Mammæ heavy, of a stony hardness; pale, but hard. hot and painful (red streaks radiate from inflammed part, Bell.).

Great thirst for large quantities, at long intervals.

Complaints: when warm weather sets in after cold days; from cold drinks or ices in hot weather; after taking cold or getting hot in summer.

**Aggravation.**—Motion; exertion; touch; cannot sit up, gets faint or sick or both; warmth, warm food; at night.

**Amelioration.**—Lying, especially on painful side; rest, cold, eating cold things.

Complementary: Alumina, Rhus tox.

**Type.**—Quotidian, tertian or quartan; periodical sweats on single parts; restless every other night. *Anticipating or postponing.*

**Time.**—All periods—time not characteristic. *Morning.*

**Cause.**—Fevers caused by getting wet (**Calc., Rhus**—sleeping in damp room or bed, **Aran.**); *in dry weather, whether hot or cold.*

**Prodrome.**—*Great thirst* for large quantities of cold water. Stretching and drawing in the limbs; *violent headache, stitching, jerking, throbbing from before backwards as if the head would burst;* vertigo.

**Chill.**—With *great thirst* for large quantities of cold water, which affords relief (**Ign., Natr. m.**—unquenchable thirst, drinks little and often, but drinking causes vomiting, **Ars.**); heat of the head and face, with flushed cheeks; **cough violent, dry, racking, with pleuritic stitching pains in chest and region of the spleen** (dry, teasing cough, *before and during chill*, without pain, **Rhus**). Stitching pain in right hypochondrium and abdomen; chill with external coldness of body and violent pains in the limbs; evening chill, frequently *only of the right side* (chill of right side, with heat of left, **Rhus**—one-sided chilliness, **Caust., Lyc.**). Shaking chill all over; hot head (internal), red, hot face and cheeks, with intense desire for cold drinks (**Arn.**). Chill begins on *lips, tips of fingers and toes;* worse in a warm room than in the open air (**Apis**); worse from moving, lessened by sitting. *Desire to lie down*, in this stage.

**Heat.**—With *increased thirst, same cough* with *pleuritic stitches* as in chill (dry cough during heat, **Acon. Ipec.**,); increased headache and vertigo; *pain in limbs aggravated by motion*; nausea and vomiting. Dry, burning, internal heat, *as if the blood in the veins was burning, or as if molten lead was running through the blood-vessels* (**Ars., Rhus**). More fever in a warm room than in the open air; *aggravation of all the sufferings during the heat.* Heat: with desire to uncover; in face with red face, with bitter taste. **Wants to be quiet and not move about in any stage.** Paleness of face. Thirst *less than in cold stage.*

**Sweat.**—**Profuse, sour, oily** (as if mixed with oil, **Cinch.**). *Easily excited by exercise* in open air (**Amm. m.**), even from slow walking, it runs in streams from his face. Sweat flowed in streams from whole body, even dropping from the hair (**Cinch.**—the least exertion puts him into a perspiration, **Psor.**). Sweat in short spells, and on single parts only (**Petr.**); profuse, at night and towards morning. Sweat on side on which he lies (on side not lain upon, Benz.).

**Tongue.**—Thick, yellow coating on the tongue; mouth and lips dry and peeling off (**Cinch., Ipec.**); everything tastes bitter. *Mouth bitter when not eating. Desires things which are refused when offered.* Aversion to food or drink (aversion to meat, **Arn.**—to pork, **Dros.**).

**Pulse.**—Full, hard and tense.

**Apyrexia.**—All symptoms of this stage are characteristic and should be carefully studied. Gastric symptoms predominate (**Ant. c., Puls., Nux v.**), but the general constitutional are almost always to be found and if present are guiding. Every spot in the body is painful to pressure. (Soreness of the part lain on, which compels him to move, although motion hurts, **Arn.**) *Feels best when lying upon painful side.*

"When fever is caused by getting wet, occipital cephalalgia, preceded by rheumatic pains in muscles of whole body; loss of appetite, eating a mouthful suffices; rotatory vertigo; redness of face, and thirst in all stages of paroxysm."—DR. HIGGINS, *N. A. J.*, p. 182.

Bœnninghausen's picture of the Bryonia fever: "Pulse hard, frequent and tense. Chill and coldness predominate, often with heat of head, red cheeks and thirst. Chill with external coldness of the body. Chill and coldness most at evening or on the right side of body. Chill more in the room than in the open air. Dry, burning heat for the most part internal only, and as if the blood burned in the veins. All the symptoms are aggravated during the heat. Much sweat: easy sweating, even from walking slowly in the cold open air. Copious night and morning sweats."

## CLINICAL.

CASE I.—Vertigo early in the morning, pressing in the whole head as if being pressed asunder. Afterwards stretching and drawing in the limbs, chilliness increasing unto a shaking chill, and chattering of the teeth; accompanied with *much thirst*, dry, sticky tongue and aversion to food and beverage; nausea and vomiting.

*Heat* after two hours, increasing with a burning, with *increase* of *headache* and *thirst*.

Profuse sweat the whole night, after the lapse of six hours. The fever (heat) was accompanied with dry, troublesome cough, violent stitches in the chest, increased by motion, asthma; stitches even during an inspiration. Cough increased by nausea, with inclination to vomit. The cough and stitches in the chest disappeared when the fever abated. No pain in the apyrexia. Bry., when the sweat broke out, and on the morning of the well day; the next paroxysm was much weaker; one more dose, cured.—*Ann. III.*, p. 43.  *Rueckert's Therap.*

CASE II.—*Tertian;* the fever *anticipates* one or two hours every day. The paroxysms are preceded by vertigo, with headache, and stitching in the chest during an inspiration. Moderate chilliness, followed by great heat. Delirium. *Unquenchable thirst*, with *dry cough*. Lastly sweat. Bry.[18] two doses, after fever. Cured.—*Hom. Clinique. Pr. Com.*, I., p. 181.

CASE III.—*Tertian fever* (this man had received large doses of Quinia under allopathic treatment). Violent chilliness for half an hour every third day at noon, preceded by violent headache; after this the skin became warmer, the pulse full and frequent, but no heat properly so called, although there was violent thirst. Sweat considerable. The apyrexia was characterized by pricking and cutting in the chest, especially when coughing; the cough being dry and troublesome. Face pale; no gastric symptoms; pulse normal; sleep tranquil. Bry.[21] soon after attack. Two days after, a feeble paroxysm. No return.—Dr. THORER, *Hom. Clinique. Pr. Com.*, I., p. 38.

These cases—although reported nearly fifty years ago, 1834—illustrate the fact that *one* or *two* doses of the properly selected remedy, even in the low potencies, given *after severity of the paroxysm had passed*, as Hahnemann advised in the *Organon*, are sufficient to cure. The single dose treatment is not new.

## CACTUS GRANDIFLORUS.

**Characteristic.**—Sanguinous congestions in persons of plethoric habit (Acon.).

Hemorrhage: from nose, lungs, stomach, rectum, bladder.

Headache: pressing, like a heavy weight on vertex; climacteric.

Headache and neuralgia: congestive, periodic, right-sided, severe throbbing pulsating pain.

Whole body feels as if caged, each wire being twisted tighter and tighter.

Constriction: of throat, chest, heart, bladder, rectum, uterus, vagina; often caused or brought on by the slightest contact.

Pains everywhere; darting, springing, like chain-lightning, and ending with a sharp, vice-like grip, only to be again renewed.

Menstrual flow ceases when lying down (Caust.).

**Aggravation.**—Motion; touch.

**Amelioration.**—In open air.

**Type.**—Quotidian. Periodicity well marked. Return at same hour each day: pains down thighs, chill, fever, pains in uterus and ovaries.

**Time.**—11 A.M. or 11 P.M.—Characteristic. *Returns at same hour every day* (**Aran., Cedr., Gels., Sab.**).

**Cause.**—After exposure to heat of sun.

**Chill.**—*Without thirst. Coldness in the back and icy cold hands* (after water in the cellar,—**Ars., Rhus**). *Chilliness which lasts three hours*, makes the teeth chatter, and does not go off although he lies down and covers himself up with many blankets. Chill not relieved *by anything, either covering* or *external heat* (**Aran.**).

**Heat.**—Burning heat of 24 hours duration (succeeding a three hours' chill), with dyspnœa and shortness of breath, and a smothering sensation so that he cannot remain quiet in bed. Great heat in the head and *flushes in the face* as if before a strong fire, which causes *horrible anxiety. Insupportable heat in abdomen; lancinating pain in heart,* suppressed urine, pains in bladder and pulsating pains in uterine region, vomiting, headache, coma, stupefaction, insensibility, terminating in very slight perspiration.

Some thirst at close of heat.

**Sweat.**—*With great thirst* (**Cinch.**). After burning heat, with shortness of breath, inability to remain lying on account of dyspnœa, a profuse sweat breaks out attended with unquenchable thirst for large quantities of cold water (**Ars., Cinch.**). Violent vomiting when perspiration fails.

**Tongue.**—Clean; taste soapy; stomach deranged.

**Apyrexia.**—From 11 P.M. till 12 M. the next day, complete apyrexia. The regularity of attack is perfect; and all stages are clearly defined. The congestive symptoms of brain and chest predominate during the heat (**Bell., Cinch., Natr. m.**). Rarely indicated, but has no substitute; effectually and permanently cures. May be compared with Aranea, Cedron or Cinchona.

Quotidian intermittent; congestion to head; flushes in face; suppressed urine; pains in bladder; lancinating in heart; violent vomiting; sweat does not appear after exposure to suns rays.

## CALCAREA OSTREARUM.

**Characteristic.**—Adapted to the leucophlegmatic; blond hair, light complexion, fair skin and blue eyes.

Scrofulous constitutions; pale, weak, timid, easily tired when walking; vertigo on ascending a height, going up-stairs, is out of breath, has to sit down (vertigo on descending, Borax); disposed to grow fat, corpulent, unwieldly.

Children, with red face, flabby muscles, who sweat easily and take cold readily in consequence; large heads and abdomens; fontanelles and sutures open; head sweats profusely while sleeping, wetting pillow far around (see Silica); diseases of dentition; during sickness or convalescence great longing for eggs.

Girls who are fat, plethoric, grow too rapidly; who begin with too early, too profuse, too long-lasting menstruation; subsequently have amenorrhœa and chlorosis with menses scanty or not appearing at all.

Women with menses too early and too profuse; feet constantly cold and damp, feel as if she had on cold, damp stockings; difficult to stop menstruating, the least excitement causes profuse return (Sulf.).

Fears she will lose her reason, or that people will observe her mental confusion.

Aversion to cold air; least cold air seems to go through and through; very sensitive to damp cold air.

Lung diseases of tall, slender, rapidly growing youth; oftener the guide to the true remedy than Phosphorus.

Disorders arising from defective assimilation; imperfect ossification; difficulty in learning to walk; have no disposition, will not try.

Longing for fresh air, which inspires, benefits, strengthens.

Feels better in every way when constipated.

Desire to be magnetised.

Complimentary: Belladonna.

**Aggravation.**—Cold air, damp winds; getting wet; ascending heights; exertion of mind or body, walking, talking, writing.

**Amelioration.**—In dry, warm weather.

**Type.**—Tertian.

**Time.**—2 P.M.—Fever without chill at 11 A.M. and 6 to 7 P.M. (11 A.M. one day, 4 P.M. the next.—E. C. PRICE.)

**Cause.**—Working while standing in cold water. Potters, brickmakers who work in wet clay; gardeners and fruit growers, handling cold vegetables and fruit (**Zinc. val.**).

**Prodrome.**—Drawing in all the joints, and great heaviness of head and body.

**Chill.**—*With thirst. Begins in scrobiculus cordis, with spasms, or fixed, cold, agonizing weight, increasing with the chill and disappearing with it.* External coldness and internal heat, or chill and heat alternating (**Ars.**). Coldness of single parts; of face, of hands, of feet, of internal organs; icy coldness in and on head; feels an inward coldness. Heat followed by chill and cold hands. Shaking chill at night. Chill in the evening in bed; was unable to get warm, though covered warmly, as though he had no warmth in his body. He was cold and his teeth chattered, though he sat over the fire. Chill with headache and drowsy fatigue of all the limbs.

**Heat.**—*Without thirst:* Followed by chill and cold hands. Frequent flashes of heat. *Severe heat in the head and great orgasm of blood.* Nightly internal heat, especially in the feet and hands; anxiety and palpitation. Frequent attacks of sudden universal heat, as if she had been drenched with hot water, with despair of life.

Heat, with inclination to uncover (**Sec., Sulf.**).

Fever at 11 A.M. *without thirst* and without *previous chill*, she felt hot and was hot to the touch, with red face.

**Sweat.**—*No thirst. Hot sweat.* Sweats during the day from the least exertion, even in the cold air (**Amm. m., Bry.**). *Profuse sweat in the morning on moderate exertion.* Sweat of palms of hands; of the feet; knees; over whole body, with severe cramp in stomach; chest; nape of neck; male organs. Clammy sweat only on the limbs. Often sleep after sweat.

**Tongue.**—Dry in the morning on awaking; coated white. Taste: bitter, sour, foul, offensive; "too fresh," like ink, like iron.

**Apyrexia.**—*Never clear.* Intermittents with spasmodic symptoms; after abuse of quinine; chronic forms with scrofula; cachectic constitutions; suppressed eruptions, or sweat; desire for eggs.

The constitutional symptoms existing or aroused by the fever, form the chief guide in selection of remedy.

## CLINICAL.

Paroxysm occurring every other day, at 11 A.M., lasting nearly an hour. Chills began in the limbs and extend toward the head; tongue quite clean; nails blue, appetite fair, bowels regular, no headache. After the chill, patient was very stupid for an hour or two, then felt well, only weak. This continued four weeks under Quinine and Gels. in large doses. I gave Eup., Nux, Natr. m. and Ars. without success. I now gave Calc. c.$^{30}$, three powders. A rash similar to herpes circinnatus appeared over arms and body, and chills and fever disappeared. The patient for some time previous to fever was very pale, and there seemed to have been a cachexia in the system for a long time.—Dr. HUTCHINS, *N. Y. S. Trans.*, 1870.

Charles R., aged 8 years, had a chill at 2 A.M., *without thirst*; fever at 6 A.M., *with thirst* and severe headache, lasting till noon; *sweat followed by profound sleep.* Paroxysm every other day. Gave Natr. m. 1$^m$, one dose. Next chill differed only in their being no headache.

In the third chill there was no other change. The mother said the child *cried for eggs to eat.* Calc. c. 1ᵐ. *No more chills,* and *no more desire for eggs.*—S. Swan, *Med. Inv.*, VII.

## CAMPHORA.

**Characteristic.**—Blondes most affected; persons very irritable and mentally weak. Catarrhal and choleraic diseases. Exceedingly sensitive to cold air. Surface cold to the touch, yet cannot bear to be covered; throws off all the covering (Secale).

Skin of the whole body painfully sensitive, slightest touch hurts.

Sudden attacks of diarrhœa and vomiting; nose cold and pointed; sweating, vomiting, purging; anxiety and restlessness; skin and breath cold. Long-lasting chill, great coldness of skin and sudden and complete prostration.

Antidotes many vegetable remedies; hence its use in the sick room is not advisable.

In most other cases the smelling of Camphor is not antidotal, but palliative by producing the symptom, "pain better while thinking of it."

**Aggravation.**—Cold air; night; motion.

**Amelioration.**—When thinking of existing complaint; warmth; warm air; drinking cold water.

**Type.**—Periodicity, not marked. Pernicious fevers: the so-called sinking or congestive stage of intermittents (**Ver. a.**).

**Time.**—At any time. All periods.

**Chill.**—*Without thirst. Long-lasting, terrible chills; icy-coldness all over; extremities cold and blue, with death-like paleness of the face* (**Verat.**). *The body generally is quite cold; coldness of the skin.* **Excessively sensitive to cold air;** *great aversion to cold air;* he is obliged to wrap himself up warmly, and even then he *is chilled through and through.* Great chilliness; excessive chill; *shaking chill* and *chattering of the teeth,* with *cold arms, hands* and *feet.* The skin of the whole body is painfully sensitive and sore to the slightest touch (**Apis**). Coldness for an hour, with *deathly paleness of the face.* Coldness increased by walking. Hands and feet extremely cold, complains of freezing, worse when walking. Chill with anxiety; pale face; unconsciousness; clonic spasm; *skin cold as marble, yet the child cannot* *bear to be covered; rattling in the throat; hot breath* (cold breath, **Carb. v.**). Frequent chilliness of back and loins (**Caps.**). Paroxysm of fever; severe chill, with gnashing of the teeth and much thirst; he sleeps immediately after the chill, with frequent wakings, almost without the slightest subsequent heat. Chill the predominant stage. Congestive chill.

**Heat.**—*Without thirst; of the whole body, which becomes excessive when walking.* Heat with *distension of the veins, increased by every motion* (relieved by motion, **Caps.**). Glowing heat, with full rapid pulse. Heat in the head, face, occiput, back, legs, lobules of the ears; body hot and sweating, but averse to uncovering.

**Sweat.**—At first warm and profuse, which relieves; then profuse cold sweat over the whole body, very weakening. Sweat most profuse during sleep, and on slightest exertion (**Bry., Cinch.**). Excessive perspiration of hands and feet. Sweat profuse, shirt and clothes drenched, having penetrated to lower side of feather-bed (**Thuj.**). Sweat often clammy and *always exhausting.* Cold sweat on face, when beginning to vomit (**Verat.**).

**Tongue.**—*Cold*, trembling, flabby, spongy, covered with a tough yellowish mucus.

**Apyrexia.**—Great weakness and exhaustion; lassitude. Convulsions may occur in children. Weak, weary and great anxiety. Face *anxious, pale, livid, haggard* and *sunken.* Yellowish, *green*, red, brown, turbid urine, of a musty odor. Terrible sinking and exhaustion.

In 1829, on the approach of Asiatic Cholera to Western Europe, Hahnemann, from a description of the disease, published in advance of its approach, that Camphor would be the remedy in the stage of collapse; and the clinical experience of each subsequent epidemic demonstrated his prediction. This power of *prevision*; the crowning glory of our school of medicine; the absolute proof that "similia" is a "*Law of Cure;*" the demonstration of the claim of Homœopathy to be ranked as *a medical science;* was first shown by Hahnemann in the fatal typhus which followed the terrible retreat of Napoleon from his Russian campaign in 1812. He published in advance that Rhus tox. would be the principal remedy, and the recognition of Homœopathy by the Austrian Government was the reward of its successful administration.

There is probably no stage of any disease that bears so close a resemblance to the collapse of cholera as the true, "pernicious" "sinking," or "congestive" stage of intermittent fever. Hence, Camphor should deservedly be placed in the front rank with Apis, Carb. v., Gels., Lach., Nux v., Verat., as one of our "sheet anchors" in this form of fever, instead of Quinine, often so indiscriminately and empirically used.

This abuse of Quinine is borrowed by the pseudo-homœopath from his allopathic brother, who has no "law of cure" upon which to rely, and is compelled to depend upon his theories (malarial and cryptogamic) to prevent the return of the paroxysm. Quinine may suppress it, as it will many simpler forms of the fever, but there are many cases *it will neither suppress nor cure*, and these are generally the fatal cases that so often occur in the practice of regular (?) medicine. The *fatal* "third paroxysm" is rarely known under the properly selected homœopathic remedy. It is a "bug-bear" of allopathic teaching and practice. No homœopath, surely, would think of giving Quinine in cholera collapse, for no better reason than that it is given by the rational (?) school of medicine. The statistics of comparative mortality of each system of practice "in cholera" ought to be convincing.

## CANTHARIS.

**Characteristic.**—Pain; raw, sore, burning, in every part of body, both internally and externally; with excessive weakness. Oversensitiveness of all parts.

Disgust for everything; drink, food, tobacco.

Drinking, even small quantities of water increases pain in the bladder.

Passage of white or pale-red tough mucus with stool, like scrapings from the intestines, with streaks of blood.

Constant desire to urinate, passing but a few drops at a time, which is mixed with blood.

Intolerable tenesmus vesicæ, before, during and after urination.

**Aggravation.**—Oil and coffee; drinking, or even sight of cold water (Hydroph., Stram.); after midnight and during the day.

**Amelioration.**—Warmth; rubbing; lying down.

**Type.**—No periodicity of fever. Many conditions or symptoms appear every seventh day.

## CANTHARIS.

**Time.**—3 P.M. till 3 A.M.—*long-lasting chill* (**Aran.**, 24 hours). At all hours in afternoon, from 1 to 10 P.M.

**Chill.**—*Without thirst*, in afternoon or evening, *not relieved by external warmth or covering* (**Ars., Ign., Kali c.**, are all relieved by external heat.—worse from external heat, **Apis, Ipec.**). General coldness of the whole body, especially the limbs. Coldness and chills *as soon as she attempts to rise, or puts one limb out of bed*, after getting warm in bed. Chill immediately *on getting out of bed*. Shivering and chill down the spine; feeling of coldness in the vertebral column (*pain all down the spine on pressure*, **Quinine**). Shaking chill beginning in, or running up the back (**Caps., Eup. purp.**). *Icy-coldness of hands and feet, with fearful pains in the urethra*. Children pass urine frequently during chill.

**Heat.**—*With thirst;* burning in the palms and soles; burning heat at night, *which she does not feel* (unbearable heat; extreme restlessness, **Ars.**). Burning on soles of feet, while hands are icy-cold. Burning, violent fever; great heat, with thirst, and redness all over the body. Great heat of abdomen (**Apis**).

**Sweat.**—Profuse, on waking at night; when walking; from every movement (**Bry., Camph.**); cold on the hands and feet; on the genitalia and external pelvic region; *smells like urine*.

**Tongue.**—Coated with thick, yellow fur; red at the edges. Taste lost; trembling tongue.

Disgust for everything. Canine hunger, especially for meat (see **Arn.**). Every paroxysm characterized by the Cantharis dysuria.

**Apyrexia.**—Irritation of the urinary organs, *difficult, frequent and painful urination*. Scanty and painful emission of blackish urine; then secretion of urine increased to four-fold the amount of liquids taken, with great thirst and **desire for meat** (aversion to meat, **Arn.**). *Very thirsty, but disgust for all kind of drinks*. Heaviness of the feet, a paralytic immobility of the limbs; *must lie in bed*.

## CLINICAL.

Cantharis[10] cured intermittent fever with catarrh of the bladder and urethra, and swelling of the penis. Chilly stage was long and mixed with heat; some sweat of urinous odor and perspiration on genitals.—*A. H. Z.*, I., p. 256.

## CAPSICUM ANNUUM.

**Characteristic.**—Adapted to the phlegmatic diathesis: persons with light hair, blue eyes, nervous, but plethoric habit; lax fibre and weak muscles, awkward, indolent, easily offended.

Children, dread the open air, are always chilly; refractory, clumsy, fat, unclean and disinclined to work or think.

Homesickness (of the indolent, melancholic) with red cheeks and sleeplessness, hot sensation in fauces.

Lack of reactive force, especially with fat, indolent persons, who are constitutionally opposed to physical exertion.

Desires to be let alone; wants to lie down and sleep.

Every stool is followed by thirst, and every drink by shuddering.

Every chill is attended with thirst and every drink with shuddering.

**Aggravation.**—From eating; drinking; cold open air. Night, after midnight.

**Amelioration.**—Warmth; during the day.

**Type.**—Periodicity strongly marked. Quotidian; rarely tertian.

**Time.**—5 to 6 P.M.; 10.30 A.M.

**Prodrome.**—*Thirst some time before chill* (**Cinch.**—*thirst and bone pains* 1 to 6 hours before chill, **Eup. perf., Natr. mur.**).

**Chill.**—With great thirst. Chill begins in the back, *between the shoulder-blades* (**Polyp.**—in lumbar region, **Eup. purp.**); worse after drinking. Shivering and chilliness after every drink. *Chill: with pain in back* and tearing in limbs, extorting cries and causing patient to bend double; *relieved* by jugs of hot water or hot irons to the back; *lessened by walking out-of-doors;* with painful swelling of spleen; contracted pupils; contraction of the limbs (**Cimex.**); anxiety, giddiness and headache; *intolerance of noise* (**Bell.**); ptyalism and mucus vomiting; in the open air, particularly in a draft, extremely sensitive to cold air (**Bar. c., Camph.**); inward burning and external chill.

*Chill followed by sweat*; or by heat with sweat and thirst (**Ant. c.**). Chill spreads gradually until extreme points are reached, then as gradually declines. During chill, coldness of chest, with a sensation of water dropping down the back.

"As the coldness of the body increases, so also does the ill-humor."
—Hahnemann.

**Heat.**—*Without thirst; lessened by motion.* Sweat and heat simultaneously (**Ant. c.**); *face alternately pale and red*; internal heat with violent burning (**Ars.**) followed by chill *with thirst during chill.* Headache with pain in the back, relieved by walking about (**Rhus**). Glowing hot cheeks, with cold hands and feet. *Heat of the ears, and hot, red tip of the nose, towards evening.* General heat; anxiety; uneasiness; dullness of the mind and *intolerance of noise.*

Fever at 11 A.M. (following chill at 10.30 A.M), lasting all night, without subsequent sweat. Fever (after very short chill at 11 A.M. or 12 M.) lasts all night with great thirst. Great sleepiness after fever (**Apis, Pod.**); especially after eating; could scarcely be prevented from going to sleep.

**Sweat.**—*Without thirst;* violent; copious; *lessened by motion.* Sweat with the heat, or *after the chill, without previous heat* (**Caust.**). Coming on soon after fever commences, and continuing with it. Sweat in axilla (**Bov.**). *Acrid sweat;* so acrid that it caused the hands of any person brought in contact with it to burn and tingle.

**Tongue.**—Burning blisters, and flat, lardaceous, spreading ulcers on the tongue. Taste sour; of putrid water. Desire for coffee, but it nauseates. Better while eating; worse after. Appetite unimpaired.

**Apyrexia.**—Clear comparatively; chill is predominant; in mucus, flabby constitutions; sometimes dysenteric diarrhœa of slimy, burning stools, attended with qualmishness of the stomach, and fullness at the epigastrium.

Intermittents attended with painful enlargement of spleen and torpidity of abdominal nervous centres. Fevers from or after abuse of Quinine.

## Capsicum.

**Time.**—5 to 6 P.M. every day. 10.30 A.M.

**Prodrome.**—Thirst, without bone pains. Thirst during chill with pain in back and limbs.

**Chill.**—Commencing in back *between the shoulders;* worse after drinking, relieved by putting jugs of hot water to back; *must have something hot to back.*

## Eup. purp.

**Time.**—Different times of day. Every other day.

**Prodrome.**—Bone pains in arms and legs. Thirst for lemonade, and acid drinks—not water.

**Chill.**—Commencing in back, *lumbar region,* passes up and down spine with bone pains, blue lips and nails. Nausea as chill is leaving.

Violent chill with *general coldness of body*.

**Heat.**—Light, transient, or mixed with sweat. *No thirst* in heat.

Headache; intolerance of n o i s e; sleepiness after.

**Sweat.**—General; copious, or alternating with heat.

Chill, heat and sweat, all relieved by motion.

Violent shaking, with comparatively *little coldness of body*.

**Heat.**—Protracted and well marked, *with thirst*.

Head light, as if *falling to left side*.

**Sweat.**—Light, mostly on forehead and head.

Neither stage relieved by anything.

Capsicum is a valuable remedy in intermittents occurring in midsummer; its symptoms are clearly defined and ought not to be confounded with any other remedy. The chill beginning in the back *between the scapulæ; relieved by hot irons or jugs of hot water* and *lessened by motion,* is characteristic. It is oftener indicated than used—just the reverse of Quinia.

Capsicum, Cinchona, Eupatorium perf. and Natrum mur. have thirst some time before paroxysm begins; "knows the chill is coming, because he wants to drink." It is a chief symptom of the prodrome in each. Both Capsicum and Cinchona are wanting in the bone pains and backache so characteristic of Eupatorium and Natrum.

"Most patients want to lie down and have jugs of hot water, hot soap-stones, hot irons, etc., *put close* to back, and cry out 'oh! how good that feels.' External heat relieves. Heat with no thirst, but with tendency to perspire."—T. D. STOW, *H. M.*, 1871, p. 163.

## CLINICAL.

Chills every morning, with shaking followed by heat, no sweat, not much thirst, little appetite, headache during the entire paroxysm, nails become blue, complexion sallow, *chills always commencing in the back.* Caps.$^2$, drop doses, three times a day. Three days after had chill every day "but did not shake." Caps.$^{200}$ one dose, another to be taken next morning. No return of chills.—R. C. SMEDLEY, *H. M.*, VII, p. 376.

I pay most attention to the apyrexia in chills and fever. A hysterical woman received Quinine for chills owing to the difficulty in getting symptoms. They stopped, but returned in two weeks. After three weeks of unsuccessful treatment, she said: "Is it not strange, every time the chill is going to come on I begin to drink." Caps.$^{200}$ one dose cured.—R. W. MARTIN, *N. E. M. G.*, vol. V.

## CARBO ANIMALIS.

**Characteristic.**—Adapted to scrofulous subjects, especially the young; or the venous plethora of elderly persons, with blue cheeks, blue lips and great debility, circulation feeble, stagnated, and vital heat sinks to a minimum.

Glands indurated, swollen, painful; in neck, axillæ, inguinal region, mammæ; pains lancinating, cutting, burning (Con.).

Benignant suppurations change into ichorous conditions.

Easily sprained from lifting even small weights; straining and overlifting easily produce great debility. Joints weak; easily sprained.

Headache at night; has to sit and hold head with both hands to prevent it from falling to pieces.

Aversion to open, dry, cold air. After appearance of menses, so weak she can hardly speak (can hardly stand, Coc.).

Complementary: Calc. phosph.

**Aggravation.**—After shaving; slightest touch; after midnight.

**Amelioration.**—From warmth; eating.

**Type.**—Periodicity not marked.

**Time.**—Evening paroxysm 5 to 8, and 11 P.M.

**Chill.**—*Without thirst. Great chilliness during the day. Chill after eating* (**Bell.**—after drinking, **Caps.**—after eating and drinking, **Asar.**). Internal chill on beginning to eat; *chill awoke her at night;* commencing *in the chest* (**Apis**), with shivering down the back; with ice cold feet; chilly when a little air entered the room (**Camph., Canth.**). Could not bear being uncovered because she immediately became chilly (**Nux v.**). Chill with goose-flesh, from 5 till 8 in the evening, afterwards at 11 P.M., waking with profuse sweat, lasting till 2 o'clock, during which she could not tolerate the bed-clothes. Great chilliness during day.

**Heat.**—Without thirst; with redness and burning of the cheeks in the evening; frequent flushes of heat in the cheeks, with redness. Heat always after a chill, mostly at night in bed. Head and upper part of the body were hot, with cold limbs; which only gradually became warm towards morning. Averse to uncovering during heat.

**Sweat.**—Offensive night-sweat; stains the linen yellow

(flies trouble him very much on account of the perspiration, **Calad.**). *Fœtid; debilitating; exhausting; profuse sweat* (Psor.); *when walking;* slightest exertion even *when eating.* Sweat in *hollows of knees;* profuse of the *feet and thighs.* Symptoms of this stage always guiding and predominant. (Bry. and Cinch. have profuse, debilitating sweat, but lack the offensiveness of Carb. an.).

**Tongue.**—Blisters on the tongue and sides of the tongue (**Canth.**), which pains as if burnt. Burning on tip of the tongue and rawness of the mouth, relieved by eating. *Ravenous hunger* (Cina, Phos.).

**Apyrexia.**—Never clear. All the constitutional troubles are aroused, and every disease is extremely prostrating. Menstruation, leucorrhœa, diarrhœa, **are all exhausting.** *Leucorrhœa stains linen yellow.*

Carb. an. will rarely be indicated, unless the fever be developed after or upon some constitutional trouble. The sweating stage is very exhausting, and out of all proportion to the chill and heat.

## CARBO VEGETABILIS.

**Characteristic.**—Best adapted to persons, young or old, who have suffered from exhausting diseases (exhausted from loss of vital fluids, Cinch., Phos.).

Ailments: from Quinine, especially suppressed intermittents; abuse of mercury, salt, salt meats, or spoiled fish, meats, fats (Cepa); getting overheated.

Diseases of venous system predominate (Sulf.); symptoms of imperfect oxidation (Arg. nit.); deficient capillary circulation causes blueness of skin and coldness of extremities; vital powers nearly exhausted; desire to be constantly fanned.

Weak digestion; the simplest food disagrees. Excessive accumulation of gas in stomach and intestines; after eating or drinking, sensation as if stomach would burst. Eructations give temporary relief.

Awakens often from cold limbs, especially cold knees.

**Aggravation.**—Generally worse in changes of weather, especially warm damp weather; or in protracted sultry heat of summer or autumn; fat food; Quinine; mornings.

## CARBO VEGETABILIS.

**Amelioration.**—From being fanned; cool air; eructations; evenings.

**Type.**—Periodicity not marked. Quotidian, tertian or quartan.

**Time.**—10 or 11 A.M.—evening.

Yearly return of paroxysm (**Lach., Sulf.**).

**Cause.**—Fevers from getting over-heated; from living in damp dwellings.

**Prodrome.**—Headache, throbbing in temples, backache, tearing toothache, and tearing pain in the limbs; cold feet; the two latter may attend the entire paroxysm.

**Chill.**—*With thirst;* at times left-sided; begins in left hand and arm (begins in right arm, **Merc. per.**). Chill with headache and unusual lassitude; *with icy-coldness of the body and cold breath (with terrible coldness as if lying on ice,* **Lyc.**—as if a piece of ice were lying on the back between the shoulders, **Lachn.**); shivering and chills in the evening, *mostly only on left side* (**Caust.**—right side, **Bry.**); evening chill with tired, weary feeling and flushes of heat. **Coldness of the knees, even in bed** (**Apis**); of **left arm** and *left leg; very cold hands and feet; finger nails blue.* Irregular paroxysm, sometimes *sweat first, followed by chill* (**Nux v.**).

**Heat.**—*Without thirst.* Sensation of heat with great anxiety in the evening, although she was cold to touch all over; flushes of burning heat in the evening, with *headache, flushed face, vertigo and nausea;* tired, aching pain in legs; pain in stomach, abdomen, spleen; oppressed breathing (**Apis, Ars.**). Heat and chill are distinct and independent; rarely heat and sweat commingled together or alternate (chill and heat are mingled, **Ars.**—heat and chill alternate, **Calc. c.**). Flushes of burning heat in evening, usually without thirst. Headache continues *after the heat* (continues *after the sweat,* **Ars., Eup. perf.**). *Loquacity during hot stage* (**Lach.** during chill and heat, **Pod.**).

"Chill with a marked degree of thirst; no thirst, or but slight during the fever, but to compensate for lack of thirst, *the patient wishes to be constantly fanned.*"—GUERNSEY.

**Sweat.**—Profuse, of a sour or putrid odor; at night; great disposition to sweat even *when eating* (**Carb. an.**). Moist on upper parts of body. Sour morning-sweat, which makes his person offensive; feet sweat when walking; sweats easily in a warm room, and is just as easily chilled. Tearing pain in the legs and teeth.

**Tongue.**—Coated with white, yellow fur; dry, fissured, lead-colored (**Ars.**); cold and contracted. Bitter taste before and after eating. Aversion to milk, which causes flatulence, to meat and fat things (longing for them **Carb. an.**—longing for coffee, sweet and salt things, **Nitr. ac.**).

**Pulse.**—Weak, irregular, intermitting, indicative of rapid sinking.

**Apyrexia.**—Prostration, paleness, weakness of memory, melancholic disposition. *Gastric symptoms;* stomach and abdomen distended with gas after eating (least mouthful *fills* up to the chin, **Lyc.**). *Sensation as if stomach or abdomen would burst after eating or drinking.* Great foulness of the excretions (**Bapt.**).

"In cachectic patients with profuse sour-smelling perspiration, *thirst only during the chill*, excitability of nervous symptoms. Patients debilitated from previous drugging, and frequent suppression of paroxysm by Quinia. *One sided chill (left) during afternoon, great prostration; with icy coldness of the body; thirst and rapid sinking; small pulse, contracted, cold and cadaverous tongue and face, with cold breath.*"—T. D. Stowe.

This picture very closely resembles a so-called "pernicious" or "congestive fever."

## CLINICAL.

Case I.—F. T., aged 14 years, had quartan fever for several months, which had resisted Quinia and all domestic remedies. *Chill* light, with *great thirst during chill*, drinking little at a time; *distinct heat* with some cephalagia; sweating, profuse and offensive. Carb. v.$^{15}$ arrested fever at once.—M. J. K., *Homœop. Clinique.*

Case II.—Excessive tearing in all the limbs, early in the morning, followed by slight chills. Profuse sweat in the afternoon without any heat, properly speaking. During apyrexia, vertigo, generally when stooping and moving about, especially on the day of the paroxysm, with heat and burning in the eyes, tearing in the nape of the neck. Yellow complexion. A number of hepatic spots in the face. Sometimes painful vesicles on the tongue. Pressure at the stomach after a meal. Quantity of flatulence. Pain in the small of the back when stooping. Every night, red stigmata make their appearance in the bends of the knees, and on the arms, violently itching and burning in the warmth, disappearing in the daytime. Pain in the left hypochondrium, the spleen is excessively swollen and hard. Carb. v.$^{30}$ removed all the febrile symptoms in eight days.—*Pr. C.,* II., p. 53.

Case III.—May, '66.—S. S. H., aged 38, tertian intermittent; *first chill*, then heat, then sweat, with pain in back and bones, and considerable thirst; preceding chill lassitude and cold feet; *chill always beginning in left hand*, thence spreading over entire body, lasting from one to two hours, followed by high fever, with pain in head, nausea, incoherent talking, no thirst. Heat followed by profuse sour-smelling perspiration, with sleep; extremely irritable and sensitive, before, during and after paroxysm; in apyrexia, feverish, irritable, easily offended, and just as easily excited to mirth. Had been treated by many Homœopathic physicians, and taken large doses of Blue Mass, Black Pepper, and Quinine since July last (10 months). Several remedies correspond to the general features of this case; but none in our Materia Medica covers this symptom so nearly—CHILL BEGINNING IN LEFT HAND—as Carb. v. See Hahnemann's *Chr. Dis.* Patient received Carb. v.$^{4000}$, single dose. No recurrence of chills to date.—A. P. Skeel's *H. M.*, II., p. 494.

## CAUSTICUM.

**Characteristic.**—Adapted to persons with dark hair, rigid fibre; weakly scrofulous persons, with excessively sallow complexion, subject to affections of respiratory and urinary tracts.

Children with dark hair and eyes, delicate sensitive skin, prone to intertrigo during dentition (see Lyc.).

Ailments: from long-lasting grief and sorrow; from night-watching (Coc.)

Melancholy, sad, hopeless; looks on the dark side of everything.

Constipation; frequent, ineffectual efforts; stool passes better standing.

Urination; involuntary, when coughing, sneezing, blowing the nose (Puls., Verat.).

Cough with inability to raise the sputa, must be swallowed; relieved by a swallow of cold water.

At night, cannot get an easy position, nor lie still a moment.

Cannot cover too warmly, but warmth does not relieve.

Cicatrices, especially burns and scalds freshen up, become sore again; patients say "they have never been well since that burn."

Paralysis of single parts; vocal organs, tongue, eye-lids, face, extremities, bladder; generally of right side.

**Aggravation.**—In clear, fine weather; coming from the air into a warm room (**Bry.**); cold air; draught of cold air; on becoming cold; getting wet; from bathing.

**Amelioration.**—In damp, wet weather; warmth; warm air.

**Type.**—Not characteristic. Left-sided (**Carb. v.**).

**Time.**—4 P.M. or midnight, with sweat at 4 A.M.

Fever *without chill,* 6 to 8 P.M.

**Chill,** *without thirst,* **lessened in bed and by drinking** (**Graph.** —increased by drinking, **Caps.**). Chilliness and coldness of *the whole left side* (**Carb. v.**); of diseased parts. Shivering, *beginning in the face,* thence extending over the body. Internal chill, followed by *perspiration without intervening heat.* (See **Caps., Cimex.**) At 4 P.M.: first, chilliness, with creeping in the legs up into the back, with weariness, lasting three hours, followed by sweat *without heat or thirst* (*without heat or sweat,* **Bov.**). *Shaking chill over the whole body; shivering chill over the whole body, without thirst or subsequent heat. He is always either chilly or in a sweat.* Shivering from the face, over the chest or along the back, down to the knees. Shivering and coldness *of single parts,* as arm, forearm, thigh, leg, abdomen, back (rest of body normal), without heat or sweat. Sensation of cold water in a small stream running across the body; of cold wind blowing upon spine between the shoulder-blades. Takes cold easily (**Baryt. c., Calc. c.**). Very sensitive to cold air, or to a draught (**Camph., Canth.**); *cold feet. Chill passes downwards.*

**Flushes of heat, followed by chill.**

**Heat.**—*Without thirst,* occurring toward morning or at night; not a clearly defined hot stage, but *mixed,* not *alternating* with chilliness. Heat of head and face; warmth and redness of face and heat in face and eyes *after eating.* Heat from 6 to 8 P.M., which is not preceded by chill or shivering—heat descending—and appears to be a secondary paroxysm of fever.

**Sweat.**—Without thirst. *Immediately after the chill, without intervening heat* (**Ant. t.**). *Profuse sweat when walking in the open air; from motion* (**Bry.**—relieved by motion, **Caps.**); *during the day when sleeping. Sour smelling night-sweat all over* (**Hep.**). *Viscid sweat of strong urinous odor.* Moisture over whole body, without heat or thirst, with yawning and stretching. Awoke at 4 A.M., with profuse sweat all over the body—without thirst—which continued 24 hours. Heaviness and roaring in the head.

"Chill predominates, much more marked than the other stages, and left sided; followed by perspiration and later by heat; all occurring towards and during the evening."—T. D. STOWE.

**Tongue.**—Not coated, dry, with painful burning vesicles on sides and tip of tongue; or coated white on both sides, red in the middle.

Desire for smoked meat; for beer. **Aversion to sweet things, which disagree.**

**Apyrexia.**—Not marked, except by previously existing symptoms, upon which *the force of the chill* is frequently expended. Previously diseased organs or parts are prone to become painful during, or the pain is renewed after the paroxysm.

Chronic cases with constitutional cachexia. One of the few remedies where sweat follows chill without intervening heat. *Left-sided chill*, most pronounced of any remedy, and a "guiding" symptom of Causticum.

## CEDRON.

**Characteristic.**—Especially adapted to women; persons of nervous, excitable temperament.

Nervous depression, and choreic attacks after coitus, more pronounced in women (debility after, more marked in male).

Sick headache every other day at 11 A.M. (Every day, Natr. m.)

Pains; tearing and twitching in limbs.

Menses: during, mouth and tongue very dry; great thirst; epilepsy, premonitory symptoms appear precisely same day that flow begins.

Before: leucorrhœa every month regularly, five or six days previous to catamenia; leucorrhœa instead of the menses (Coc.).

After: profuse ptyalism.

Removes roaring in ears, produced by Quinine.

**Aggravation.**—Movement renews chill; before a storm.

**Amelioration.**—Warm drinks; warm room.

**Type.**—Quotidian; tertian. *Periodicity marked;* attacks occur with clock-like regularity (**Aran.**). Intermittent headache, neuralgia, prosopalgia. At same period of pregnancy, tendency to miscarry.

**Time.**—*Evening at 6 or 6.30 P.M.; 4 A.M. and 4 P.M.*

(3 A.M., Thuja); 3 P.M. till evening (Apis).

**Prodrome.**—At noon, *preceding feverish paroxysm,* depressed spirits, dullness of senses, and pressive headache. For 20 to 40 minutes mental excitement; exaltation of vital energy; florid, animated face and a sensation of general heat.

**Chill.**— *With thirst.* Regular paroxysms, commencing by chills in the back and limbs, coldness in the feet and hands. Chill severe; shakes the whole body. Mouth dry, great thirst for cold water. *General coldness,* shivering in the back, ice-cold feet, burning hands, sensation in the eyes as after much weeping. Shivering all over at 3 A.M., with malaise and inclination to lie down (**Thuja**); shiverings are *renewed by every movement* (**Nux v., Cinch.**); coldness of the hands, feet and nose; flushes of heat in the face; toward 6 P.M. face constantly hot, with smarting in the eyes, especially when closing them. Chilliness of the back and legs; unusual paleness of the hands, red face, heaviness of the head; chilliness followed by severe frontal headache, red eyes, and itching of the eyelids internally and externally, icy-coldness of the hands and *of the tip of the nose,* rest of the face hot and burning hot. During chill, hands, feet and nose cold, with congestion of the head, palpitation and hurried respiration. Cramps and painful feeling, with tearing, twitching pains in upper extremities, feet and hands icy-cold. Chills and shivering of whole body. Chill predominates (**Petr.**).

**Heat.**— *With thirst* for warm drinks (**Casc.**). "Cannot drink anything but hot drinks during fever." Dry heat during the night; dry heat of entire body; animated face and profuse perspiration; chattering of the teeth and shaking of the whole body; great desire and longing for warm drinks (rarely wants cold drinks), and emission of large quantities of pale urine. Desire to sleep as heat passes off (**Apis**). "Numb, dead feeling in the legs; they feel enlarged. Entire body feels numb" (hands and feet feel dead, **Cimex**—fingers feel dead, **Sep.**).

**Sweat.**— *With thirst. Dry heat, followed by profuse perspiration* (**Cinch.**), preceded by cramps, these followed by contracting, tearing pains in upper and lower extremities, with a cold sensation in the hands and feet; mouth dry, great thirst and desire for cold water; chills and shivering, sometimes very strong shivering of the whole body; *palpitation and hurried respiration; urine scanty and high colored.*

**Tongue.**—Coated yellow even to the tip, on rising in the morning. At 5 P.M. intolerable pricking-itching of the tongue, she had to keep rubbing it against the palate. At 5.30 P.M. pricking of the tongue, half an hour later chilliness, with heat of the face, pale hands; *feet and tip of the nose cold.* Pricking of tongue early in the morning; goes off after eating.

**Pulse.**—Weak and depressed during chill, quick and full, with animated red face, in heat.

**Apyrexia.**—Lasted from 15 to 17 hours, after which, and in about the same time as previous day, the paroxysm was repeated; restless; very nervous; cold and pale; weakness, yet return of appetite; transient pains are felt in the joints, principally in right elbow, which seems to perspire; general malaise; great debility; body heavy; mind depressed. Roaring in ears, deafness at night.

The debility is almost as marked as in Cinchona, but appears to be due more to the action on the brain and nervous system than to the effect of the profuse perspiration which is so characteristic of the latter. Said to be adapted to the intermittent fevers, occurring in *low, marshy regions*, particularly *in warm seasons* and *in tropical countries.* Ought to be the first remedy thought of in "Panama" fever.

The chill or chilliness predominates, but no stage of the paroxysm is "clear cut" or well marked, as in Cinchona, Eupatorium and some other remedies. *With the chill* there is chilliness and heat, or hot flushes, or hot hands, or red face and congestion of the head, particularly of the meninges. During heat, shivering, shaking, cold hands and nose. During sweat, coldness and heat, and heat and sweat irregularly intermingled.

Were it not for "its clock-like periodicity" Cedron would be much better adapted to remittent than intermittent fevers, if we were treating a name along. Has been used with more success in Southern States and tropical climates than in higher latitudes, where it has fallen into disuse of late years from frequent failures, though appearently indicated.

## CHAMOMILLA.

**Characteristic.**—Adapted to persons, especially children, with light or brown hair, excitable, nervous temperament; oversensitive from use or abuse of coffee or narcotics.

Peevish, irritable, oversensitive to pain, drives to despair (Coff.); cannot return a civil answer.

Child exceedingly irritable, fretful; quiet only when carried; impatient, wants this or that, becomes angry when refused, or when offered petulantly rejects it; "too ugly to live."

Patient cannot endure anyone near him, is cross, cannot bear to be spoken to, answers snappishly.

One cheek red, the other pale.

Oversensitive to open air, aversion to wind. Complaints from anger, especially chill and fever.

Pains; spasmodic, distressing, wants to get away from them.

**Aggravation.**—Evening, before midnight; heat; anger.

**Amelioration.**—From fasting; warm, wet weather.

**Type.**—*Quotidian;* regular stages in afternoon. Anticipates, usually two hours every day.

**Time.**—11 A.M.—4 *P.M. lasting till* 11 *P.M.* Fever without chill, 9 A.M. to 12 M. *with redness of one cheek and paleness of the other.*

**Cause.**—Spring fevers (**Canch.**) in nervous, sensitive persons, especially residents of cities; from abuse of coffee or opium.

**Chill.**—*Without thirst;* slight shiverings frequently creep over the body, alternating with heat of face. *Shivers, when uncovering or undressing* (**Hepar**); in the cold air; in some portions, in the face, on the arms, over back and abdomen. Shivering of single parts and heat of others (sweat and heat of single parts, **Bry.**). Shivering and heat intermingled, **mostly with one red and one pale cheek.** *Chill only on posterior with heat of anterior portion of the body,* or vice versa; *returns in paroxysms.* Cold limbs, with burning heat of the face, in the eyes, and burning hot breath. Coldness over the whole body, with burning heat of the face, **which comes out of the eyes like fire.** Chill and coldness of the whole body, with burning heat of the face and hot breath.

**Heat.**—*With some thirst. Long-lasting heat, with violent thirst, and frequent startings in sleep. Heat and shivering intermingled,* with **one cheek red, the other pale.** Burning heat in lightly covered parts, though almost cold when not covered. Heat and sweat of the face when eating and drinking (**Anac., Bell.**). *Great agitation, anxiety. Very irritable, can hardly answer one civilly* (**Bry.**—*exceedingly irritable, everything makes him angry,* **Anac.**).

**Sweat.**—*Hot perspiration, especially of the face and head;* sweats easily. *Profuse sweat on covered parts* (**Cinch.**—affected parts sweat profusely, **Ant. t.**). Profuse sweat at night; on walking the sweat ceases, and returns on falling asleep (see **Sab.**). Sweat frequently of sour odor and with smarting of the skin (**Caps.**). Relief of pain, after sweat not during.

**Tongue.**—Coated yellowish; or white at the sides and red in the middle (reverse of **Ant. t.**). Blisters on the tongue. Taste—bitter, sour, putrid.

**Apyrexia.**—Never clear; constitutional and mental symptoms of this stage are usually guiding. Patients suffer from bad digestion.

In consequence of anger or vexation, we often have instead of the usual fever paroxysm, violent colic, bilious bitter vomiting and diarrhœa. Chamomilla vies with Cina and Arsenicum in the treatment of intermittents occurring in children.

## CLINICAL.

Mrs. T., a large, fleshy lady, 30 years of age. Slight chilliness, lasting for three hours, with red cheeks, no thirst. Fever high, *with one red cheek and vomiting of bile.* She was so cross as to be uncivil to me. Considerable sweat. Paroxysm in forenoon, with anticipation of two hours. Cham.$^{200}$, every three or four hours during apyrexia. Cured. A. L. FISHER, *A. J. H. M. M.*—V., p. 177.

## CHELIDONIUM.

**Characteristic.**—Adapted to thin, spare, irritable persons; light complexion, blondes; subject to hepatic, gastric and abdominal complaints (Pod.).

Constant pain under the lower and inner angle of right scapula (under left, Sang.).

Ailments renewed on change of weather.

Periodic orbital neuralgia (right side) with excessive lachrymation, tears fairly gush out (Rhus).

Constipation; stool hard; round balls (Opium, Plumb.).

Diarrhœa; at night; slimy, grayish, yellowish, watery, pasty.

Debility and lassitude after eating, wants to lie down.

Face, forehead, nose, cheeks, remarkably yellow.

**Aggravation.**—Morning (**Bry.**, **Nux v.**).

**Amelioration.**—Evenings (worse, **Puls.**).

**Type.**—Variable. Periodicity not marked.
**Time.**—*Hour*, not characteristic.
Afternoon and evening paroxysm.

**Chill.**—Without thirst, over whole body, *beginning in hands and feet* (**Gels.**), when walking in open air; passes off in the room. Shaking chill in the evening in bed. *Shaking chill, with shivering, chattering of the teeth, as if dashed with ice-cold water.* (**Amm. m., Ant. t., Sab.**) Shaking chill, with nausea; worse on hands and feet; *with distension of veins of hands and arms* (enlargement of veins of arms and legs during heat, **Chin. s.**). Right leg and foot as far as knee, icy-cold (coldness of right limb as if standing in cold water, **Sab.**). Coldness of nose; face; cheeks; occiput; pit of stomach; abdomen; hands and feet; intestine, after drinking water; in open air; running down the back (**Meny., Petr.**).

**Heat.**—Burning heat of hands, face, cheeks, eye-lids, head, ears, tip of nose, forehead. Flushes of glowing heat of different single parts of body; on scapula; in hip-joints. Burning cheeks, of a dark red circumscribed color (**Sang.**—of a mahogany color, **Eup. perf.**). Heat of the cheeks, with red swollen face (**Cact.**).

**Sweat.**—During sleep; towards morning; better after waking. Sweats when pain disappears (pains relieved by profuse sweat, **Arn., Natr. m., Eup. perf.**).

**Tongue.**—Coated thickly, white or yellow, with red margin; shows imprint of teeth (**Mer., Pod.**). Taste: bitter; insipid; bitter saliva collects in mouths. *Desire for milk, which agrees now,* (which causes flatulence, **Carb. v.**). Pain in stomach; *relieved by eating* (**Anac., Petr.**)

**Pulse.**—During chill, small and quick; after paroxysm, slow.

**Apyrexia.**—Never clear; liable to run into a remittent or continuous fever. Stitching pains in region of liver, shooting toward the back. Left hypochondrium sensitive to pressure.

Arsenicum follows well and will often be required to complete the cure.

## CINCHONA.

**Characteristic.**—Adapted to stout, "swarthy" persons; to systems once robust, which have become debilitated, "broken down",

## CINCHONA.

from exhausting discharges; ailments from loss of vital fluids, especially hemorrhages or excessive lactation.

After climacteric with profuse hemorrhages; acute diseases result in dropsy.

Pains are darting or drawing-tearing; in every joint, all the bones, periosteum as if strained, sore all over, obliged to move limbs frequently as motion gives relief (see Rhus tox.); renewed by contact, and then gradually increase to a great height.

Great debility, trembling, aversion to exercise; nervous; sensitive to touch, to pain, to draughts of air; unrefreshing sleep.

Excessive flatulence of stomach and bowels; belching gives no relief (see Lyc., Pod.—gives relief, Carb. v.).

Colic: at a certain hour each day; from gall-stone, worse nights, after eating; better bending double.

Labor-pains cease from hemorrhage; cannot bear to be touched, not even her hands.

Hemorrhages from mouth, nose or bowels; longing for sour things.

Hemorrhages; blood dark, or dark and clotted, with ringing in the ears, fainting, loss of sight, general coldness and sometimes convulsions.

**Aggravation.**—From slightest touch; every other day; draught of air; milk; at night; after the chills; bending double; mental emotion.

**Amelioration.**—Warmth; during rest.

**Type.**—Variable. *Tertian* or double tertian; quotidian or double quotidian; double quartan. Anticipates from two to three hours each attack (**Quinine**).

"Paroxysm every seventh day, anticipating about three hours each succeeding chill."—W. J. HAWKES.

**Time.**—Not characteristic; may begin at any hour of day; generally toward midday; *never at night*. 5 P.M., 5 A.M. *Paroxysms return every seven or every fourteen days* (**Ars., Puls.**).

**Cause.**—Paludal fevers have always been considered its special domain. A change of theory may revolutionize the cause to which Cinchona is now supposed to be especially adapted; but thanks to *similia* it will not in the least affect its homœopathic indications.

**Prodrome.**—Great thirst (**Caps., Eup., Puls.**—thirst and bone pains, **Eup. perf.**); *canine hunger; nausea; anguish;* headache;

debility; *palpitation of the heart*, with anxiety; sneezing when exposed to cold air; oppressive colic; and a general feeling of illness.

" *Restless sleep night before the paroxysm.*"—HAHNEMANN.

**Chill.**— *Without thirst\** (with thirst, **Caps., Ign., Quin.**). *Thirst ceases as soon as chill begins.* **General shaking chill over whole body,** beginning in the legs below the knees, *increased by drinking. Shivering or chilliness, with goose-flesh, after every swallow of drink* (abstains from drinking because every swallow increases the chill, **Eup. perf.**—because drinking causes vomiting, **Ars.**—shuddering and chill after every drink, **Caps.**—drinking makes headache and all symptoms unbearable, **Cimex**). Thirst *before* or *after*, but *not during* the chill. *Coldness and shivering* when walking in the open air at 5 P.M., *disappearing in the room;* an hour afterwards, *great heat,* especially in the face, *increased on motion and on walking* (**Bry.**); *thirst follows an hour after* the disappearance of the heat. Wants to be near the stove, but it increases the chill (**Ipec.**—relieved by heat of stove, **Ign.**—relieved by external heat, **Ars.**). *Internal and violent chill, with icy-cold hands and feet,* and congestion of blood to the head. Chill with pain in the liver. Shaking chill and *internal coldness* for several hours; shivering over the whole body *without thirst; coldness of the hands and feet even in a warm room;* chill alternating with heat, skin cold and blue (**Camph., Carb. v.**—hands cold, nails blue, **Nux v.**). Sensation of internal coldness in upper abdomen, *after every swallow of drink,* and renewed on every inspiration. Coldness over whole body *as if dashed with cold water* (**Ant. t., Rhus**). Paleness and icy coldness of the hands and feet, aggravated by walking; vertigo and paleness of the face.

**Heat.**— *Without thirst.*† *General heat, with distended veins, congested headache, desire to uncover, but chilly when uncovered* (chilly when

---

\* *Observation by Hahnemann.*—In all my observations I have found that the Cinchona fever is characterized by the thirst not appearing during the cold stage, either shuddering or chilliness; that, on the contrary, thirst came after the cold stage, or, which is the same thing, that thirst came *shortly before* the hot stage set in.

† *Observation by Hahnemann.*—There is likewise no thirst in the Cinchona fever during the hot stage, except some burning of the lips, or some dryness of the parts, which dryness accounts for the symptom; sensation of slight thirst during the hot stage; "the thirst accompanying flushes of heat." In the Cinchona fever thirst sets in after the hot, or, which is the same thing, during the sweating stage.

uncovered in any stage of paroxysm, **Nux v.**). *Canine hunger* or aversion to food, pain in the region of the liver, back, chest, limbs; dryness of mouth and dry, burning lips, with redness of face and often delirium. *Long-lasting heat, with sleep.* Cough dry, spasmodic, fatiguing, with pain in both hypochondria and at pit of stomach (with stitching pain in chest, **Bry.**). Heat of the whole body, *externally and internally, with swollen veins of the arms and hands*, without sweat or thirst. Heat of the whole body, aggravated by walking (relieved by walking, **Caps.**). Sensation of heat in abdomen as of hot water running down. The cheeks are red and hot *to the patient*, although *they are not warm*. *If he eats in this stage, sleepy after eating.* *On the least movement an unpleasant sensation of heat in the head and stomach.*

"Entire absence of thirst during the paroxysm."—AD. LIPPE.

**Sweat.**—**With great thirst.** The first indication of its approach is the return of the thirst which preceded the chill, but which was absent during the cold and hot stages. Intense thirst during chill and especially during heat, positively contra-indicates **Cinch.** **Sweating during sleep.** **On being covered** *he sweats profusely all over;* this he cannot avoid, although very troublesome, he is so sleepy he cannot get up. Partial; cold; greasy, or as if mixed with oil; *profuse and debilitating* (profuse, but not debilitating, **Samb.**); sweat on the back or side on which he lies (sweat on the side not lain upon, **Benz.**). Profuse sweat over the whole body *when walking in the open air* (**Bry.**). Easily excited sweat during sleep and motion (excited by motion only, **Bry.**—relieved by motion, **Caps.**). *The sweat parboils the skin* (**Canch.**—parboils the fingers, **Ant. c.**). Often slow in becoming established, and frequently out of all proportion to the intensity of the cold and hot stages (see **Eup. perf.**).

"The patient sweats profusely, especially on the back and neck, when he sleeps."—HAHNEMANN.

**Tongue.**—White or yellow; thick, dirty coating. Taste: too acute. *Bitter taste in the mouth.* Indifference to all food, even when thinking of it. Toothache, especially when infant nurses (see **Sil.**).

**Pulse.**—*Quick, hard* and *irregular* during chill and heat; slow and feeble in apyrexia.

**Apyrexia.**—*Sweats easily; great debility* and *exhausting* night-sweats continue, *followed by ringing in the ears*, and constricting sensation over vertex from ear to ear. A saffron yellowishness of the skin of scalp, face, neck, chest and abdomen (**Chel.**); with the characteristic anæmic and cachectic appearance, once seen, never forgotten. There is swelling of both hypochondria, which are painful to pressure and worse by motion, bending, or coughing. Swelling, pain and pressure of epigastric region, with hypertrophy of spleen. Entire loss of appetite, with sinking feeling in stomach, or hunger easily satisfied. Bitter eructations and bitter vomiting (sour eructations and sour vomiting, **Lyc.**). The urine is scanty and turbid, with a yellow or brick-dust sediment; and general dropsical symptoms are often present. Bloated or tympanitic abdomen, and hard spleen or liver in nursing children, with profuse sweating and great weakness (without profuse sweating, **Ars.**).

This constitutes the paroxysm *of Cinchona.* But Cinchona has also another, an exception to the rule (probably a secondary reaction) which is often confounded with Arsenicum; hence its notice in this place. It has only two differential stages—Chill and Heat.

**Chill.**—With thirst (*no thirst* in regular chill). *Febrile chill over the whole body from time to time during the day*, especially upon forehead, which has cold sweat upon it; *violent thirst a quarter of an hour after the first chill.* (No thirst during *chill* or *heat*—which is long-lasting—in first paroxysm.) Cold hands in the evening, with hot cheeks; one hand is icy cold, the other warm; ice-cold feet, with warmth of rest of body. (This alternate heat of one part and coldness of another at same time belongs only to this paroxysm.)

**Heat.**—*With thirst* (*no thirst in previous heat*). Heat over the whole body, with fine, needle-like stitches in the skin, especially of the throat, together with *great thirst for cold water.* Heat alternating with the chill; *some thirst for cold water* with the chill; heat follows half an hour or an hour after the chill. A very transient sensation of heat over the whole body, with *thirst for cold water.* Sensation of flushes of heat, *with thirst for cold drinks.* Warmth and redness of the face, while the rest of the body was cold. The right hand is warm, the left cold; the hands are now warm, now cold; heat, with *burning lips and thirst*, followed by sweat; chill, *with thirst;* then heat, *with thirst; the thirst continues even during the apyrexia. Violent desire for cold drinks,* accompanied with stinging in various parts of the skin.

"*The fever heat, accompanied with stinging over the whole body, seems to form an exception.*"—HAHNEMANN.

The symptoms occurring *before the chill* and *during the sweat and apyrexia* are alike in both paroxysms. The *thirst during the chill*, with alternate warmth and coldness of different parts at same time; the *thirst during heat*, with stinging or fine, needle-like stitches in skin, with heat of one part and coldness of another, are the characteristics of this paroxysm.

## CLINICAL.

CASE I.—Mrs. M., æt. 20, recently married, complained of pain in head, back and extremities; loss of appetite, furred tongue and general prostration. At 8 A.M. she was seized with a severe chill, lasting one hour, when fever and perspiration followed in their turn. During the greater part of which time she was *dull and drowsy, had severe headache, flushed face,* full throbbing pulse (120), and *resembled one whose brain was congested.* She seldom asked for water, but when it was offered would drink large quantities at a time. She preferred rather not to be disturbed, as *she was so tired and weak; desired to doze,* and *was at times slightly delirious.* This, with the fact that she was worn out with the fatigue of travelling, made a perfect picture of the Cinchona disease. Waiting until the fever had entirely subsided, I gave her one drop of Cinchona$^{100}$, on a powder of Sac. lac., every two hours during the day, for two days. There was no return of either chill or fever. I have never witnessed a more prompt cure of this or any other disease.—C. PEARSON, *U. S. M. & S. J.*—I., p. 207.

CASE II.—Mrs. B., æt. 45, large, weighing 180 pounds, leuco-phlegmatic temperament. Feeling of coldness every night at 12 o'clock, followed by light fever and sweat. Cinchona$^{30}$ produced amelioration. I thought I was not curing fast enough, and gave Quinine with no effect whatever. I again resorted to Cinchona$^{200}$. Three powders, one daily, made a permanent cure.—G. B. SARCHET, *U. S. M. & S. J.*—VII., p. 365.

CASE III.—B., a boy of 12 years, had already had two paroxysms every other day when I was called. Light chill, followed *by heat for* 12 *hours,* with *severe headache; profuse sweating, with great thirst.* Cinchona$^6$, every two hours, after fever had subsided. No more attacks.—Dr. SCHAB, *Homœp. Clinique.*

## CHININUM SULFURICUM.

**Characteristic.**—Adapted to persons of dark complexion, bilious temperament.

Whirling in the head like a windmill.

Ringing in the ears, especially the left (especially the right, Cinch.).

" It will change an intermittent or remittent into a continued fever," and I have known it to cause typhoid and pneumonia (by suppressing the original disease)."—Hale.

Great weakness, especially of lower extremities.

**Aggravation.**—Contact (dorsal vertebræ); when covered (sweats profusely).

**Type.**—*Tertian;* rarely quotidian. Every fourteen days. Each attack anticipating from one to three hours (**Ars., Bry., Cinch., Nat. m., Nux v.**). A perfect regularity both in the invasion and progress of the paroxysm, is always guiding.

**Time.**—10 or 11 A.M.; 3 and 10 P.M.

**Cause.**—Marsh miasm; malaria. Acute intermittents of supposed malarial origin.

**Chill.**—*With thirst.* **Decided shaking chill at 3 P.M. (Apis, Ced.)**; chilliness, with paleness of the face, pain in the forehead and temples, and ringing in the ears at 11 A.M. *Violent shaking chill followed by heat, then sweat for several hours.* Violent chill with *trembling in the limbs,* so that she could scarcely walk; after going to bed she had *violent heat with frequent yawning* and sneezing, which was followed by a *copious sweat.* Violent paroxysm with *shaking chill* and *severe pain in left hypochondrium;* chilliness for an hour, with *blue lips and nails* (**Cinch., Nux v.**), paleness of the face and **pain in the middle dorsal vertebræ**; increased hunger and constipation.

**Heat.**—*With excessive thirst.* Intense heat over the whole skin, with *redness of the face.* External heat, with dryness of the mouth and fauces, obstinate constipation. Heat which passes over into sweat; over whole body, *which gradually breaks into sweat,* **while perfectly quiet (Staph.).** *Delirium during heat.* Flushes of heat in the face, with thirst at 4 P.M. "Great enlargement of veins of arms and legs."

**Sweat.**—*With thirst.* Sweat breaks out over the whole body from time to time, even during perfect quiet. Profuse sweat on the least motion (**Bry.**). Sweat during the morning sleep, so profuse that the bed was soaked with it. Profuse, exhausting sweats; nightly diarrhœa (nightly diarrhœa before the paroxysm, **Puls.**). Thirst often begins in latter part of hot stage, and relieves all symptoms of head and chest. (**Natr. m.**—sweat relieves all symptoms but headache, which is increased, **Eup. perf.**). Drinking is grateful and affords relief. Most perspiration on parts pressed by clothing, back, axillary and perineal regions.

**Tongue.**—Flabby; white or yellow coating in the centre, pale on the margin (reverse of **Ant. t.**). Taste bitter, with clean tongue.

**Pulse.**—Large; full during chill and heat. Weak and trembling at close of paroxysm, ranging from 50 to 60 per minute.

**Apyrexia.**—Constant excessive thirst during the entire apyrexia, which in daily fever is short, the paroxysm closely resembling a remittent or continuous fever. But whether it be short or long, always distinguished by great debility and prostration (**Ars.**); the perspiration is exhausting (all the discharges are debilitating and weakening, **Carb. a.**). Canine hunger more marked, if possible, than in Cinchona, even in nervous enfeebled patients. Light exercise readily produces palpitation. Obstructions of the portal system are especially marked, and the spleen swollen and painful. Ringing and burning in the ears, accompanied with vertigo and a sensation of enlargement of head. Hiccup may become a troublesome symptom in any stage, but especially in apyrexia. Urine fatty and deposits a straw-yellow, brick-dust sediment; urates in large quantities. *Spine painful on pressure in all stages of paroxysm.* The sensitiveness of the spinous processes of the dorsal vertebræ should be borne in mind, for Quinine acts specifically upon the spinal cord and the nerves proceeding from it.

## Cinchona.

**Time.**—All periods, except night. Variable type. Every fourteen days. Anticipating one to three hours.

**Prodrome.**—*Great thirst* and canine hunger; headache and debility.

**Chill.**—*Without thirst.* Chill increased by drinking. External and internal coldness.

**Heat.**—*Without thirst.* General, with distended veins, congestive headache, desire to uncover, but chilly when uncovered.

**Sweat.**—*With great thirst.* Sweats profusely on being covered. Night-sweat very profuse.

**Apyrexia.**—With *no thirst.* Sweats easily. Pain and soreness of hypochon-

## Chininum sulf.

**Time.**—10 A.M., 3 and 10 P.M. Regular paroxysms, tertian type. Anticipates two and a half hours every day.

**Prodrome.** — Premonitory symptoms are wanting.

**Chill.**—*With thirst,* paleness of face, lips and nails blue. *Dorsal vertebræ painful on pressure.*

**Heat.**—*With thirst,* hot, dry skin, dry mouth and fauces; flushed face; delirium. *Pain in spine on pressure.*

**Sweat.**—*With great thirst.* Sweats profusely during perfect quiet; morning sweat. *Pain in lumbar vertebræ, and sacrum on pressure.*

**Apyrexia.**—With *great thirst.* Apyrexia short; sweat hardly ceases before

dria, worse on pressure and motion. Hepatic region swollen and sensitive. Jaundiced.

Different *stages* of paroxysm follow in regular succession.

Contra-indicated where there is much thirst during cold and hot stages. Perspiration *always profuse*, or Cinchona is contra-indicated.

chill begins again. *Pain all down the spinal column on pressure.* Spleen swollen and painful.

Cold stage may be long, light, irregular, or wanting in acute cases.

*Contra-indicated where there is no thirst during cold or hot stages.* Perspiration must *succeed the heat*, or will be contra-indicated.

Where the indications for any remedy are not very clear, the paroxysm incomplete but regular, Chin. sulf. 30th or 200th may clear up or cure the case.

"In recent intermittents, there may or may not be a chill, but there must be fever, and it *must be followed by sweat*—and it generally is profuse and exhausting—or Quinine will be utterly useless." "As a rule, chronic, long-lasting intermittents are only aggravated by Quinine."—BURT.

The *cachexia* produced by long continued massive doses of Chin. sulf., such as rheumatism of the extremities, chronic diarrhœa, ascites and organic disease of the liver and spleen, although now a constitutional malady, requires antidotal treatment. This may be most speedily removed by Arn., Ars., Carb. v., Fer., Lach., Natr. m., Puls., as indicated by symptoms of each individual case.

Samuel Swan, M.D., of New York, has reported some bad cases of quinine cachexia, cured with Chin. s. 10 m. and c. m. potency.—See last paragraph *Hahnemann's Chronic Diseases*, Vol. I, p. 195–196, as authority.

Chin. s. is often indicated in intermittent fever, and when indicated will cure more promptly and more safely in the potencies than in the crude form. There is little doubt that it is *oftener prescribed* than *indicated*, and that it will, in a majority of cases, suppress the paroxysm—without reference to *time of appearance*, whether *with* or *without chill, heat, sweat, thirst*, etc., etc.—there is as little doubt. But Morphine will also suppress pain and diarrhœa, quite as effectually as Quinine will the fever paroxysm, and the homœopathic physician, half-read or not read at all, in his Materia Medica, "borrows both the theory and the Quinine from his allopathic brother, for the same reason that he borrows his hypodermic syringe and morphine," with which to relieve the pain and diarrhœa, viz., it is a "short cut" to palliate the pain, relieve and thus retain his patient, and avoid the necessity of studying the case. There is a wide difference between *suppressing* and *curing* a fever paroxysm, or any other disease. The homœopath *can* and *ought to cure*, not "break up the chill," "suppress" or "cover up" the disease. Leave the "breaking up of the paroxysm" to the allopath who invented the phrase; "rational (?) medicine" can do it "scientifically."

Prof. John Ellis, M.D., when in Cleveland College, in treatment of "congestive chill," advised : " That 25 or 30 grs of Chin. s. given during the intermission, will rarely fail to prevent a return, or to rescue the patient from death." " Not that Quinine *may be given* in such cases, but that it *must be given*." Also, " That in recent cases of 'pernicious' fever, two-thirds of our patients will die in spite of any known homœopathic remedy or remedies in the ordinary doses."—College Note Book.

L. M. Jones, M.D., of Michigan, who has had an extensive experience in the treatment of "congestive chill," on the other hand, says: " It has fallen to my lot to treat a number of cases of 'congestive chills,' first and last. In my early practice I treated a few cases with Quinine, but it was not satisfactory ; and since then I have relied on the attenuated homœopathic remedy, and never lost a case. Nux v. has been more frequently indicated in the cases I have met with than any other remedy."—Priv. Com.

Dr. Lippe says : " I lived for ten years in the country, where ague prevailed, and **never** resorted to Quinine. I **cured** my cases. I have always been of the opinion that a physician who professes to be a homœopath **must** cure **all** his cases of intermittent fever with homœopathic potentized remedies, under the law of the similars."

I am convinced that **every case of "congestive chill,"** like Asiatic cholera, can be cured more safely and speedily by the potentized remedy than in any other way, if it can be cured at all; and the mortality under homœopathic treatment will never approach 66 per cent.

## CLINICAL.

CASE I.—I have recently made several satisfactory cures with Chin. s. Two or three of them, with one dose each of the 200th and as many others with the 6th. I think this is an important remedy with us, and that it succeeds *better in attenuation* than in the crude form. *The crude drug never gave me such satisfaction.* Some of the indications in a number of recent cases were *clear intermissions, regular paroxysms, clean* or *tolerably clean tongue,* and *profuse sweats.*—H. V. MILLER.

CASE II.—Mrs. A., aged 25, blue eyes, auburn hair, mirthful temperament. Nov. 15th, '69, after treatment from June 16th, under homœopathic and allopathic medication, was partially, but not completely, suppressed by large doses of Quinia. Now presents following symptoms: *Before chill,* a little thirst, uneasy sleep, and a little night sweat. The *chill* lasted only about one-half an hour, and the heat from two to three hours, which passed off with a gentle sweat. During apyrexia a pretty good appetite, and she felt pretty well, though weak and nervous, and a little exercise gave her palpitation. Chin. s. $^{200}$, a dose every other day for a week, cured.—*Anon., Med. Ind.,* VII., p. 296.

## CICUTA VIROSA.

**Characteristic.**—Adapted to persons of a highly nervous organization. Women subject to epileptic and choreic convulsions; spasms of teething children.

Convulsions, with frightful distortions of the limbs and of whole body.

Epilepsy: with swelling of the stomach as from violent spasms of the diaphragm; screaming; red face; trismus; hiccup; loss of consciousness and distortion of the limbs; frequent, during the night; recurring at first at short, then at long intervals.

Puerperal convulsions: frequent suspensions of breathing for a few moments; upper part of body most affected.

**Aggravation.**—From tobacco smoke (**Ign.**).

**Amelioration.**—In open air.

**Type.**—Quotidian; periodicity not marked.

**Time.**—Afternoon (2 to 3.30 P.M.) paroxysm.

**Chill.**—And chilliness, with desire for warmth and to go to the warm stove (**Lach.**). The chilliness begins in the chest and extends down the legs and into the arms, *after which follows a disposition to stare at one point.* Icy-coldness of the whole body; ears cold; cold sensation streams through lower legs, especially the right. The whole abdomen was cold. *They all long for a warm stove* (**Bov., Ign., Lach.**).

**Heat.**—Without thirst; general of whole body; of single parts and special organs; in the chest and abdomen; in both legs. Sensation of hot water in the chest, arms, legs and ears; hot internally and externally. Burning and redness of the face. Constant desire for open air.

**Sweat.**—*On the abdomen;* at night, and in the morning hours. Feels invigorated after.

**Tongue.**—Swelling of the tongue. Thirst, with inability to swallow (**Cimex**).

The conditions calling for Cicuta are liable to occur during or following epidemic spinal meningitis.

## CIMEX.—(Acanthia Lectularia.)

**Characteristic.**—Affects the right side most. Violent headache during the chill, which almost deprives him of the power of thinking; worse when he drinks.

Pain in liver as if strained; painful when touched and coughing.

Constipation: stool dry, like small nuts, and only able to pass a small piece with each effort.

Cough: with gagging, belching, or vomiting; with purulent sputa; in daily attacks with fever paroxysm.

Irresistible drowsiness and sleepiness.

**Aggravation.**—Drinking: every movement, especially extending a limb, produces pain in extensor tendons; suffers the thirst rather than move.

**Amelioration.**—By abstaining from drinking.

**Type.**—Tertian or quartan.

**Time.**—All periods, day or night.

**Prodrome.**—Thirst; *can drink before the paroxysm begins.* Heaviness in lower limbs five or six hours before chilly stage begins (thirst, with pains in bones of limbs one to three hours before chill begins, **Eup. perf.**).

**Chill.**—*Without thirst.* Chill commencing in the feet, which first become cold; clenching of hands; violent raging; cold shuddering, as if cold water were poured over her (**Cinch., Rhus**); stretching, yawning; great drowsiness during chilly stage, he is unable to resist sleep (**Opium**); hands and feet feel dead (fingers feel as if they were dead, **Sep.**—all the body feels numb, **Cedr.**). During chill, pain in all the joints (pain in ankles and wrists, **Pod.**), *as if tendons were too short, contracted,* so that the legs cannot be stretched, *particularly the knee joints, which he is unable to extend.* Oppression of the chest; must take a long breath frequently (oppression of chest; he must be raised up in order to breathe, **Apis**). Chill terminates with a feeling in the legs as if tired by walking, obliging constant change of position of limbs. *After the chill* (instead of fever), *thirst; but when he drinks, violent headache, which almost deprives him of the power of thinking;* with tickling in the larynx, causing dry, uninterrupted cough; oppressed breathing; heaviness in the middle of chest and anxiety. Tormented *with thirst*, yet he abstains from drinking, because it makes headache and all the above symptoms unbearable (see **Ars.**, **Caps.**, **Eup. perf.**).

**Heat.**—*Without thirst*, but desire to drink nearly all day, on account of dryness of throat (**Nux m.**). When the dry heat sets in, the uneasiness disappears, in place of which she feels *a pressure and gagging in the œsophagus, affecting whole chest and impeding respiration;* when she drinks for the purpose of putting a stop to the gagging, *the water can only be swallowed at intervals, as if the œsophagus were constricted* (**Cic.**). The *gagging does not cease until hot stage terminates*, after which ravenous *hunger* (hunger before chill, **Cinch.**—hunger during entire paroxysm, **Cina**). If he drinks during heat, is obliged to urinate soon after; urine hot and brown, depositing much sediment; continues hot even 24 hours after fever.

**Sweat.**—*Without thirst;* relieves all the other symptoms (**Natr. m.**). Musty-smelling, sour sweat; the odor is very offensive to him (**Carb. an.**). Light sweat, mostly on head and chest, *with continued hunger* (**Eup. perf.**).

**Tongue.**—Coated white; saliva collects on middle of tongue and tastes of iron; tongue, gums and palate feel burnt or scalded. Throat dry, causing drinking.

**Apyrexia.**—A good deal of thirst in this stage, in which, like before the chill, he can satisfy his thirst, without headache, gagging or œsophageal constriction.

## CLINICAL.

A well marked chill, and afterwards thirst, but no fever; when the patient drank, *she lost her breath, gagged, had dyspnœa and a gagging cough.* Cured with Cimex.—T. D. STOWE, *H. M.*, p. 162.

## CINA.

**Characteristic.**—Adapted to children with dark hair; very cross, irritable, ill-humored; wants to be carried, but carrying gives no relief; does not want to be touched; cannot bear you to come near it; averse to caresses; desires many things but rejects every thing offered; uneasy, distressed; rubs or picks the nose all the time; pitiful weeping when awake; starts and screams during sleep; suffer from worms.

Face is pale; sickly appearance around mouth and eyes; dark rings around the eyes.

Canine hunger; hungry soon after a full meal.

Child is afraid to speak or move for fear of bringing on a paroxysm of cough (Bry.).

Intermittents of nervous, weakly, scrofulous children.

**Aggravation.**—At night.

**Type.**—Quotidian; quartan; tertian; regular; periodicity pronounced.

**Time.**—1 P.M., afternoon or evening. *At same hour every day. Evening;* fever lasting all night (nursing children).

Daily fever (without chill) at same hour.

**Cause.**—Intestinal worms.

**Prodrome.**—*Ravenous hunger,* nausea, vomiting of food, and diarrhœa, and vomiting of bile (when the stomach is empty); pale face, with blue margins around the eyes.

**Chill.**—*Without thirst. Febrile shivering over the whole body, with hot cheeks, without thirst.* Chill extends from upper part of body to head, *even by the warm stove. Shivering-creeping over the trunk, so that he trembles even by a warm stove, not relieved by external warmth* (chill increased by external heat, **Ipec.**). *Coldness of the pale face,* with warm hands; *cold face; cold cheeks; cold sweat on forehead,* nose and hands. Evening paroxysm of nursing children, *heat with hunger and thirst continue all night.*

"Predominance of coldness, with cold sweat and *continued hunger.*"
—J. S. Douglas.

**Heat.**—*With thirst;* mostly in face and head (with red face and bursting headache, **Bell.**); *face puffed, pale especially around the mouth* *and nose, with red cheeks; picks and bores in the nose with the fingers; rubs the eyes; restless sleep; starts and screams as if frightened;* pupils dilated. **Rising heat and glowing redness of the cheeks, without thirst, after sleep.** *Burning heat over the whole face,* with *redness of the cheeks,* and *thirst for cold drinks.* Daily fever at same hour, with very short breath. Fever daily in the afternoon. Violent fever, with *vomiting and diarrhœa* (**Verat.**—see **Elater.**). Fever; vomiting of food, followed by chill all over, and then heat with great thirst. *Canine hunger.* Heat worse at night; with thirst; with anxiety. *Picking finger ends.*

**Sweat.**—*Without thirst; generally light; cold sweat on the forehead,* around the *nose* and on the *hands.* After the sweat, *vomiting of food* and *canine hunger,* at the same time (hunger after paroxysm, **Eup. perf.**).

**Tongue.**—**Always clean** (**Psor.**).

**Apyrexia.**—*Never clear.* *Hunger* even in this stage, though not so marked, or so constant. The child had a craving appetite for some time previous to fever, then loss of appetite and desire only for dainties, with vomiting and whitish diarrhœa. General "*worm symptoms*" predominate; restless, frightened sleep; *urine turbid, turns milky and semi-solid after standing.*

The vomiting during prodrome, often during and always after the paroxysm, succeeded by canine hunger with *clean tongue,* should always call attention to *Cina.* In *Antimonium crud.* the same condition may be present but the tongue is covered with a thick, whitish coating. In *Ipecacuanha* the tongue is sometimes clean, but there is nausea, and the vomiting predominates over the diarrhœa. The prostration of *Veratrum* is wanting, and the mental symptoms are entirely different.

" *The child is very whining, peevish and complaining; weeps piteously if one goes to handle or lead him.* Great earnestness and sensibility; cannot take a joke. Indifference to all impressions. Restlessness. Greediness. *Cannot be composed by things at other times agreeable, or by caresses.*"—CARROLL DUNHAM.

"Cina is frequently the epidemic remedy for children when adults require other drugs. Is always to be thought of in patients between two and ten years of age."—A. MCNEIL.

## CLINICAL.

A chill in afternoon not mitigated by heat; heat mainly in the face; vomiting during chill. The child was pale and puny; abdomen bloated; breath foul; an occasional thin, whitish diarrhœa; rubbing of the face, ears, nose, and perinæum; wetting the bed; starting in sleep; lying on the belly; restlessness at night; continually rolling over and about; throwing away everything given it, and crying at nothing. Cina, two prescriptions, cured.—T. D. STOWE, *H. M.*, p. 162.

## COCCULUS.

**Characteristic.**—For women and children with light hair and eyes; prone to seasickness from riding in a carriage, railroad car, or boat, or even looking at a boat in motion.

Diseases peculiar to drunkards.

Attacks of paralytic weakness, with pain in the back.

Great lassitude of the whole body; it requires exertion to stand firmly.

Vertigo, as if intoxicated, when rising up in bed; must lie down (Bry.—worse sitting than walking, and extreme when lying down and closing the eyes, Apis).

Sensation in abdomen of cutting and rubbing, as of sharp stones, on every movement.

During the effort to menstruate she is so weak she is scarcely able to stand (see Alum., Carb. an.) from great weakness of lower limbs.

**Aggravation.**—Drinking, eating, sleeping, smoking, talking, riding in a carriage, cold air, motion of carriage, swing or ship.

**Amelioration.**—At night, after sweat.

**Time.**—8 A.M. Afternoon or evening.

**Chill.**—*Without thirst.* Chilliness alternating with heat. Shaking chill for half an hour at 8 A.M., without thirst, and without subsequent heat. (**Caust.**) Shaking chill over the whole body in the afternoon, or in the evening. Chill, **with severe colic,** *not relieved by a warm stove;* with lameness of the small of the back; chill more in the back and on the legs; in afternoon or evening; with shivering through the whole body; not relieved by external warmth. Continuous chilliness with hot skin. Nervous, spasmodic symptoms. The cold stage is predominant.

**Heat.**—Without thirst. Dry heat during the night. Flushes of heat, with burning cheeks and cold feet. *Intolerance of both cold and warm air* (of cold air, **Bar. c., Camph.**). Burning heat in the cheeks, which are *glowing hot*, with coldness of whole body, or only of the feet (**Caps.**). Now one hand, now the other, is alternately hot or cold (**Dig.**—see **Caust.**—one foot hot the other cold, **Lyc.**). Vertigo and nausea on raising the head.

**Sweat.**—Of the body from evening till morning, which is *cold only on the face.* Sweat in the morning, especially on the chest. Cold sweat, now on one, now on the other hand. *Sweat over the whole body during the slightest motion* (**Bry.**). Sweat of the affected parts (**Amb., Ant. t.**).

**Tongue.**—Coated white, edges dry. Metallic taste. Tobacco tastes bitter. Aversion to sour things (desire for pickles, **Ant. c.**).

**Apyrexia.**—When the fever threatens to assume a slow, "sneaking," nervous form, attended with vertigo; dull pains in the head, general weakness and physical depression; anorexia, with a tongue comparatively clean, but a marked tendency to nausea—as if the stomach was always nauseated, *Cocculus* should be thought of.

## COFFEA.

**Characteristic.**—Over-sensitiveness; all the senses more acute, sight, hearing, smell, taste, touch (Bell., Opium).

Ailments, the bad effects of pleasurable surprises (fright).

Pains are felt intensely; seem almost insupportable; driving to despair (Cham.).

Sleepless, wide-awake condition; ecstacy, full of ideas, no sleep in consequence; physical excitement through mental exaltation.

Headache: from over mental exertion, thinking, talking; one sided, as from a nail driven into the brain (Ign., Nux, Verat.); as if the brain were torn or dashed to pieces, worse in open air.

Unusual activity of mind and body.

Intermittent, jerking toothache; relieved by holding ice water in the mouth, but returns when water becomes warm (Bry.).

**Aggravation.**—Excessive joy; cold open air.

**Amelioration.**—Warmth; during rest; evening until midnight.

**Type.**—Simple; quartan (?).

**Time.**—3 and 8 P.M.; fever usually without chill.

**Chill.**—Without thirst. Coldness and chilliness running all through the limbs. *Chills running down the back.* Chilly feeling, with external and internal warmth (**Cinch.**). Internal shivering, with external heat of face or whole body. Chills ascend from the fingers and toes to nape of neck, thence to vertex; increased by exercise (relieved by exercise, **Caps.**). Great sensitiveness to cold (**Bar. c.**). Cold hands and feet. Flushes of heat, or currents of cold air down the back. *Ecstacy.*

**Heat.**—*With thirst.* External, dry heat of the skin. External heat, with thirst, and shivering in the back after lying down at night. Dry heat at night, with hot flushes to the face, hot cheeks, and delirium. *Dry warmth of the face.* Feeling of heat when in bed, yet avoids being uncovered (**Acon.**—must uncover, **Bell.**). One cheek hot and red, with constant shuddering (**Cham.**). *Ecstacy.*

**Sweat.**—*With thirst.* Morning sweat. General over whole body, most on palms of hands, and in the face, with internal shivering. Extremely sensitive and nervous.

## CLINICAL.

E. S., æt. 32, had ague of eighteen months' standing, contracted in the army. Paroxysms every four days, leaving two well days intervening. Had taken large doses of Quinine without benefit. Several remedies were given without result, when he complained of great restlessness, lying awake most of the night and tossing about in bed. Coffea tr., three drops to be taken every two hours. Reported in four days that he had been able to sleep since last prescription, and his last chill was lighter. Completely cured in two weeks, and no return for two years.—J. D. CRAIG, *Hom. Obs.,* IV., p. 442.

## COLCHICUM AUTUMNALE.

**Characteristic.**—Adapted to the rheumatic, gouty diathesis; persons of a robust vigorous constitution. Old people.

External impressions, such as bright light, strong odors, contact, misdeeds of others, make him quite beside himself.

Pains are drawing, tearing, pressing; superficial during warm weather; affect the bones and deeper tissues when air is cold. From left to right.

Smell painfully acute; the odor of cooking food causes nausea.

Autumnal dysentery, discharges from bowels contain white, shreddy particles in large quantities.

Affected parts very sensitive to motion and contact.

**Aggravation.**—At night; mental emotion or exertion. Motion: if the patient lie perfectly still the disposition to vomit is less urgent. Every motion renews it (Bry.).

**Amelioration.**—During rest.

**Type.**—Not marked.

**Time.**—Hour not marked. Epidemic or autumnal intermittents.

**Chill.**—And shivering, running down the back, through the limbs; even in a warm room. Nose, cheeks, and **extremities cold.** Chilly shivering in stomach and abdomen. Coldness in evening relieved by warm covering, but returning on going to bed as a chilliness, with chattering of the teeth, disappearing after a short time while lying still; it threatened to return on motion.

**Heat.**—External dry heat the whole night, with violent, unquenchable thirst. Internal with attacks of flushes of heat, or short flushes of heat intermingled with chilliness, even near the warm stove. *Great heat of the face,* of the hands and feet.

**Sweat.**—Wanting or *suppressed;* or profuse, easily produced; *sour-smelling sweat.*

**Tongue.**—Heavy, stiff, insensible; bright red; covered with a **downy white fur** (milky white coating, Ant. c.). Desire for, or aversion to food, with loathing when merely looking at it, *and still more when smelling it;* the smell of broth nauseates, and that of fish, eggs, or fat meat, almost makes him faint.

Nausea with great restlessness; on assuming the upright position, great inclination to vomit.

**Apyrexia.**—Never clear. The gastric symptoms which come to the surface during this stage are usually characteristic.

In Colchicum we frequently find the *genus epidemicus* for the intermittents so often met with late in autumn, when epidemic dysentery prevails.

## CONIUM MACULATUM.

**Characteristic.**—Especially suitable for diseases of old men, old maids; women with rigid muscles; persons with light hair who are easily excited.

Glandular indurations of stony hardness; of mammæ and testicles in persons of cancerous tendency; after contusions and bruises.

Breasts sore, hard and painful during menstrual period; hysterical symptoms and vertigo increased.

Vertigo, particularly when lying down or turning in bed.

Cough: in spasmodic paroxysms, caused by dry spot in larynx (dry spot in throat, Actea); itching in chest and throat (Iod.); worse at night; when lying down; during pregnancy.

Frequent urination; flow intermits.

Dreads being alone, but avoids society (see Bis., Kali c., Lyc.).

Bad effects of celibacy and excessive indulgence.

**Aggravation.**—At night; lying down; cold air; rising up in bed.

**Amelioration.**—In the dark; moving; when walking.

**Type.**—Quotidian; simple.

**Time.**—4 or 5 A.M.—3 to 5 P.M. Very ill-humored from 5 to 6 P.M.

**Chill.**—With trembling in all the limbs, and *constant desire for warmth*, especially **for heat of sun** (for heat of stove, **Lach.**—relieved by covering up, **Nux v., Rhus.**—warm air seems cold, **Thuja**). Chilliness in the back, with cold hands and blue nails. Internal chill in the morning; with shivering in the afternoon. Extremities and whole body were icy cold. Shivering over the body.

**Heat.**—With thirst, and redness of the face. *Great internal and external heat, with great nervousness. Heat, with* **profuse sweat at same time.** Uneasy sleep, great trembling, and short, rapid, snoring respiration.

**Sweat.**—*Day and night,* **as soon as he sleeps, even when closing the eyes** (*sweats when awake, dry heat when he sleeps*, **Samb.**). Sweat over whole body, with redness of face. Sweat while sitting in a chair and dozing. Night-sweat with offensive odor; smarting the skin (**Canth.**). Profuse sweat on limbs, perinæum, genitals (**Hepar, Thuja**). "Eruption during sweat" (what kind?).

**Tongue.**—Stiff and painful; taste bitter; saliva thready; lips and tongue *dry and sticky* (**Nux m.**). Craves coffee, salt, or sour things.

**Apyrexia.**—Complete; sometimes with vertigo on lying down.

## CURARE.

**Aggravation.**—*Dampness, damp weather, change of weather, cold wind,* or *the least movement.*

**Amelioration.**—After *the first mouthful of food.* (Compare with **Aran.**).

**Type.**—Quotidian.

**Time.**—2 or 3 P.M., *every day, and continuing well into the night.*

**Chill.**—Without thirst. Coldness commencing on the abdomen and spreading all over. Sensation of shivering, starting from the stomach and spreading over the whole body.

**Heat.**—With thirst, especially in the head, on the back and legs; burning in the hips; great weakness and prostration, crampy pains on the least movement. Fever with thirst and great hunger; yawning and stretching, hot head and hands, convulsive paroxysms and fainting. Daily fever, commencing at 2 or 3 P.M., and continuing well into the night; burning heat, accompanied by partial and transient chills, incoherent speech, and often by paralysis of the extremities. *Pernicious fever, with constant chilliness* (**Petr.**), heat increased at night or in the open air; less in the morning.

**Sweat.**—*Cold and bloody,* especially at night.

**Tongue.**—Deep red, cracked and bleeding.

Neither our provings nor clinical experience of Curare have yet been sufficient to warrant us in saying what is characteristic.

## DIGITALIS.

**Characteristic.**—Suitable for sudden flushes of heat, followed by great nervous weakness and irregular, intermitting pulse, occurring at climateric; worse by least motion.

Sensation as if heart would stop beating if she dared to move (fears that unless constantly on the move, her heart will cease beating, Gels.—See Fer.).

Faintness or sinking at the stomach, feels as if he were dying.

Great weakness of chest, cannot bear to talk.

At night frequent waking in a fright, as from a dream, as if he fell from a height or into the water.

**Aggravation.**—Lying down; motion; in a warm room.

**Time.**—No periodicity. *Pulse,* characteristic.

**Chill.**—Commencing in the fingers; palms of the hands, soles of the feet, thence over the whole body. Coldness first of hands and arms (of extremities, **Gels.**—of arms, **Bell., Hell.**—in fingers, toes and lips, **Bry.**). *Great coldness of skin. Great sensitiveness to the cold* (**Bar. c., Camph.**); chilliness and shivering over the whole back; internal chill with external heat; chill and heat in alternation; *cold extremities;* excessive coldness of the hands and feet, with cold sweat. Chilliness over the whole body with heat and redness of the face.

**Heat.**—Without thirst. Sudden flushes of heat, followed by weakness of all parts. General violent heat, with swollen veins and rapid pulse. *One hand hot, the other cold* (**Lyc.**). Heat of body, with cold sweat of face. Heat in the head, face and ears, hands, with redness of the cheeks.

**Sweat.**—Immediately after the chill (**Bov., Caust.**—heat with profuse sweat at same time, **Con.**). Night-sweat, generally cold and clammy. *Covered with a copious perspiration, without relief of heart symptoms.* Cold sweat on body, warm sweat on palms of hands. Sweat on upper parts of body; on the face.

**Tongue.**—Clean or coated white. Taste: desire for sour drinks and bitter food; bread tastes bitter; want of appetite, or hunger. Constant ptyalism.

**Pulse.**—*Third, fifth* or *seventh* beat, *intermits. Extremely slow* when at rest; *accelerated, full and hard from every motion.*

Digitalis should not be followed by Cinchona in any form, as according to Hahnemann, Cinchona increases the anxiety caused by Digitalis to deadly anguish.

## DROSERA.

**Characteristic.**—Whooping-cough; in violent paroxysms, which follow each other so rapidly he is scarcely able to get his breath.

Cough, aggravated: by warmth; drinking; singing; laughing; weeping; lying down; after midnight.

Clergymen's sore throat (see Arg. n., Arum.); with rough, scraping, dry sensation deep in the fauces. Constriction and crawling in larynx, hoarseness and yellow or green sputa.

**Aggravation.**—After midnight; warmth; during rest.

**Type.**—Quotidian; tertian.

**Time.**—Before 9 A.M., *every morning.*

**Cause.**—Frequently called for where fevers occur during prevalence of epidemic pertussis, then it often becomes the genus epidemicus.

**Chill.**—*Without thirst.* Chill with *icy cold hands, blue nails, cold, pale face* (**Nux v.**), *and cold extremities;* must lie down. *Febrile shivers over the whole body, with heat of the face and icy coldness of the hands,* and sometimes bilious vomiting. He always feels too cold, he cannot get warm (**Calc. ost.**); he feels cold at night in bed; shivering during rest, but not during motion (chill, heat and sweat all relieved by motion, **Caps.**); even in bed he is unable to keep from shivering and feeling cold, though body is warm to touch (**Bar. c.**). Spasmodic cough with violent pressing, pulsating pains in the head. After midnight, coldness of the *left half of the face,* with sticking pains in it; the right half hot and dry (see **Caust.**). Constant chilliness, *cannot get warm* (**Aran.**).

**Heat.**—*Without thirst. Heat at night, chilly during the day.* Heat *worse after midnight.* Heat almost exclusively on face and head. Increased warmth of upper body, evening. After chilliness, slight thirst, heaviness of head, throbbing pain in the occiput, and heat of face, usual warmth of rest of body, lasting till 3 P.M. Feels well in the evening.

**Sweat.**—Cold sweat on face, feet, *abdomen.* Warm sweat, particularly just after midnight; *most profuse on* **face and abdomen.** Sometimes general sweat, particularly *at night,* attended with *a spasmodic cough, which brought on retching and nausea.*

**Tongue.**—Clean (**Cina**). *Food has no taste* (**Eup. perf.**). Bread tastes bitter.

"*Profuse discharge of watery saliva during febrile stage.*"—HAHNEMANN.

"Intermittent fever, with sore throat and nausea."—LIPPE.

**Apyrexia.**—Usually clear, though gastric symptoms may be present at times (clear with good appetite, **Canch.**). *Coughs more than in sweating stage.* As in Aranea and Bovista, the chill predominates, the other stages being light, sometimes only partially developed.

## CLINICAL.

In several cases of intermittent fever, Drosera has been very useful, when the heat was intense, followed by cold face, with icy coldness of hands and feet with bilious vomiting; when heat was accompanied with violent pressing and throbbing pains in the head and spasmodic cough. Gastric symptoms were present in apyrexia. In fevers occurring at same time when whooping-cough was epidemic.—Case 1504, *Homœop. Clinique.*

## DULCAMARA.

**Characteristic.**—Adapted to persons of phlegmatic, scrofulous constitutions; restless, irritable; subject to catarrhal, rheumatic or skin affections, brought on or aggravated by cold, damp, rainy weather.

The skin is delicate, sensitive to cold, liable to eruptions, especially urticaria, every time patient takes cold, or is long exposed to the cold.

Anasarca; after ague, rheumatism, scarlatina, measles.

Dropsy after suppressed sweat, or suppressed skin diseases, from cold air or damp dwellings.

Diarrhœa from taking cold, in damp places or damp weather.

Catarrhal ischuria in grown up children, with milky urine, from wading with bare feet in cold water.

Cannot find the right word for anything.

Complementary to Baryta c.

**Aggravation.**—Evening; during rest; cold, damp weather (see **Aran.**)

**Amelioration.**—From moving; warm, dry air.

**Type.**—Double quotidian; tertian; double tertian; double quartan.

**Time.**—Irregular hours.

**Cause.**—Fevers occurring during cold, damp, rainy weather; worse when weather suddenly becomes colder.

**Chill.**—With violent thirst. Commencing in or spreading from the back; not relieved by warmth (relieved by hot applications, **Caps.**); shaking, with a feeling of coldness, or actual coldness over the whole body, so that he could not get warm near the hot stove, with shuddering from time to time. Chilliness of the back, without thirst, in the open air, but especially in a draught (**Canth.**). Chilliness mostly toward evening, over the back, nape of the neck, occiput, with a feeling as if the hair stood on end (**Bar. c.**).

**Heat.**—General, dry, burning heat all over. Dry heat over whole body; heat and burning in the back. Burning in the skin of the whole back as if he were sitting by a hot stove, with sweat in the face and moderate heat.

**Sweat.**—*Offensive sweat*, night and morning, over the whole body; during the day more over back, in axillæ, and palms of hands. *Badly-smelling sweat*, with profuse discharge of transparent urine. Often wanting.

**Tongue.**—Dry; swollen, as if paralyzed with cold. Bitter taste. Ptyalism; the gums are loose and spongy; saliva tenacious, soap-like. *Great desire for cold drinks.*

Like Aranea, the fevers to which Dulcamara is adapted, are rare. They are caused by rheumatic exposure, living in damp rooms, sleeping in a damp bed; during cold, rainy, changeable weather; but the fever of Aranea comes on with great regularity, while that of Dulcamara has no reference to time.

## ELATERIUM.

**Characteristic.**—Cholera morbus-like attacks; copious liquid dejections.

When chills were suppressed, urticaria appeared over the whole body. Unlike Apis, Hepar, Ign., Rhus, in which the urticaria appears during different stages of the paroxysm.

**Type.**—Quotidian; double quotidian; tertian; double tertian; quartan. When suppressed by Quinine or "ague cures," prone to appear under some other type, or even assume the double type. *Frequent change of type*

**Time.**—12 M.—1 P.M.—*Twice a day*, every third day.

**Prodrome.**—Chilliness with continued gaping and quivering; headache and soreness of the limbs, and pains in the bowels.

**Chill.**—With thirst, increased pain in the head and limbs and continued gaping and stretching. Pain under shoulder-blades; in small of back, left side, and cramps in the legs and soles of the feet. Yawning and gaping, with a sound resembling the neighing of a horse; lachrymation and profuse coryza.

**Heat.**—With intense thirst; violent, tearing pains throughout the head, more especially on the vertex. Increased cutting pains in bowels, and pains in extremities; the pains *shooting to the very tips of the fingers and toes*, and then shooting back again into the body. *Nausea, vomiting and copious discharges from the bowels of a frothy character.*

**Sweat.**—Copious perspiration, with gradual relief of all the symptoms.

**Tongue.**—Coated with a dirty brown fur; taste bitter.

**Apyrexia.**—Urticaria; relieved by rubbing.

" If urticaria appear all over the body after suppression of intermittent fever, Elaterium is the remedy."

## CLINICAL.

CASE I.—" Commencing with quotidian ague, which was repeatedly suppressed for a few days, and when he called upon me was of the tertian type. The paroxysms were preceded by much gaping and attended with much thirst, pain in the abdomen and great pain in the extremities, darting down into the fingers and toes."

CASE II.—Intermittent fever contracted in Virginia eighteen months since, and suppressed every one, two or three weeks by the use or abuse of Quinine. Paroxysm at 1 P.M., preceded by headache; pains in the bowels; soreness of the limbs; continued gaping and stretching. In the *chill*, slightly increased pain in the head and limbs. During *heat*, violent tearing pains throughout the head, worse on the vertex; increased pain in the bowels and extremities; and pains shooting to the very tips of the fingers and toes, and then shooting back into the body; with intense thirst. Elater.[2] cured these cases promptly.—DR. JEANES, *S. C.*,—I, p. 692.

CASE III.—Quartan ague of six weeks standing, the paroxysms occurring about 12 M., when an attack resembling cholera morbus supervened; after this period *severe and copious discharge of frothy fluid matter*, frequently dejected from the bowels, with cutting pains at intervals and vomiting. Verat.[3] was given with only partial relief. Elaterium[2], every two or three hours, effected in a few hours an entire cure of the symptoms of cholera; and when the period arrived for the recurrence of his ague, the patient found he was also cured of that, and has remained well.—C. B. MATTHEWS, *S. C.*;—I, p. 692.

CASE IV.—Obstinate ague for *five years*, which was contracted while residing in Virginia. Suppressed by Chin. sulf. in large doses, but always recurred at longer or shorter periods. When the chills were suppressed she was generally attacked with urticaria over the whole surface, and she was frequently afflicted with a disordered state of the mind, characterized by an irresistible propensity to wander from home even in the night and range the woods. The chill occurred every third day, twice in the day, continuing two hours; pains in the head; under the shoulder-blades; in the left side, in the calves of the legs and small of the back; yawning and gaping with a sound resembling the neighing of a horse; running at the nose; cramp in the legs and soles of the feet. The chill was followed by high fever, which ended in copious perspiration. Elater.[2] cured. *Urticaria:* After the ague had subsided in the above case, urticaria appeard, with tendency of mind as above stated. A continuance of the Elaterium for a few days entirely and permanently removed this latter affection and she has had no recurrence. —*Ibid.*

The Elaterium urticaria, like Rhus, has intolerable itching, but, unlike Rhus, is relieved by rubbing.

## ELAPS.

**Characteristic.**—Vertigo with tendency to fall forward. Weight in the stomach after eating. Canine hunger, yet unable to eat. Fruits and drinks lie on the stomach like ice (see **Ars., Verat.**).

**Type.**—Quotidian.

**Time.**—8 and 10 P.M., every day.

**Chill.**—Without thirst, followed by dry heat and burning redness of the face. *Chilliness and heat alternately* (**Ars., Calc. ost.**) at 8 P.M.; *chilly for a few minutes,* then *heat for a quarter of an hour. Shaking chill,* felt internally as if *in the bones,* followed in half an hour by *burning heat;* the skin hot, with thirst, the fever lasted whole night until 10 A.M. next day. Coldness *aggravated by drinking cold water* (**Caps.**); after a drink, shivering from head to foot with chattering of the teeth. Terrible coldness after drinking, and as if ice water were rising and falling through a cylindrical opening in left lung. Great sensitiveness to cold. Right leg up to knee, cold as ice. Arms cold by putting hand in cold water.

**Heat.**—With thirst, *alternating with chilliness. Dry heat* from 7 to 9 P.M., followed by *chill till* 10 *P. M.* Fever at 7 P.M., with less chill, more violent heat, but little sweat; sleep interrupted by heavy dreams (of dead people), with difficult breathing the whole night. *Flushes of heat, with redness of the face and ears.*

**Sweat.**—All over. Sweat cold and profuse. Sweat on forehead and nape of the neck.

**Tongue.**—Deep red, clean, or swollen and black.

## EUPATORIUM PERFOLIATUM.

**Characteristic.**—Adapted to diseases of old people; worn out constitutions, especially from inebriety.

Pains; osteocopic, affecting the back, limbs, head, chest, particularly the wrists as if dislocated, the eyeballs; the more general and severe the better adapted. Like Bryonia, they are accompanied by headache, constipation and pain in hepatic region, but here the similitude ends.

In Bryonia, the perspiration is profuse, easily excited by motion, and the pains compel patient to lie still upon the painful side.

In Eupatorium the sweat is scanty or wanting, the pains cause restlessness without any relief from motion, and there is entire inability to lie on left side.

Pains as if broken; come quickly and go away as quickly (reverse of Stan.).

Vertigo: sensation as if falling to the left (cannot turn the head to the left for fear of falling, Col.).

Followed well by Natrum mur. and Sepia.

**Aggravation.**—Motion; drinking; uncovering.

**Type.**—Tertian; double tertian; rarely, double quartan, and then only when changed from original type by Quinine. All types may be cured by it. Anticipating.

**Time.**—7 A.M.; 7 to 9 A.M.; 7 to 9 A.M. one day, lighter chill at 12 M. next day; 10 A.M.; 12 to 2 P.M.; 5 P.M. Will cure without reference to time, when totality of symptoms are present.

**Prodrome.**—Insatiable thirst, *but drinking causes nausea and vomiting, and hastens the chill. Sick stomach and thirst night before the paroxysm.* Thirst, sometimes for warm drinks (Casc., Ced.), *from one to three hours before the chill;* he knows the chill is coming because *"he cannot drink enough"* (knows chill is coming because she is thirsty, **Caps., Cinch., Natr. m.**); yawning, stretching, *pain in back, especially above right ilium, and the bones of extremities as if broken.* Colicky pain in the upper abdomen (**Coc.**); *painful soreness of the eyeballs.* Must *be covered*, before and during chill (covered during entire paroxysm, **Nux v.**). *Hungry* (Cina).

**Chill.**—*With intense thirst; but drinking water* increases the nausea, and *causes bitter vomiting* (drinking causes vomiting, **Ars.**—drinking increases the chill, **Caps.**). Chilliness with excessive trembling and nausea (from the least motion). *Chilliness in the morning, heat throughout the whole day,* **but no perspiration.** Chill may leave for a few minutes and return again, but *no heat in the interval* (reverse of **Ars.**, which has alternate chill and heat). Shivering increased by motion; intense, throbbing headache; pain in back and bones of extremities; moaning with pain; distressing pain in stomach and spleen. Yawning and stretching; more shivering than the degree of coldness warrants. Must be warmly covered (Nux v.). Begins in or *may spread from the back,* or *runs up the back* (begins in back between the shoulders, **Caps., Polyp.**—begins in lumbar region, **Eup. purp.**). *At close of chill, nausea and vomiting of bitter fluids and bile, aggravated by drinking,* or *after every draught vomiting* (Caps.—sour vomiting at close of chill, Lyc.).

**Heat.**—Preceded by *thirst,* which is often felt most between chill and heat (**Ars., Cinch.**), or there may be little thirst, when cephalalgia and bone pains are increased; trembling, faint from motion; great weakness; cannot raise the head while fever lasts; cheeks mahogany red; throbbing headache; internal soreness from head to foot, all over the body (Arn.); sleep with moaning. Seldom any nausea during this stage, but bitter vomiting (sour vomiting, **Lyc.**) occurs at close of heat if absent at close of chill. Heat and lachrymation. Much shivering even during heat. "*A swallow of water will make him shiver*" (will make him shudder, Caps.). Pain in scrobiculus cordis. Fever in the forenoon, preceded by thirst early in the morning, but no chill; attended by fatiguing cough, and not followed by perspiration.

**Sweat.**—Generally scanty, or absent altogether, in which case *the headache continues for several hours after fever is gone* (**Ars.**). When there is much perspiration, *it brings relief of all pains except cephalalgia,* **which is increased** (sweat relieves all pains **Natr. m.**). *Coldness during nocturnal sweat.* Perspiration; at night giving no relief; during sweat the slightest movement of patient, or jar of bed, will cause a transient chill to run through the frame, especially along the back on uncovering (Nux v.); not debilitating if profuse (reverse of **Cinch.** and **Carb. v.**). *When chill is severe, sweat is light or wanting* and *vice versa.*

**Tongue.**—Coated white or yellow. Taste, insipid, bitter; food has no taste (**Dros.**). Desire for ice cream; thirst. Paleness of mucous membrane of mouth (**Fer.**). Cracks at the commissures of the lips (**Natr. m.**). Canine hunger after Quinine.

**Apyrexia.**—*Imperfect; very little remission.* Jaundiced hue of skin and conjunctivæ; *loose cough;* if any sweat, it is attended with chilliness and worse from motion and uncovering. *Bone pains are present in every stage, and only gradually disappear with disappearance of sweat.* Feels worse morning of one day, and afternoon of next. The severity of vomiting has relation to time of eating; the nearer the meals the surer to vomit; first of ingesta, afterwards of bile, which is usually bitter.

"Eupatorium has been a favorite remedy with the most successful practitioners where remittent and intermittent fevers have prevailed epidemically *in miasmatic districts, along rivers, at fisheries, on marshes,* and their several neighborhoods."—C. J. HEMPEL, *S. C.*, I., p. 696.

"*Eupatorium perf.*, both by its pathogenesis and clinical verification in practice, is one of the most valuable of the Materia Medica in the treatment of western intermittents."—J. S. DOUGLAS.

To this statement I would add that its efficacy is not bounded by latitude. Sometimes it corresponds to the genus epidemicus, and will alone cure nearly every case, particularly if occurring in autumn. It vies with Arsenicum, Cinchona and Natrum mur. as one of our sheet anchors in this disease; its symptoms are "clear-cut" and well defined; its action prompt and decisive. It has cured in all potencies from tinct. to cm.

## Arsenicum.

**Type.**—Quotidian; tertian; quartan; double tertian and quartan. Anticipating. Every fourteen days. Irregular both in type and stage (Nux v.).

**Time.**—Characteristic; 1 to 2 P.M., 12 to 2 A.M. Afternoon paroxysm predominates.

**Prodrome.**—*No thirst.* Headache, with vertigo and pale face; pain in bowels and watery diarrhœa. Debility; great weariness; must lie down. Malaise.

## Eupatorium.

**Type.**—Tertian; double tertian, rarely double quartan. Anticipating. All types may be cured with Eupatorium.

**Time.**—7 A.M. or 7 to 9 A.M.; 7 to 9 A.M. one day, lighter chill at 12 M. next day. Forenoon predominates.

**Prodrome.**—*Insatiable thirst.* Drinking hastens chill and causes vomiting. Know chill is coming because "he cannot drink enough." Yawning, stretching, backache, and bone pains in extremities.

**Chill.**—Irregular; mingling of chilliness and heat; or chills and heat alternate; *ameliorated by external heat.* Thirst is not always present; if present, drinks little and often, but generally for hot drinks. Thirst, except for hot drinks, contra-indicates.

**Heat.**—Intense, dry, burning, long-lasting heat, pungent to the touch, and *insatiable thirst for cold water. Great restlessness.* Must be uncovered. Heat as if hot water were coursing through the blood-vessels.

**Sweat.**—*With unquenchable thirst for large quantities of water,* which causes vomiting. Cold, clammy. Great weakness and prostration. Previous symptoms relieved during sweat.

**Tongue.**—Tip red, sides furred, with red streaks down middle; brown-blue. Desire for acids, brandy; water tastes bitter; *aversion to food.*

**Apyrexia.**—*Never clear. Great weakness and prostration.* Face pale, sallow, sunken or bloated. Debilitating, watery diarrhœa. General anæmic appearance.

Fevers contracted at sea-shore watering-places, appear in autumn, or "wintered over" and come on in spring.

**Chill.**—*With great thirst.* Begins in back; with *yawning, stretching, backache and bone pains.* May leave and return, but no heat in interval. Must be covered warmly (Nux v.). Bitter vomiting at close of chill. More shivering than coldness warrants.

**Heat.**—Great weakness; cannot raise the head while heat lasts. Rarely any thirst; cheeks mahogany red, and intense throbbing headache; a swallow of water produces shivering. Body sore from head to foot.

**Sweat.**—Scanty or absent. If much, is more profuse at night and then cold. Relieves all pains except cephalalgia, *which is increased.* When chill is severe, sweat is light or wanting, and vice versa.

**Tongue.**—Coated white or yellow pale; food tasteless, insipid, bitter. Desire for ice cream. Canine hunger after Quinine. Commissures of lips cracked. (Natr. m.)

**Apyrexia.**—Imperfect, very little remission. Jaundiced hue of skin and conjunctivæ; loose cough. Bone pains in every stage, unless relieved by sweat.

Fevers of miasmatic, marshy regions; autumnal; often the genus epidemicus. Apt to become remittent.

## CLINICAL.

CASE I.—Dr. Neidhard reports two cases in which was: *Violent thirst before the chill* and slight during it; *nausea and sickness* of the stomach (in which case vomiting) at the commencement of the heat, with violent throbbing headache; *tastelessness of food; want of appetite; tongue coated yellow;* the chills set in *in the morning* and lasted for one or two hours; heat during rest of the day, and slight perspiration in the evening; type tertian. In one case Quinia had been given without preventing recurrence of paroxysm. Eup. cured.—*S. C.,* Vol. I, p. 696.

CASE II.—The chill generally began *at* 9 *A.M.*, lasting four hours, followed by heat for seven hours, and rarely perspiration. Next day a lighter paroxysm *at* 12 *M.*, and ceased about same time in evening as the heavier one on the day preceding. The paroxysms continued alternately thus for twenty-three days, notwithstanding my unceasing efforts to arrest them with a number of remedies. Dec. 12th, chill commenced *at* 9 *A.M.; lasted four hours, with great shivering and trembling; raging thirst before the chill, and during chill and heat; vomiting of ingesta and bile,* with distressing *pain at epigastrium;* distracting *headache during the heat;* heat ceased about 8 P.M. and was followed by *inconsiderable perspiration.* Eup. perf. 1st, in water, a teaspoonful every hour in apyrexia, cured the case without the recurrence of another paroxysm. —DR. WILLIAMSON, *S. C.*, Vol. I, p. 696.

CASE III.—Aug. 1st, 1878, saw (in consultation) Miss W., aged 50, corpulent, resident of New York, very sick since last April from attacks of intermittent fever and *scientific* (?) treatment. The attacks had been suppressed at times by Quinia, Fer., "Blue mass," administered by the most prominent allopathists in New York, always to return sooner or later, with added new sufferings. Her debility and nightly restlessness were so great that Dr. C. C. Smith, her physician, gave her Ars. (high), which very much relieved her and brought out the old suppressed attacks of chills and fever. The cold stage came on in the afternoon, each alternate day an hour earlier; never amounted to a chill; *thirst before and during cold stage,* which lasted three hours; *vomited much bile after drinking;* muscles painful, worse in cold stage, followed by intense heat, with perspiration; hot stage lasted six to eight hours, with thirst. During attack she would be warmly covered, then profuse perspiration, without heat, continued during sleep all night. Great debility, even when free from fever. Liver much enlarged and very sensitive to touch. *Urine extremely scanty, turbid and of an offensive odor.* No appetite for some time. Eup. per $^{50m}$ (Finke) in water, one teaspoonful every two hours for twelve hours, during apyrexia. Next paroxysm was most severe she had ever had, but she had passed *a large quantity of limpid urine.* No medicine. Succeeding paroxysm very mild and short; *urine continued profuse.* Fourteen days after, a slight attack; a single dose of Eupatorium at the end of it; since then no chills and fever, general health good; no signs of hypertrophy of liver. AD. LIPPE (see comments in), *Organon,* April, 1879.

CASE IV.—A boy, æt. 8, had a chill every other day at 2 P.M. Cold for an hour and a half; shakes part of that time. Thirsty *before the chill, vomiting of food as the chill passes off;* wants to be warmly covered when in the chill; appetite good, pain at pit of stomach, back of neck, between the shoulders. More thirst with chill than heat; *stretches and yawns;* fever for three hours, followed by perspiration; sweat till midnight. *Cold perspiration at night.* Eup. perf. cm., cured.—J. H. P. FROST, *H. M.*, Oct., 1874.

CASE V.—Mrs. A. T., 22, *chilliness* with thirst in middle of the night, but before chilliness, was awakened out of sleep by severe pains, like cramps in the lower limbs—a sense of numbness, as if the flesh were falling off the bones, followed by cold sweat on them. **Heat**, with thirst, then perspiration. Nausea and inability to vomit, with both chills and heat. Chills frequently during the night at irregular intervals, attended with pain in the limbs. Eup. $^6$ cured in a few days.—*Ibid*

CASE VI.—Mrs. A., four months pregnant, has the following: *Thirst before the chill; chill at 6 A.M.; very thirsty for warm drinks; vomiting as the chill passed off.* **Heat**, *with thirst for warm drinks;* very weak during fever; very nervous; no sweat after fever, but some during the night; *good appetite immediately after the fever.* Eup. perf., $^{1m}$ one dose, cured all but the lassitude and debility. They were removed by same remedy in $^{10m}$ potency.—S. SWAN, *Med., Inv.*, VIII, p. 73. In the provings of Eup. we find "thirsts *for cold drinks*" and "*hunger before the chill.*" Are the opposite symptoms in above case secondary, and cured because the remedy was given high? Bone pains may not be present and the patient may prefer warm to cold drinks, and yet Eup. cure the case.*

CASE VII.—A strong, fleshy man, about 27 years of age, has had one attack. All the forenoon very thirsty; at 10 A.M. violent, sharp, colicky pain in upper abdomen; headache; *pain in back and legs;* no chill. This was soon followed by *high fever*, with *nausea, horrid headache and bone pains*, but colic was relieved. Fever lasts four hours; is followed by profuse sweat, with relief of pains *except headache*. After sweat, soreness of the scalp. Eup. perf. $^{200}$ in water every three hours during the apyrexia. No return.—A. L. FISHER, *A. J. H. M. M.*—V, p. 177.

CASE VIII.—Mrs. P. had severe chill every morning at 7 o'clock, lasting an hour, with terrible bone pains in extremities and lumbar region. Thirst begins some time before the chill and continues during chill and fever. Chill terminates in bilious vomiting, and as fever passes off falls into deep sleep, during which she has profuse perspiration. Eup. perf. $^{200}$ in water, a teaspoonful every three hours while awake. Next day paroxysm much lighter; medicine continued every six hours, and no return of the chill.—H. C. ALLEN, *Homœopathist*, Dec., 1878.

CASE IX.—Several weeks ago I gave three doses of Eup. perf. $^6$ in a case of intermittent fever, characterized by much thirst before chill and during chill and heat; chill about 8 A.M.; during chill bitter (bilious)

---

* The true explanation, probably, is that our knowledge and our provings of Eupatorium are obtained from the tincture and gathered from clinical experience. If we had provings made with potencies, from 30th to 1$^m$, the finer characteristics of the remedy might be brought out. This is the reason why we often cure or remove many symptoms, not found in the provings, where a high potency is given, on some guiding indication.

vomiting and headache, backache, and pain in bones. The patient lives in a malarious region, and now reports that he has had no more paroxysms and is well.—H. V. MILLER, *Priv. Com.*

## EUPATORIUM PURPUREUM.

**Characteristic.**—Has been praised as a preventive. All symptoms worse on left side.

Sensation as if falling to the left; persistent, cannot get rid of it.

Weak, tired feeling in every organ of the body; cannot move without making a desperate effort.

Rheumatic pains go from below upward (Ledum—shoot downward, Kalmia); change places frequently.

Sleep, restless, disturbed with frightful dreams.

Mechanical dysuria; from displaced uterus; jolting ride during pregnancy.

Constant desire to urinate; no matter how often he voids urine, bladder still feels full.

Incontinence of urine in children.

Chronic cystitis; uneasy; deep aching; dull pain and soreness in bladder; smarting and burning in bladder, urethra, on urinating.

**Aggravation.**—Motion; changing position.

**Type.**—*Double tertian*; double quartan.

**Time.**—Different times of the day; hour not marked. (3 to 5 P.M.)

**Prodrome.**—Bone pains in arms and legs (bone pains with intense thirst, **Eup. perf.**). Dry, hacking cough in spells.

**Chill.**—*With thirst; begins in small of back—lumbar region* (interscapular region, **Caps.**, **Polyp.**), passing up and down, thence extends over the body. *Longing for lemonade, cold acid drinks*, with *violent bone pains, blue lips* and *nails* (**Natr. m.**, **Nux v.**), extremities cold, and *frontal headache. Violent shaking, with comparatively little coldness* (Eup. perf.). *Nausea, but no vomiting*, as the chill is leaving (vomiting at close of chill, **Eup. perf.**, **Lyc.**). Nervous, restless, hysterical mood. Numbness of the legs *after* or *in conjunction with* the severe bone pains.

**Heat.**—*With thirst. Long-lasting heat*, with bone pains, nausea and vomiting. *Hunger*, with desire to eat immediately after the fever (hunger before chill and during sweat, **Cinch.**). Frightful dreams. *Longing for hot drinks* (**Casc.**, **Cedr.**).

## EUPATORIUM PURPUREUM.

**Sweat.**—Without thirst; slight, mostly about forehead and head; *of upper parts of body.* Chilly down the back, *when changing position ever so little.* Very rarely, sweat is profuse (same as its congener, **Eup. perf.**).

**Tongue.**—Heavily furred, brown along the centre; bitter, pappy taste with the chill.

**Apyrexia.**—Passes more urine than normal, with frequent desire; scalding on urinating. Profuse flow of clear, limpid urine; weak, tired and faint after urinary symptoms. Vertigo, with "a dizzy feeling" all over, and a persistent sensation of *falling to the left* (of falling, **Gels.**).

### Eup. purp.

**Type.**—Double tertian.
**Time.**—Different times of day.

**Prodrome.**—Bone pains in arms and legs. Dry, hacking cough in spells.

**Chill.**—*No thirst*, or thirst for lemonade and acid drinks. Chill begins in lumbar region, thence extends over body. Nausea as the chill is leaving, but no vomiting.

**Heat.**—Long-lasting; thirst, bone pains, and hunger as the heat is passing off (Cina, Cinch.).

**Sweat.**—Chilly, when changing position ever so little during sweat.

**Apyrexia.**—Vertigo, with falling to the left.

Urine, profuse, urging, scalding.

### Eup. perf.

**Type.**—Tertian.
**Time.**—7 A.M., or 7 to 9 A.M. one day; 12 M. next day.

**Prodrome.**—*Thirst* several hours before, with bone pains and pains in back.

**Chill.**—Great thirst for cold water. Chill, with bone pains, pains in back, gaping, stretching, throbbing headache. Bitter vomiting at close of chill. Drinking hastens chill and causes vomiting.

**Heat.**—With sleep; moaning, increased headache. "A swallow of water will make him shiver" (Caps.).

**Sweat.**—Bone pains disappear with disappearance of sweat.

**Apyrexia.**—Jaundiced hue; great weakness; anæmia. Light chill and profuse sweat, or shaking chill, and light or wanting sweat.

## CLINICAL.

CASE I.—Intermittent from a miasmatic district, paroxysm comes at different times in the day; *chill commences at the small of the back*, spreading up and down the trunk, finally reaching the extremities. Lips and nails blue. *Violent shaking, with comparatively little coldness.* No thirst during the chill, but considerable pain across the forehead. This lasted several hours, when some fever set in; not very severe, merging in about three hours into a moisture not amounting to sweat.

Chill two and a half years.—H. N. MARTIN, *Am. Jour. of Mat. Med.*, p. 17.

CASE II.—For several days headache and thirst, followed in a few minutes by coldness of feet and hands; chill along the back, *beginning at the lower dorsal region and running up the back.* Chills not amounting to regular shakes, commence every day about 4 P.M., lasting twenty minutes, followed by excessive thirst, flushed face; skin hot and dry; nausea and vomiting; chills. Hot stage protracted for several hours during the night, followed by moisture of skin, not amounting to a sweat, *principally about the forehead and head.* Previous to attack, a spell of dry, hacking cough, continuing throughout the paroxysm.—J. G. HOWARD, *Am. Jour. of Mat. Med.*, p. 16.

CASE III.—Miss C., æt. 20, had been suffering for seven or eight days with following symptoms: During the morning headache, distressing pain in the lumbar region, pain in the arms and legs and occasionally pain in left side of the throat, causing much pain during the act of deglutition, which would disappear entirely in a few hours and return again the following day. These symptoms would continue until about 3 P.M., after which the following would set in: *Chilly feeling in the lumbar region,* extending up the back as far as between the scapulæ, coldness of the hands and feet; finger nails turned blue and general coldness of the whole body ensued, never amounting to a real shake, still, well-marked coldness of surface; pain in upper and lower extremities. These symptoms would last from one to three hours, and then fever would begin with flushed face, suffusion of eyes with lachrymation; running at the nose and great heat; constant thirst; desire for cold and acid drinks; hands and feet cold; loss of appetite; restless sleep with frightful dreams. As the fever abated, a perspiration, not amounting to sweat, but rather profuse about the forehead, appeared. The fever and sweat continued from three to five hours. Eup. purp. 3x cured.—C. H. VON TAGEN. *Ibid.*

## FERRUM.

**Characteristic.**—Adapted to persons of sanguine temperament; pettish, quarrelsome, disputative, easily excited, least contradiction angers; women who are weak, delicate, chlorotic, yet have a very red face.

General hemorrhagic diathesis.

**Extreme paleness of the face, which becomes red and flushed on the least pain, emotion, or exertion.**

"Have cured intermittents where these face symptoms were prominent."—W. J. Hawkes.

Erethic chlorosis, worse in winter.

Red parts become white.

Menses: too soon, too profuse, too long-lasting, with fiery red face; ringing in the ears; intermit two or three days and then return; flow pale, watery, debilitating.

Vertigo; with balancing sensation as if on the water; on seeing flowing water; when walking over water, like when crossing a bridge (Hydroph.); when descending (Borax).

Headache; for two, three, or four days, every two or three weeks; hammering, beating, pulsating pains, must lie down in bed; with aversion to eating or drinking.

Complementary to Alumina, Cinchona.

**Aggravation.**—While at rest; sitting still.

**Amelioration.**—Walking slowly about.

**Type.**—Tertian. *Morning chill. Afternoon fever.*

**Time.**—7 A.M.—12 M.—3 P.M.

Fever, without chill, 3 to 8 P.M.

Intermittent fever after abuse of Quinine; congestions to head and face; veins distended; vomiting ingesta; swelling of spleen; anæmia marked by pseudo-plethora; skin transparent when it is not earthy. The totality of the characteristic symptoms.

**Prodrome.**—Vomiting of ingesta as the chill is coming on. Loose stool in early morning (**Sulf.**).

**Chill.**—*With thirst.* Chilliness with headache in the morning. General coldness of the body, hands and feet very cold. Chilliness and trembling all over. Chilliness in frequent short attacks. In the afternoon, violent chill for half an hour, then thirst, must go to bed, followed by heat with perspiration. *During the chill his face got glowing hot* (Arn.). *Hands and feet cold and numb* (**Cedr., Cimex, Sepia**), chilly all over, does not go off by walking. Feet *cold* and *numb* all night, as after skating. *Feet very cold, toes cold as ice, fingers stiff.*

**Heat.**—*Without thirst.* Heat in the body, with *red cheeks*, but the head is free (but head aches, **Bell.**). Sensation of heat all over the body, *which was cold to the touch*, with sensation in the face and around the eyes, as if swollen and bloated (reverse of **Bar. c.**, coldness of body which was hot to the touch). Flushes over the whole body, as if perspiration would break out. Heat of head, feet cold. Great heat of *palms of hands* and *soles of feet*. Heat in the stomach (relieved by eating), vomiting of the ingesta. Dry heat, worse towards evening; inclination to uncover (Sec.); better by moving about, eating, speaking. *Face very red.*

**Sweat.**—*From early morn till noon every other day, preceded by headache.* Sweat *profuse, long-lasting,* whether by day at every motion, or night and morning in bed. *Strong-smelling, clammy, debilitating nightsweat.* Sweat *stains yellow,* and is fœtid on going to sleep. All the symptoms *are worse* while sweating (all the symptoms *are relieved* by sweating, **Natr. m.**). "Nausea during sweat."—Pearson.

**Tongue.**—Coated white. *Lips, gums, tongue,* and *mucous membrane* of entire buccal cavity *pale* and *bloodless* (**Sec.**). All food tastes bitter, dry, woody and insipid. Taste like rotten eggs (**Acon., Arn.**). Anorexia; extreme dislike to all food.

**Pulse.**—Hard and full at beginning of paroxysm; or weak, small and scarcely perceptible during apyrexia.

**Apyrexia.**—*Prostration, debility* and *great loss of muscular power.* Anæmia. Œdema of feet and face, especially upper and lower eyelids (**Apis, Ars.**—of upper eyelids, **Kali. c.**). Headache; vertigo; *swelling of the cutaneous veins;* splenic region swollen and sore on pressure (**Apis, Arn.**). *Vomiting of everything eaten without being digested.* Constipation or chronic diarrhœa with lienteria. Cadaverous, jaundiced complexion. Yellow spots on the face (Sep.). Very weak and tired, but always better when *walking slowly* about (better from being perfectly still, **Bry.**). Cases maltreated by Quinine.

"Iron is evidently one of the most precious remedies against the cachectic condition: but I admit that its action is due to neither the chemical reasons that have been imagined and which have been current even on the lips of our school, nor the massive doses which naturally flow from these considerations; it is by its dynamic virtues that Ferrum acts and confers all its benefits.—A. Charge.

## CLINICAL.

Paroxysm every other day. Headache; pressing in the forehead, followed by violent chilliness, lasting three-quarters of an hour, with increased headache and much thirst. Afterwards moderate heat and sweat. Bitter taste. Loss of appetite. Constipation. Yellowish complexion. Great weakness. Moderate headache during the apyrexia. Ferrum acet. Another dose in three days. Cured.—*Rückert's Therapeutics,* p. 458.

## GAMBOGIA.

**Characteristic.**—The conditions calling for Gambogia are apt to occur especially toward evening or night.

Frightful vomiting and purging attended with fainting (Elat., Verat.).

Stool: profuse, watery, with colic and tenesmus; dark green mucus, offensive, corrosive, discharged with a single, somewhat prolonged effort; great relief after stool as though an irritating substance were removed from the bowels.

**Aggravation.**—Evening and night; while sitting.

**Amelioration.**—During motion in the open air.

**Type.**—*Quotidian*, tertian; double tertian; intermittent often becomes remittent. Postponing oftener than anticipating.

**Time.**—7 P.M.; EVENING 6 TO 8 P.M., lasting all night (Lyc., Puls., Rhus, Sarac., last all night).

**Chill.**—*Violent shaking at 7 P.M., beginning in the back*, with external coldness of whole body, *continues till 4 A.M.* (chill lasts 12 hours, **Canth.**—24 hours, **Aran.**). *Internal and external coldness*, at 6 to 8 P.M., lasting from a quarter to two hours, or the whole night to 5 A.M. Sensation of chilliness and elongation of incisor teeth. Chill for two hours with chattering of the teeth, with violent thirst; the skin is warm to the touch. Sudden shaking chill at night, waking him from sleep, and as suddenly disappearing.

**Heat.**—Increased warmth, with anxiety and flushes of heat. Always slight, often wanting.

**Sweat.**—Over whole body on waking at 4 A.M. Early morning sweat.

The fevers of Gambogia occur while diarrhœa is prevalent. The paroxysm consists almost wholly of the cold stage; the others being light or wanting.

## GELSEMIUM.

**Characteristic.**—Adapted to children; young people; women of a nervous, hysterical temperament; irritable, sensitive, excitable; onanists, both sexes.

Desire to be quiet, to be let alone, does not wish to speak, nor have any one near her for company, even if the person be silent (Ign.).

Complaints: from exciting or bad news (from pleasant surprises, Coff.); sudden emotions; the anticipation of any unusual ordeal; general depression from heat of sun or summer.

Vertigo: spreading from the occiput; with diplopia, dim vision, loss of sight; seems intoxicated when trying to move.

Children: fear of falling, seize the nurse.

Lack of muscular co-ordination; giddy, confused; muscles refuse to obey the will.

Headache: beginning in cervical spine; pains extend over the head, causing a bursting sensation in forehead and eyeballs (Sang., Sil., begin in same way, but are semi-lateral); worse from smoking.

Sensation of a band around the head above the ears; scalp sore.

Fears that unless constantly on the move, the heart will cease beating (would cease beating if she moved, Dig.).

**Aggravation.**—Damp weather; before a thunder storm; sudden emotions; bad news; rest. Smoking tobacco.

**Amelioration.**—In the cold, open air.

**Type.**—Quotidian; tertian; same hour of the day with every paroxysm (**Aran., Cedr., Sabad.**). Periodicity extends throughout its entire pathogenesis; all its fevers are of a regular type, but characterized by disorders of innervation. *Simple, uncomplicated cases.* When the remittent takes on the intermittent type (reverse of **Bapt., Eup. perf., Quin.**).

**Time.**—Afternoon and evening paroxysm 2, 4, 5 and 9 P.M. Fever without chill at 10 A.M. (**Bapt., Natr. m.**).

**Prodrome.**—Sudden mental emotions, the anticipation of any unusual ordeal, fright, grief, bad news, may hasten chill or produce diarrhœa. Could tell when chill was about to return, as incontinence of urine would set in. Thirst, but does not drink much; hurts to swallow.

**Chill.**—*Without thirst.* Chill commences in the hands and feet (in recent cases—in old chronic cases, **Natr. m.**). Chill ascending from feet; *chill and chilliness, especially along the spine; running up the back from loins to nape of neck,* and following each other in rapid wave-like succession from *sacrum to occiput* (running *up and down* the spine, **Eup. purp.**). Chilliness with cold hands and feet, headache, and heat of head and face. Chilliness with tired, languid feeling in back and limbs; wants to avoid all muscular exertion. Feet feel as if in very cold water. Coldness is so severe as to be painful. Sleepy as chill is leaving (**Apis**). Nervous chill, the skin is warm; wants to be held that he may not shake so much. Child wants to be held so that he will not shake so hard (**Lach.**).

**Heat.**—Without thirst; **intense burning**. General heat. mostly about the head and face. Warmth over the whole body, as if sweat would break out, then chilly down the back. Directly after the chill comes a flying heat and pricking in the skin, rapidly followed by perspiration, which at times is profuse, and lasting from twelve to twenty-four hours (**Caust.**). *Heat in the face, sleep or sleepy*, stupid, besotted; with half-waking, muttering delirium; tired, *wants to lie still* (**Bry.**), or great nervous restlessness; sensation of *falling, in children; child starts and grasps attendant or crib*, and *screams out from fear of falling*. Semi-stupor; cannot open his eyes or think correctly; vertigo, staggers as if intoxicated. Sensitive to light or noise (**Bell.**—intolerant of noise, **Caps.**). Long-lasting heat; far into night; pain in one leg; jerking of the limbs.

**Sweat.**—Profuse, which relieves the pain. Sweat coming gradually and moderately, always relieving the pains (sweat relieves all the symptoms, **Natr. m.**). Sweats freely from slight exertion (**Psor.**). Perspiration, sometimes profuse and continuing from a few hours to twenty-four hours, with langour and prostration. Sweat most profuse on genitalia.

**Tongue.**—Coated yellowish-white, or nearly clean, or with white centre and red margins. If coated thickly, breath fœtid. Taste: bitter, foul, with blood-colored saliva.

**Pulse.**—Irregular, intermitting, yet full (**Dig.**). Small, weak, feeble, almost imperceptible.

**Apyrexia.**—*Often wanting*, or *very short*. Heat and perspiration are so extended that many fevers are more remitting than intermitting. *Great prostration of whole muscular system.* Headache, aggravated by smoking tobacco (Ign.—relieved by smoking, **Aran.**). Patient is nervous, irritable, easily angered (**Cham.**—very irritable, **Anac., Bry.**).

Intermittent fever: Patient wants to be held during the chill (**Lach.**); sleep throughout heat; thirst during sweat; muttering delirium when half awake; absence of all gastric and hepatic symptoms.

"For intermittents or remittents which are contracted at summer watering places and 'wintered over,' making their appearance in early spring, Gelsemium is a remedy of great value."—R. LUDLAM. (See Ars., Eup. perf.).

Gelsemium is one of the few remedies that has the regular periodic fever, *without chill*. It divides the honors equally with Arsenicum in the treatment of children's intermittents, from which it is distinguished by the regularity of the paroxysm, absence of thirst, and the burning fever and restlessness. The child is neither so weak and prostrated nor pale and feeble as in the Arsenicum fever. Sensation of falling is a genuine symptom, often occurring in children. Gelsemium is always to be thought of in recent uncomplicated cases, where chill begins in extremities (in chronic cases, **Natrum mur.**). Also where a remittent takes on the intermittent type, or *vice versa*.

## CLINICAL.

CASE I.—Ida R., æt. 3 years, "has always had ague," the mother says. Many times suppressed with Quinine, only to re-appear.

*Chill*, every day 4 or 5 P.M.; slight with "goose-flesh;" lasts three-quarters of an hour; with thirst.

*Heat*, long, severe, may last till nearly time for next chill. The sweating short, most marked. Much debility during apyrexia. The curious feature was that every time the chills had been suppressed, the mother could tell when they were about to return, as *eneuris would invariably set in*. Gels. 3x cured in two weeks.—W. P. POLHEMUS.

CASE II.—Lady, age 19, red hair. Quotidian intermittent every afternoon at 1 o'clock.

*Prodrome*, with thirst, but not much drank, as it hurts to swallow.

*Chill*. Shaking begins in hands, with thirst, headache, vertigo; pains in back, limbs, knee, with cramps.

*Heat*, with some thirst, begins in head; headache, vertigo; pains continue; heat and chill together, shivers up the back; red cheeks, hot face.

*Sweat* comes gradually and relieves all the symptoms. Tongue clean; pulse quick, soft, irregular. Must be covered in all stages of paroxysm. Had four paroxysms before I saw her. Gels. 1x cured.—A. J. WILLIAMS.

## GRAPHITES.

**Characteristic.**—Adapted to women inclined to obesity, who suffer from habitual constipation, and whose history reveals a tendency to delaying menstruation.

"What Pulsatilla is at puberty, Graphites is at the climacteric."

Morning sickness during menstruation; very weak and prostrated.

Leucorrhœa: acrid, excoriating, occurs in gushes day and night; before and after menses (before, Sepia; after, Kreos.).

Hard cicatrices remaining after mammary abscess, retarding flow of milk.

Unhealthy skin; every injury suppurates (Hepar); eruptions, behind the ears, on various parts, from which ooze a watery, transparent, sticky fluid; nails brittle, crumbling, deformed; painful and sore, as if ulcerated.

Cracks or fissures of ends of fingers and nipples, labial commissures, of anus, between the toes (see Nit. acid).

Burning round spot on top of head (Calc., Sulf.—cold spot, Sep., Verat.).

Constipation; stool large, knotty (Sulf.).

Cataleptic condition; conscious, but without power to move or speak.

Takes cold easily; sensitive to draught of air (Borax, Hepar), suffering parts emaciate.

Hears better when in a noise; when riding in a carriage.

Complementary: Causticum, Hepar, Lycopodium. Follows well after the latter.

**Aggravation.**—Cold or becoming cold; night; during and after menstruation.

**Amelioration.**—Eructations (Carb. v.); while walking.

**Type.**—Quotidian; double quotidian.

**Time.**—6 or 7 A.M.; morning in bed; afternoon, 4, 5, 6, 7, 8 P.M.

**Chill.**—Without thirst, in the morning in bed; from 4 P.M. till evening; chilliness and coldness of whole body at 5 P.M., with icy-cold feet. Violent febrile chilliness morning and evening, the heat followed by sweat. Shaking chill every day, in the evening; after an hour, hot face and cold feet *without subsequent sweat*. Chill in evening, with headache and tearing in the limbs, great thirst, and profuse perspiration after midnight, lasting till morning. Chill *worse after meals; better after drinking and in the open air* (Caust.—worse after drinking, **Ars.**,

Caps., Cimex.); *better in open air* (Apis, Ipec.—worse in open air, Ign.). Icy-cold feet, alternating with burning.

**Heat.**—At night; with restlessness; unable to sleep, or remain in bed on account of it; when riding in a carriage. Dry heat every evening and night, lasting till morning, with headache on vertex and in nape of the neck till noon. Hands and soles of the feet hot and burning.

**Sweat.**—Profuse at night; from the slightest motion; on front of body and centre of chest (sternum); stains yellow; is sour and offensive smelling (Hep., Lyc.). Profuse sweat on the feet; they smell and become sore (Iod., Sil.). Entire inability to sweat (Hep.).

**Tongue.**—Coated white and sensitive. Taste sour, salty, bitter; like rotten eggs. Rotten odor from mouth. Breath smells like urine. Lips and nostrils sore and cracked, as from cold. Averse to meat, fish, cooked food, salt.

**Apyrexia.**—Excessive hunger, or no appetite, with great distension of abdomen, as from accumulation or incarceration of flatulence. Constipation. Urine turbid, and deposits white sediment.

## HEPAR SULFURIS CALCAREUM.

**Characteristic.**—Suitable for torpid, lymphatic constitutions; persons with light hair and complexion, slow to act, muscles soft and flabby. Like Sulfur, Hepar is adapted to the psoric scrofulous diathesis.

In Sulfur the skin affections are dry, itching and not sensitive to touch, in fact, relieved by scratching and rubbing; while in Hepar the skin is unhealthy, suppurating, even slight injuries suppurate and maturate, and are extremely sensitive to touch, the pain often causing fainting.

Diseases where suppuration seems inevitable.

Diseases where the system has been injured by the abuse of Mercury.

Patient is peevish; angry at the least trifle; hypochondriacal; unreasonably anxious; hurried speaking and drinking.

Extremely sensitive to cold air; must be wrapped up to the face even in hot weather (Psor.); cannot bear to be uncovered (Nux v.—

## HEPAR SULFURIS CALCAREUM.

cannot bear to be covered, Camph., Sec.); coughs when any part of the body is uncovered; croup or cough from exposure to dry west wind (Acon.).

Eyeballs: sore to touch; pain as if they would be drawn back into head (Oleander, Paris).

Sensation of a splinter, fish-bone or plug in the throat.

**Aggravation.**—Lying; painful sore feeling on the side on which he lies, at night, must change position (see **Kali c.**); cold air; uncovering; touching the parts.

**Amelioration.**—Warmth; wrapping up warmly (Silicea).

**Type.**—*Simple.* Quotidian. Period the same every day.

**Time.**—Morning at 2, 6 or 7 A.M. The evening paroxsym, like Graph., Lyc., Puls. and Rhus, is most severe. **6 or 7 P.M.**—4, 5, 6, 7 or 8 P.M.

Fever, without chill, 4 P.M., lasting all night. Morning fever preceded by bitter taste in mouth, returning twice a day.

**Prodrome.**—Itching, stinging, nettle-rash. Bitter taste in the mouth, for hours before chill.

**Chill.**—Without thirst. **Great chilliness in open air;** *must get to warm stove;* heat feels agreeable but does not relieve (must get to warm stove as soon *as chill begins*, **Bov.**—must get to warm stove, *and lie down*, **Lach.**). **Great sensitiveness to open** *air, with chilliness* (excessively sensitive to open air, **Camph.**—chill aggravated by least draft of air, **Bar. c.**). *Violent chill every morning, at 6 or 7 o'clock, without subsequent heat* (without subsequent *heat* or *sweat*, **Bov.**). *Violent chill*, with chattering of the teeth, lasting a quarter of an hour, with *coldness of the hands and feet,* followed by heat with sweat, especially on the chest and forehead, and slight thirst. *Violent shaking chill* with chattering of the teeth, *icy-coldness* and *paleness* of the *face, hands* and *feet, unconsciousness* and *coma* (**Bell., Opium**). *Febrile chill*, from 4 to 8 P.M., or in the *night, could not get warm,* with *aggravation of all complaints* (**Ars.**); *without subsequent heat.* Chill at 2 A.M., with febrile shivering and hot, dry skin. **Nettle-rash, with violent itching** *and* **stinging,** *disappears as heat begins* (nettle-rash appears as the chill is passing off, **Apis**—during sweat, **Rhus**—during heat, **Ign.**).

**Heat.**—*With thirst. Burning, febrile heat, with almost unquenchable thirst, distressing headache* and *slight delirium, lasting from 4 P.M. all* *night,* without chilliness. Larynx much affected, hoarse, weak voice. *Heat light* in comparison with the chill, though he was obliged to uncover himself (**Puls.**). Dry heat of body at night, with sweaty hands which cannot *tolerate being uncovered* (**Bar. c.**). Febrile paroxysm during the day, chilliness alternating with heat, *with photophobia.* Violent fever, with flushing heat in the face and head. **Fever blisters around the mouth** (**Ign., Natr. m., Nux v., Rhus**).

**Sweat.**—*With flushes of heat.* **Sweats profusely day and night without relief. Perspires easily on every motion, however slight,** *mental exertion, even on writing a few lines* (**Psor., Sep.**); or, at first, no sweat at all, then sweats profusely. *Profuse, sour-smelling sweat at night,* which is often clammy (**Lyc.**). *Sweat of perinœum, groins, and inside of thighs* (sweat most profuse on the genitalia, **Gels.**). **Constant offensive exhalations from the body.** Sometimes thirst with night-sweat.

**Tongue.**—*Tip painful and sore;* back of tongue coated *like dry clay.* Taste: bitter; putrid; metallic; of rotten eggs. Offensive odor from the mouth, which he notices (which he does not notice, **Puls.**). Longing for acids, strong-tasting things. Aversion to fat. Stomach out of order.

**Apyrexia.**—Characteristic: Never clear. Constitutional symptoms always present, and always guiding. Unhealthy skin, with itching, apt to be developed by the fever.

"Intermittent fever; first-chills, then thirst, and an hour later, much heat with interrupted sleep. Violent chill at 8 P.M. with chattering of teeth; hands and feet cold; followed by heat with perspiration, especially on the chest and forehead, with slight thirst."—LIPPE.

## HYOSCYAMUS.

**Characteristic.**—Adapted to persons of sanguine temperament; who are irritable, excitable, nervous, hysterical.

Diseases with increased cerebral activity but of a non-inflammatory type, as in hysteria or delirium tremens.

Convulsions: of children from the irritation of intestinal worms (Cina); of labor; or during the puerperal state.

Delirium: with restlessness, jumps out of bed, tries to escape;

makes irrelevant answers; thinks he is in the wrong place; talks of imaginary wrongs, but has no wants, makes no complaints.

In delirium, Hyoscyamus occupies a place midway between Belladonna and Stramonium; lacks the constant cerebral congestion of the former, and the fierce rage and maniacal delirium of the latter.

Fears: being left alone; poisoned; bitten; sold; to eat; to take what is offered.

Bad effects of unfortunate love; with jealousy, rage, incoherent speech, or inclination to laugh at everything; followed by epilepsy.

Lascivious mania.

Dry, spasmodic, nocturnal cough; worse when lying down, relieved by sitting up.

Spasmodic affections are apt to be epileptoid in character.

Intense sleeplessness of irritable, excitable persons, from business embarrassments, often imaginary.

**Aggravation.**—Evenings; night; during menses; mental affections; jealousy, unhappy love.

**Amelioration.**—Stooping (head); sitting up (cough).

**Type.**—Tertian; quartan.

**Time.**—11 A.M.—alternate days.

**Chill.**—Without thirst. Commencing in *the feet* and running up the spine to nape of neck. Coldness runs from small of back to the nape of the neck (commencing in *hands and feet*, and running up the spine to nape of neck, **Gels.**). *Chill from feet upward.* Shivering over the whole body, with burning redness of face, and cold hands. *Whole body cold*, with *burning redness of face*; *chill alternating with heat* (**Bell.**); **cannot bear to be talked to** (**Cina, Sil.**), or **hear the least noise** (**Caps., Gels.**). Sudden chilliness; coldness of spine; body cold and stiff, cannot get warm in bed; *congestive chills with cold extremities.*

**Heat.**—With thirst. *Burning heat all over, skin hot and dry to touch, with distended veins* (**Bell., Cinch.**). Heat over whole body; much thirst, lips sticky. Burning heat without external redness; *the blood burns in the veins* (**Ars., Rhus**). The skin burning hot to the examining hand, which leaves a burning in place touched (**Bell.**). Heat along the whole spine, which runs up the back. **Epileptiform convulsions** (**Stram.**). **Sleeplessness.**

**Sweat.**—Profuse, general perspiration, mostly on legs. Sweats during sleep. Sweat on back and pit of the stomach. Sweat cold, sour.

**Tongue.**—Coated brown or red, partially paralyzed, protrudes it with difficulty (Lach.). Taste bad, putrid, offensive. Thirst, drinks but little at a time. Dread of water (Hydroph.).

**Apyrexia.**—Extreme weakness; illusions of vision, spots before the eyes; mouth dry, difficult to swallow liquids, hiccough, nausea; vertigo and pressure in the head.

## IGNATIA (Strychnos).

**Characteristic.**—Especially adapted to the nervous temperament; women of a sensitive, easily excited nature; derk hair and skin, but mild disposition; quick to perceive, rapid in execution. In striking contrast with the fair complexion, yielding, lachrymose, but slow and indecisive Pulsatilla.

The remedy of great contradictions; symptoms often, and suddenly, directly opposite (continually changing, no two attacks alike, Puls.).

Mental conditions rapidly, in an almost incredibly short time, change from joy to sorrow, laughing to weeping.

Persons mentally and physically exhausted by long concentrated grief; involuntary sighing, and a weak, empty feeling at pit of stomach, not relieved by eating.

Bad effects of anger, grief, or disappointed love; broods over imaginary trouble in solitude.

Children: reprimanded, scolded, sent to bed, get sick, are convulsed in sleep.

Headache, as if a nail were driven out through the side, relieved by lying on it.

Cannot bear tobacco.

In talking or chewing, bites inside of cheek.

Sweat on the face, of a small spot only, while eating.

Prolapsus ani from moderate straining at stool.

Hemorrhoids: prolapse with every stool, have to be replaced. Stitches up the rectum (Nitr. ac.).

Cough: dry, spasmodic; after warm drinks; every time he stands still during a walk; the longer he coughs the more the irritation to cough increases.

Roaring in ears relieved by music.

Pain; in small circumscribed spots; oversensitive to.

In most cases Ignatia should be given in the morning.

**Aggravation.**—Tobacco; coffee; brandy. Contact; motion; strong smells; mental emotions, grief, etc.; cold air.

**Amelioration.**—Warmth; hard pressure; lying on the back.

**Type.**—Quotidian; tertian; quartan. Irregular; continually changing, especially by the abuse of Quinine (Eup. perf.).

*Postponing* or anticipating; the former the rule, the latter the exception (postpones or anticipates, Gamb.).

The attacks are irregular both in periodicity and evolution of their stages.

**Time.**—**Irregularity of hour,** *characteristic.* Paroxysm at sunset, late in afternoon or evening; then fever heat nearly all night. **At all periods.**

**Prodrome.**—Violent yawning and stretching; sometimes terrible shuddering.

**Chill.**—*Always with* **great thirst** *for large quantities of water* (same, but in all stages, **Bry.**—before and during chill, **Caps., Carb. v., Eup. perf.**), **only during chill** (if thirst in any other stage, it is light and in short spells). Chill commences in *upper arms* and spreads to back and chest (in both arms at once, **Bell.**—in hands and feet, **Gels.**—*chill begins in and spreads from arms;* goose-flesh; hot face; drowsy; worse, motion, getting out of bed, **Hell.**). Chilly at sunset; chilly in cool air; very cold all over, with one-sided headache. **Shaking chill, with redness of the face,** *in the evening.* Coldness and chilliness of whole body, or *only of posterior portions,* **relieved at once in a warm room or by a warm stove (Kali c.).** Chilliness on the back, and over upper arms, with *heat of ears;* about the knees, which are cold externally; in the face and on the arms, with chattering of teeth and goose-flesh; feet and legs, thigh and forearm; *chill* of single parts *only* (*chill and heat* of single parts, **Bell, Rhus**); *proceeding from the abdomen* (most severe in abdomen, **Meny.**,—from the stomach, **Cal. c.**—running to and terminating in the stomach, **Arn.**). During the chill: ill humor, colic, nausea, vomiting of food, mucus and bile (rare); great paleness of face; pain in back; lameness of lower limbs. Chill and coldness aggravate the pains. External coldness, internal heat, or internal chill with external heat.

"*The febrile coldness relieved by external warmth is characteristic of Ignatia.*"—HAHNEMANN.

**Heat.**—*Without thirst.* **Heat of the whole body in the afternoon, without thirst, with sensation of dryness of the skin. External heat and redness, without internal heat.** Sudden flushes of heat over the whole body. *External warmth is intolerable* (**Puls.**); *must be uncovered* as soon as heat begins (**Acon., Sec.**). *One ear, one cheek, and side of the face* **red and burning** (*one cheek* red and hot, the other cold and pale, **Cham.**); hot knees with cold nose; heat of the face, with coldness of the hands and feet; continuous quick alternations from heat to cold. Heat and coldness of single parts (**Apis, Bell.**). **Deep snoring sleep during heat (Apis, Opium); frequent sighing;** beating headache; vertigo, delirium; pain in stomach and bowels; vomiting of ingesta, with coldness of the feet and spasmodic twitching of the extremities. *Urticaria over the whole body, with violent itching,* **easily relieved by scratching,** which disappears with the sweat (itching, stinging, nettle-rash before and during chill, **Hepar,**—during chill and heat, **Rhus**—see **Dulc.**). Patient is hungry after the fever (**Eup. perf.**).

"The heat of Ignatia is almost always *external;* also, there is very seldom thirst with this heat, even in intermittent fever; hence Ignatia is able to cure *homœopathically* and *permanently in the smallest dose, intermittent fever which presents thirst during chill but not during heat.*"—HAHNEMANN.

**Sweat.**—*Without thirst;* warm perspiration of extremities; usually light, though general. *Fainting during sweat,* or as the heat passes into sweating stage. Sweat when eating. Sensation as if sweat would break out over the whole body, which, however, does not follow. Warm perspiration on the hands, or on the inner surface of the hands and fingers, in the evening; at times cold, but generally warm and sour-smelling.

**Tongue.**—Clean. Saliva has a sour taste. Food tasteless

**Apyrexia.**—Complete. The face is pale; *eruption on the lips and in the corners of the mouth;* lips dry and chapped; hungry about 11 A.M. (Sulf.), but little or no appetite at time of meals; aching pain in pit of stomach; colic, with hard stools and ineffectual urging; pain in back and limbs; languor, apathy, giving away of the knees, starting in sleep, or sound sleep with snoring. The sleep usually continues from the heat during and through sweating stage, into apyrexia. All pains and headache aggravated by tobacco and coffee.

"*During the chill, thirsty, seeks external warmth; during the fever heat, no thirst, external warmth very pleasant; sitting up relieves the chill.*" —HAHNEMANN.

Ignatia is adapted to recent mild cases, or long-lasting and complicated ones, particularly those occurring among women and young people of a highly nervous organization. No remedy has *thirst during chill* and in no other stage, chill relieved by external heat, and heat aggravated by external covering, so prominently marked as Ignatia. The Ignatia patient is able to resume his occupation as soon as paroxysm is over. Ignatia is indicated if the tertian type has become quartan after taking large doses of Quinine.

## Gelsemium.

**Time.**—2 P.M., 4 to 5 P.M., and 9 P.M. Regular—every day at same hour.

Morning fever, without chill.

**Prodrome.**—No symptoms.

**Chill.**—*Without thirst;* commencing in hands and feet. Chills follow each other in wave-like rapid succession up the spine from sacrum to occiput.

**Heat.**—Without thirst. Flying heat and flushes followed by perspiration.

**Sweat.**—Profuse, coming on gradually, relieving all the pains.

**Tongue.**—Yellowish-white, breath fetid. Saliva blood-colored.

**Apyrexia.**—Often wanting or very short. Intermittents often become remittents.

## Ignatia.

**Time.**—Not characteristic, chill late in afternoon or evening. Irregular—anticipates or postpones.

Morning fever, with chill.

**Prodrome.**—Yawning and stretching.

**Chill.**—*With great thirst;* commencing in upper arms *and spreads* to back. Shaking chill with red face, *relieved at once in warm room or by heat of stove.*

**Heat.**—Without thirst. External heat and redness, without internal heat.

**Sweat.**—Light, warm, chiefly on extremities, or of the face only.

**Tongue.**—Clean. Saliva has a sour taste. Food tasteless.

**Apyrexia.**—Complete. Face is very pale. One type frequently changes to another.

## CLINICAL.

CASE I.—Dr. McManus, of Baltimore, once related a case to the author, that had for months resisted the best directed efforts of allopathy, and for a long time baffled his skill. The young lady was cured by Ign.$^{200}$ The "guiding symptoms," *thirst only during chill, no thirst in heat or sweat.*

CASE II.—A lady who had a constantly returning ague each spring for several years, which was annually suppressed by large doses of Quinine, consulted me after a second chill. She was faithless in regard to my small doses, so my cure can hardly be said to be one of the imagination. The symptom that governed me in my prescription was, *thirstlessness in the hot stage, and thirst while the chill was on.* I gave her Ignatia and she had no more chills.—G. N. BRIGHAM, *Homœopathist*, Oct., 1878.

CASE III.—J. C., a young man, had been about ten months under different treatment from a number of medical men. Chills occasionally checked for a few days by large doses of Quinine, only to return with renewed severity in another form. No regularity in occurrence of paroxysm, assuming all types—quotidian, tertian, quartan, anticipating or postponing, and coming on at all hours of the day or night. Chill severe and pronounced, lasting usually about an hour, *with intense thirst only during chill. Chill relieved by external heat.* As soon as chill began, although the thermometer was registering "the nineties," he would go at once to the kitchen stove, and "over a hot fire drink the hydrant dry," as he expressed it. Fever always well developed with much headache and vertigo, *but no thirst.* Very rarely any perspiration, and with the exception of some vertigo felt well during the apyrexia. Thanks to similia and the guiding symptoms, I had little difficulty in this obstinate case in selecting the remedy. Chill, *relieved by external heat*, belongs to Arsenic. and Ignatia; and thirst only during chill to Capsicum, Carbo veg. and Ignatia; but the whole case was so well covered by Ignatia that I confidentially assured him of a cure. He received twelve powders of Ignatia$^{200}$, one every four hours while awake. Had a slight chill two days after, *without thirst*, fever heat lasted two hours without the usual headache and vertigo, and that was the last of it. Well ever since, now two years.—H. C. ALLEN, *Homœopathist*, Dec., 1878.

CASE IV.—Ignatia, four doses, removed a quotidian fever with violent thirst at the commencement of the violent and continuous chills, accompanied with still and taciturn disposition.—*A. H. Z.*,—I., p. 107.

CASE V.—Violent thirst during the chilly stage, diminishing when the hot stage set in, vomiting of food, bile or mucus during the chilly stage. Ignatia$^{12}$, after the paroxysm, cured.—*Arch.* VIII.,—I, p. 32.

CASE VI.—Paroxysm every other day, preceded by violent yawning and stretching, violent chill in the afternoon, especially along the back and arms, *with thirst*, for an hour; followed by heat of the whole body, with cold feet; accompanied with internal shuddering, not disappearing until the sweat has broken out, the sweat lasting several hours. *No thirst* during the *hot* or *sweaty stage*. Dull, aching pain in the pit of the stomach; heaviness in the limbs, with pain in the joints. During apyrexia great weariness and bending of the knees. Sleep sound, with snoring breathing, Taciturn, indifferent, starting. Tongue coated white; lips chapped and dry. Countenance pale. Ignatia$^9$, one drop cured.—*Ann. I.*,—p. 168.

## IODUM.

**Characteristic.**—Persons of a scrofulous diathesis, with dark hair and eyes; a low cachectic condition with profound debility and great emaciation.

Great weakness and loss of breath; on going up stairs (Cal.); during the menses (Alum.).

Eats freely, yet loses flesh all the time (Natr. m.).

Empty eructations from morning till evening, as if every particle of food was turned into air.

Itching: low down in the lungs, behind the sternum; causing cough. Extends through bronchi to nasal cavity (Coc. c., Con., Phos.). Hypertrophy and induration of the glands.

Palpitation, worse from least exertion (from least motion, Dig.).

Sensation as if the heart were squeezed together (see Cac.).

Iodum and Lycopodium are complementary.

**Aggravation.**—Warmth; wrapping up the head; cannot bear hat on.

**Amelioration.**—Cold air; washing in cold water.

**Type.**—Quartan; tertian.

**Time.**—Any hour; often at night.

**Chill.**—Shaking chill, or unusual chilliness, even when in a warm room. Hands, nose, feet icy-cold; cold feet the whole night. Chill frequently alternating with heat.

**Heat.**—*Quartan fever*, **with a constant diarrhœa on the days free from fever** (with urticaria when fever has been suppressed, Elat.). Hot flushes of heat over the body (**Fer., Sep.**). Internal heat, with coldness of the surface. Burning heat of the hands (burning heat of palms of hands and soles of feet, with cold feet, **Sulf.**). Fever with dry skin, weak and rapid pulse, twitching of the muscles, and more coldness than heat of skin.

**Sweat.**—With thirst. Debilitating, sour sweat all over in the morning hours, with great weakness of the limbs. Profuse, cold, viscid sweat at night. Palms of hands sweat continually. Cold feet sweat easily; so acrid that it corrodes the skin (**Graph.**).

**Tongue.**—Thickly coated, brown in centre, white at the edges. Salivation: salty or sour taste.

**Apyrexia.**—Countenance *sallow; distressed look;* **ravenous hunger, must eat every few hours; left hypochondriac region hard and acutely sensitive to pressure.** Emaciation, debility, restlessness. Gets anxious and worried if he does not eat, *yet loses flesh all the time while eating freely.*

## IPECACUANHA.

**Characteristic.**—Adapted to cases where the gastric symptoms predominate (Ant. c.).

In all diseases, as well as intermittent fever, the constant and continual nausea is guiding.

Nausea; profuse saliva; vomiting of white, glairy mucus; with distended abdomen; sleepy afterwards; worse from stooping.

Stomach feels relaxed as if hanging down (Staph.).

Stool: grassy green; white mucus, bloody; fermented; preceded by griping, pinching pain about the umbilicus, as from a hand, each finger seemingly pressing sharply into the intestines, aggravated by the slightest motion.

Hemorrhage: bright red from all the orifices of the body; uterine, profuse, clotted, heavy oppressed breathing during; stitches from navel to uterus; cutting across from left to right (from right to left, Lyc.); large accumulation of mucus in the bronchi, difficult to raise (Ant. t.).

Intermittent dyspepsia, every day or every other day at same hour.

Oversensitive to heat and cold.

Complementary to **Cuprum.**

**Aggravation.**—Slightest motion; worse in winter and dry weather; warm, moist south winds (Euph.); warm room; night.

**Amelioration.**—Rest; closing the eyes.

**Type.**—Quotidian; tertian; quartan. Apt to postpone and become irregular.

**Time.**—9 or 11 A.M. (10 to 11 A.M., Natr. m.) and 4 P.M.

Fever, without chill, at 4 P.M.

**Cause.**—Irregularities and indiscretions in diet. Cases drugged with Quinine and Arsenic.

**Prodrome.**—Violent retching; yawning, stretching, backache, headache, and profuse flow of saliva. *Nausea.*

**Chill.**—Without thirst. Chilliness; he is always *worse when in a warm place. External coldness with external heat.* Chill **worse in a warm room**; or **from external heat** (**Apis**—relieved by external heat, **Ars., Ign.**), *lessened by drinking and in the open air* (**Caust.**—aggravated by drinking, **Caps., Cinch., Eup. perf.**). *Shivering; then chilliness, with coldness without thirst,* at 4 P.M. The hands and feet are icy-cold, and wet with cold sweat, with *redness of one cheek* and *paleness of the other.* Chill short and usually not severe, with or without nausea and vomiting. Paroxysm begins by an internal chill, *made worse by external heat.*

**Heat.**—*With thirst; usually long-lasting,* over whole body, with alternate *coldness* and *paleness* of face; *nausea* and *vomiting;* anxious, *oppressed breathing,* and *dry, hacking cough,* often exciting nausea and vomiting (cough with pleuritic stitches, **Acon.**—dry, teasing cough, before and during chill, **Rhus**—cough during chill and heat, **Bry.**); cold hands and feet. Sudden heat about 4 P.M., with sweat on arms and back; heat of entire body in the evening. External heat without internal heat (see **Ign.**). One hand cold, the other hot (Dig., Lyc.). Heat about head and face, sometimes with, often without, redness of cheeks, with dilated pupils and prostration of body and mind.

**Sweat.**—Sudden attacks of sweat in a room; on upper parts of body; increased by motion and in the open air (**Bry.**—lessened by motion, **Caps.**); by being out of doors; cold on the forehead; *sour sweat with turbid urine;* stains yellow. Nausea and vomiting may be present. Always *worse during sweat; better after it* (relieved by sweating, **Eup. perf., Gels., Natr. m.**). *Light sweat* in uncomplicated cases, but *may be sour. Sweat becomes profuse* **only after abuse of quinine.**

May cough in sweating stage. Sweat may only amount to a cold, sticky, clammy feeling of the skin in some cases.

**Tongue.**—At first clean; then coated yellowish or white; pale in all cases. Taste bitter, sweetish, like rancid oil. Desire for sweets, dainties.

**Apyrexia.**—Never clear; disturbed by more or less gastric trouble (**Ant. c., Puls.**); loss of appetite, nausea and vomiting. *Stomach feels relaxed and seems to hang down loose* (Staph.). Aversion to food (aversion to meat, **Arn.**); bad taste in the mouth, languor and debility, with absence of sleep. Bitter taste of everything eaten (Bry.—everything tastes bitter except water, **Acon.**); profuse secretion of saliva, and vomiting after eating.

"*Short chills; long fever; cold hands and feet;* great *oppression of* the chest, he *can hardly breathe*. Always after previous *drugging with quinine.*"—N. A. Roth, *H. M.*, 1874.

" Intermittent fever; nausea and vomiting predominate; slight chills are followed by much heat, with thirst and no subsequent perspiration. Fever consequent upon abuse of Quinine; slight chilliness without thirst, afterwards violent heat, with thirst, nausea and vomiting, dyspnœa, stitches in the chest, finally copious perspiration."—Lippe.

**If paroxysm has been suppressed by Quinine, Ipecacuanha is all the more indicated.**

*Relapses from improprieties in diet* always an additional indication for Ipecacuanha. This is a very common cause of a return of paroxysm and one frequently overlooked by physicians.

**The persistent nausea,** which does not always amount to vomiting, that is usually present in every stage, is the "*guiding symptom*" of Ipecac, although it may be and often is indicated when neither nausea nor vomiting is present. When fever returns in another form, after *suppression by Quinine,* and symptoms do not clearly point to any remedy, *if nausea or vomiting were present in first onset of disease,* Ipecac. will often cure.

Chill not marked and distinct, being either a chilliness up and down the back or a mingling of chills and heat; half an hour the longest. If thirst in chill, may continue during chill and heat, although rarely so severe in heat. *Great lassitude and weariness during chill.* Chill usually followed by nausea and vomiting, first of contents of stomach, afterwards of bile. *Hot stage* lasts four or five hours, and even all night. *Sweat* light, partial, on single parts (**Bry.**), sour. If mixed with Quinine cachexia, *profuse, sour, and soaking the bed through.*

In the irregularity of the different stages of the paroxysm, as well as the universality of its indication, Ipecacuanha resembles Arsenic.; and should always be thought of where indiscretions in diet may have been the cause of original attack, or have produced a relapse. The *greatest prostration occurs during chill* (the prostration of Arsenic. is greatest after heat).

In his " Forty Years' Practice," Jahr places Ipecacuanha at the head of the list of remedies in the treatment of intermittent fever, and recommends its administration in commencing the treatment of every case. He says: " I almost always commence the treatment with Ipecac.[30], unless some other remedy is distinctly indicated. I give a few globules in water, a teaspoonful every three hours, beginning immediately after the chill. By pursuing this course I have cured many cases of 'fever and ague' by the first prescription, thus saving myself a good deal of necessary seeking and comparing. If it does not help altogether, it changes the character of the fever so that Arn., Ars., Ign., Nux v., etc., will complete the cure."

This advice is also given by J. S. Douglas in his work on Intermittent Fever, p. 80; and a number of our closest and most successful prescribers have adopted it, with apparent success. H. V. Miller says: " I am apt to give Ipecac. when I do not clearly see the indications for another remedy. Then it serves to clear up the case and prepare the way for some other remedy to complete the cure."

I cannot endorse the above indiscriminate use of Ipecac., *on principle;* it is empiric practice, and will certainly be attended with many mortifying failures. That it is infinitely superior to the more prevalent, empiric and indiscriminate use of Quinine; and attended with less failures and less constitutional derangements, I have no doubt at all. If the attack can be traced to dietetic irregularities, this advice of Jahr is undoubtedly sound; the best proof being its success at the bedside. A case like the following very often occurs in practice:

A messenger is sent many miles for some medicine for " ague;" and that is all the information we can obtain. If we do not prescribe some one else will; and rather than lose a patient and have it said that we cannot cure " so simple a thing as ague" we make a " chance shot," and, unless we have found the "*genus epidemicus*" of the season, are as apt to fail as to cure.

This is, in my opinion, the opportunity to follow Jahr's advice and exhibit Ipecac.; and it would be infinitely better for *our patient, our school of medicine,* and *our professional reputation,* if we did so instead of sending Quinine. Ipecac. covers a much larger range of symptoms than Quinine, and, in a case like the above, will cure more patients.

In regard to this routine habit of prescribing Ipecac., Dr. Chargé says: "I have known practitioners, highly commendable in other respects, who always began with Ipecac., under the pretense that, after it, the case was better outlined and the choice of the true specific was consequently easier. This is simply an encouragement to indolence. Ipecac. presents itself to us with so clearly defined features, that it is impossible with a little attention not to recognize at once the cases which call for it."

## CLINICAL.

Case I.—Mrs. ——, a lady about 35 years of age, had been sick with chills and fever for nearly two weeks. No regularity of paroxysm; *chill* light and of short duration, though so weak she must go to bed during chill; heat long but not very violent; no thirst during chilly stage, but much thirst all through the heat; tongue thickly furred with a white, pappy coating; complete loss of appetite; and great weakness and prostration during apyrexia. Constant nausea and occasional vomiting were marked symptoms from the outset. For the last four days was compelled to keep her bed. Had taken two grains Quinine three times a day, and was taking Gelsemium and Arsenicum in alternation every two hours. Ipecac.[3] relieved promptly. No more chills.—H. C. Allen in *Advance,* Dec., 1878.

Case II.—Miss Alice B., æt. 11, black hair and eyes, had long been subject to attacks of ague, for which Quinine had been successfully given, without preventing recurrence of paroxysm with every new provocation. *Chill* every other day, she shivers awhile, then *shakes for twenty minutes.* Headache, hands first cold. Nausea as the chill goes off; *nausea all the time.* No thirst with the chill. *Heat* following the chill; thirst with the heat. Perspiration when the fever passes off. Found her covered upon the sofa shaking with a chill when I visited her. Blank powders to take during the afternoon and Ipecac.[1m] (Fincke) to take at bedtime. Was in bed next day most of the time; following day at play. Cured.—J. H. P. Frost, *H. M.,* Oct., 1874.

Case III.—A Swede girl, 26 years old, has had ague three years, always treated with Quinine. Has a hard chill every other day at 1 or 2 P.M. *Continual nausea and vomiting of bitter, bilious matter, and everything taken into the stomach. Chill very violent, with great thirst,* drinking only a little at a time. Towards the last (of cold stage) has chills and flushes of heat, then great heat and profuse sweat, but *the nausea and vomiting persist through all stages.* Saw her when fever was at its height. Ipecac. cm. (Swan) in six teaspoonfuls of water, one every hour. No return after lapse of several weeks.—GEO. H. CARR, *Organon,* April, 1879.

CASE IV.—Mr. T., a woodcutter, had ague for years, every spring and fall. Was treated nine weeks with Quinine without effect. First paroxysm at 10 A.M., while in the woods. Aching in bones and pain through the temples, with heaviness in forehead. Chills up and down the back, with *great thirst,* lasting fifteen minutes. Was not a "regular shake;" accompanied by great languor and weakness, so that "he fell down in a bunch." Then came nausea and vomiting, followed by a burning fever, which lasted until 2 P.M. Thirst and throbbing headache during the fever, followed by profuse sour sweat. Paroxysm had postponed until it now came on at 5 or 6 P.M. A second paroxysm now occurred at 9 A.M., which became more and more severe. Feb. 8th, Ipecac.[3]. Feb. 10th, the P.M. paroxysm had disappeared, and on the 11th the morning one also. Well to date.—STERLING MORRISON, *H. M.,* May, 1879.

CASE V.—Patient, brown hair, blue eyes, light complexion. *Chill* at 9 A.M.; teeth chatter; nails and lips blue; no thirst. *Fever* next; slight thirst; moaning, sighing; slight heat; restlessness; pulse large and soft; tongue coated white and thick; frontal headache; diarrhœa, stools yellow and painless; internal heat with external coldness; *drinks little; much nausea and vomiting;* albuginea yellow; perspiration stains linen yellow. Ipecac. cured.—T. D. STOW, *H. M.,* V.,—p. 237.

## KALI BICHROMICUM.

**Characteristic.**—Adapted to fat, light haired persons, who suffer from catarrhal, syphilitic, or scrofulous affections; fat, chubby, short-necked children, disposed to croupous inflammations.

Affections of any of the mucous membranes—eyes, nose, mouth, throat, bronchi, gastro-intestinal and genito-urinary tracts—discharges of a tough, stringy mucus which adheres to the parts, and can be drawn out into long strings. Complaints in hot weather.

Pains: in small spots can be covered with point of finger (Ign.); shift rapidly from one part to another (Puls.); appear rapidly, disappear suddenly (Bell.); neuralgia every day at same hour.

## KALI BICHROMICUM.

Nose: pressive pain in root of nose; discharge of "clinkers," plugs; mucus tough, ropy, green, bloody; in clear masses, and has violent pain from occiput to forehead if discharge ceases; ulcers and scabs on or ulceration of septum (Alum., Sep., Teucr.).

Diphtheria; pseudo-membranous deposit, firm, pearly, fibrinous, prone to extend downwards to larynx and trachea (from bronchi to throat, Brom.); bladder-like appearance of uvula, much swelling, but little redness (Rhus).

Cough: hoarse, metallic in croup (membranous or diphtheritic), with expectoration of tough mucus or fibro-elastic casts; in morning on awakening, with dyspnœa relieved by lying down (cough on awakening, with dyspnœa **when** lying down, Aral., Lach.); sputa tenacious, expectorated but cannot be easily detached, sticks to throat, mouth, lips (tenacious, frothy, detached with great difficulty, but easily expectorated, Aral.).

Sexual desire absent, in fleshy people.

Prolapsus uteri, seemingly in hot weather.

**Aggravation.**—Morning; after eating.

**Amelioration.**—Heat; skin symptoms in cold weather (rev. of Alum., Pet.).

**Type.**—Complaints appear periodically (dysentery every year in the beginning of summer; headache in the morning) at the same hour daily. Pains intermit.—LIPPE.

**Time.**—Afternoon or evening paroxysm.

Fever, without chill, 4 and 5 P.M.

**Chill.**—Without thirst. Coldness and shivering of arms, shoulders, back, with sleepiness; seeks a warm place. Shivering, alternating with flushes of heat. Chilliness commencing in feet and legs and extending upwards over whole body, with sensation *as if vertex or pericranium* were constricted (**Sil.**), occurring in frequent paroxysms; an hour after chill, heat and dryness of mouth and lips, had to be frequently moistened, followed by great thirst next morning, but no sweat. Ill-humor. Chilliness, especially on the extremities, and flushes of heat alternating with general sweat. Feet and hands cold.

Chilliness, with giddiness and nausea, followed by heat, with sensation of cold and trembling; periodical pains in the temples; no thirst.

**Heat.**—With thirst. General heat over whole body at night.

Flushes of heat in the face. Face and hands glowing hot, while arms were cold and deep internal chilliness continued. Sudden flushes of heat in the face which came on at 4 and 5 P.M.

**Sweat.**—**Profuse while sitting quietly** (profuse on least motion, (**Bry., Sep., Sil., Sulf.**). Sweat on forehead; *rest of face dry*. Hands cold and *bathed in cold sweat* (Sec.). General sweat, alternating with flushes of heat.

**Tongue.**—Broad, with indented edges (Merc.). Thick, yellow coating, coppery taste; *saliva stringy, ropy;* desire for acids (**Ant. c.**), for beer. Aversion to meat (Arn.).

## KALI CARBONICUM.

**Characteristic.**—Adapted to diseases of old people, dropsies and paralyses; dark hair, lax fibre, inclined to obesity (Graph.).

After loss of fluids or of vitality, particularly in the anæmic (deficient vitality, lack of susceptibility to medicinal action, Carb. v.).

Pains; stitching, darting, worse during rest and lying on affected side (stitching, darting, better during rest, and lying on painful side, Bry.).

Cannot bear to be touched; starts when touched ever so lightly, especially on the feet.

Great aversion to being alone (Ars., Bis., Lyc.—desire to be alone, Ign., Nux v.).

Bag-like swelling between upper lids and eyebrows.

Weak eyes; after coition, abortion, measles.

Stomach distended, sensitive; feels as if it would burst; excessive flatulency; everything she eats or drinks appears to be converted into gas (Carb. v., Iod.).

Feels badly week before menstruation.

"Persons suffering from ulceration of the lungs can scarcely get well without this antipsoric."—Hahnemann.

Complementary to Carbo vegetabilis.

**Aggravation.**—From 2 to 4 A.M., nearly all ailments, especially those of throat and chest; cold air; becoming cold; rest, and lying on painful side.

**Amelioration.**—Warmth; getting warm; eructations.

## KALI CARBONICUM. 155

**Type.**—Quotidian; same every day. Intermittent fevers with whooping-cough (Dros.).

**Time.**—9 A.M., 12 M. 5 to 6 *P.M.*

Fever, without chill, 9 A.M.

**Chill.**—With thirst; *great chilliness* **after eating,** and *towards evening* (**Nux v.**). Chilliness *on every motion, even in bed* (**Nux v., Hep.**). Chilliness, then heat, then chilliness again. Chill towards evening, *relieved near the warm stove and after lying down* (relieved by external heat, **Ars., Ign.**—increased by external heat, **Apis, Ipec.**). Chill with the pains (**Puls.**—all symptoms worse during chill, **Ars.**); *increased out of doors* (increased while going from a warm room into the open air, **Puls.**). Constant chilliness; violent thirst from internal heat; hot hands, and aversion to food; with oppression of breathing; constriction of chest; pain in right hypochondrium. After the chill, nausea and vomiting of bile.

"Violent chill towards evening for some minutes; he must lie down; followed by nausea, vomiting and spasmodic pain in the chest through the whole night, with short breath and much internal anxiety and much perspiration."—HAHNEMANN.

**Heat.**—Without thirst, with *long yawning, stitching pains in head and chest, pulsations in abdomen. Internal heat, external chilliness* (chills intermingled with heat, **Ars.**—external coldness and internal heat **Arn., Cal. c., Thuja.**). *Chill and heat,* with dyspnœa. Dry heat of the cheeks and hands, *with shortness of breath.* Redness and heat in the face, with icy coldness of the feet (**Sep.**).

**Sweat.**—**All night without relief** (**Hep.** — sweat relieves, **Lach.**). Sweat of *axilla* and *perinæum;* of upper parts of body; after eating; *perspires easily on least exertion.* **Sweat on every mental exertion,** *reading, writing,* etc. (**Sep.**—on least physical exertion, **Bry.**). Profuse warm sweat, with much heat, from 12 to 3 A.M.

**Tongue.**—Coated white; tip of tongue sore. Taste bad; bitter; flat.

**Apyrexia.**—Chest feels constricted; *right hypochondrium painful and tender to touch.* Excessive aversion to food, especially bread. Intense thirst, morning, noon and night. In the morning bad taste in the mouth; want of appetite; aversion to food, especially bread; and agglutination of the eyelids.

## CLINICAL.

Case I.—Mr. T., æt. 60, chill severe, shaking him dreadfully for two hours; after the chill, nausea and vomiting of bile; during the chill and fever he breathes very quick, from oppression of the chest; cannot well talk on account of the oppression. Is not restless, but suffers from anguish; lays quiet, has much thirst; no sleep, but perspires all night; no appetite, but pain in the liver, which seems to be smaller than usual. Kali carb.$^{200}$ Cured.—A. Lippe, *H. M.*,—I., p. 122.

Case II.—Chill every morning till noon, slight perspiration at night. Headache, stitch-pain and pressure of head down into eyes; pain deep in eyes with photophobia and lachrymation; the pain is first pressing, then stitch-like and causes to cry; flashes like lightning and sparks in the eye; staring look; half an hour afterwards, foggy and dark before eyes; *upper eyelids swollen*, face red and hot; headache wakens him in morning out of sleep, increased by coughing and sneezing. Urine, red-yellow; sweat on every mental exertion; stools hard and dry. Kali carb.$^{200}$ Cured in five days.—J. Schelling, *A. H. Z.*, p. 82, 1869.

## KALI IODATUM.

**Characteristic.**—Adapted to scrofulous persons of lymphatic temperament; victims of mercurial, syphilitic or lead poisoning.

Chronic periosteal rheumatism of a syphilitic or mercurial origin; the nocturnal bone pains become intolerable at night, driving the patient to despair.

Before menses; frequent urging to urinate; the menstrual pains are felt most acutely in the thighs as if squeezed. (See Con., Nux m.)

Glandular swellings; interstitial infiltration.

**Aggravation.**—At night, the bone pains become unbearable; cold air; rest.

**Amelioration.**—Motion.

**Time.**—4 to 8 p.m. (**Hep., Lyc., Mag. m.**); 10 p.m.

**Type.**—Simple.

**Chill.**—With thirst. Chilliness from the p.m. till the next morning. *Chilliness* **with sleepiness,** beginning by creeping up the back and extending over the whole body, from 6 to 8 p.m. Chill from 4 to 7 p.m., with shaking; *was able to get warm in bed, but* **not by heat of stove** (**Pod.**—relieved by heat of stove, **Ign., Sab.**). *Shaking chill at night,* sleepy with frequent waking; *so chilly at night that she could not get warm.* Shivering fit; feels frozen; cannot get warm with any amount of clothing. *Sleepy* and *drowsy.* Coldness of the feet with anasarcous swelling (**Apis, Ars.**).

**Heat.**—Great heat with thirst (as after exertion) followed by excessive coldness with trembling. Flushes of heat with dry skin; at times chilly; at others profuse sweat. Heat of head with burning redness of the face, alternating with coldness, languor, and sometimes sweat.

**Sweat.**—Scanty; or occurs during hot stage.

All the preparations of Kali have febrile conditions marked by **hot flushes**, particularly **Kali c.** (same as **Sep., Sulf.,** etc.).

## LACHESIS.

**Characteristic.**—Suitable to persons of a choleric, melancholy temperament, dark eyes and a disposition to low spirits and indolence.

Women of choleric temperament, with freckles and red hair. (See Phos.)

Better adapted to thin and emaciated than to fat persons; or adapted to those who have been changed both mentally and physically by their illness.

Climacteric ailments; hemorrhoids, hemorrhages, hot flushes, burning vertex headaches; especially after the cessation of the flow (Sang.).

Drunkards; with headaches, hemorrhoids; prone to erysipelatoid inflammations.

Left side principally affected; diseases begin on the left and go to the right.

Great sensitiveness to touch; throat, stomach, abdomen; can bear nothing tight around the waist; cannot bear bedclothes or nightdress to touch throat or abdomen, not because sore or tender as in Apis or Bell., but the clothes cause an uneasiness. (See Agar.)

Extremes of heat and cold cause great debility.

All symptoms, especially the mental, worse after sleep, or the aggravation wakes him from sleep; unhappy; distressed.

Mental excitability; ecstasy, with almost prophetic perceptions; great loquacity.

Catamenia at regular time; but too short, too feeble; pains all relieved by the flow; always better during menses (Zinc.).

Great physical and mental exhaustion, would constantly sink down from weakness, worse in the morning (Sulf.).

Epilepsy; comes on during sleep, from loss of fluids, onanism, jealousy.

Hemorrhagic tendency; small wounds bleed much (Phos.); blood dark, non-coagulable.

Boils, carbuncles, ulcers; dark bluish-purple appearance; tend to malignancy.

Complementary to Lycopodium.

Natrum mur. follows well when type changes.

**Aggravation.**—After sleeping; from acids, alcohol, cinchona, mercury; contact; morning and evening; extremes of temperature.

**Amelioration.**—Warmth.

**Time.**—Periodicity strongly marked. 12 M. to 2 P.M. Afternoon or evening chill; fever lasting all night.

**Type.**—Quotidian; tertian; quartan. Every fourteen days. **Annually returning paroxysm every spring (Carb. v., Sulf.)**, after suppression by quinine the previous autumn. This is guiding.

**Cause.**—Especially useful when paroxysms of fever are sure to return after taking acids.

**Prodrome.**—Thirst, then shuddering (shuddering after drinking, Caps.).

**Chill.**—Without thirst; **commencing in the small of the back** (**Eup. purp.**), runs up the back to the head (**Gels.**), lessened in a warm room. *Violent chill in the evening, with chattering of the teeth,* soreness of chest, and **longing for the fire. Wants to be near the fire and lie down;** *heat makes him feel better,* but *his chill continues as long as if he were in bed (heat of stove relieves the chill.* Chill does not amount to much; *if he can sit near a hot stove he gets warm,* **Ign.**). Pain in the limbs; pleuritic stitches, oppression of the chest; convulsive movements; and *in children, convulsions.* **Child must be held firmly to relieve the pain in head and chest, and prevent shaking (Gels.). If held firmly or pressed down, feels relieved.** "A lady wanted her daughter to lie with her full weight across her during chill; a boy wanted a sack of flour put on him to keep him from shaking." *Chill and heat alternating and changing from place to place.* Nausea and vomiting accompany paroxysm when severe, with some thirst. Coldness in one side of the head. Icy-cold feet, with oppression of the chest. After icy-cold calves, shaking chill with warm sweat; then strumming through the limbs, intermingled with flushes of heat.

**Heat.**—With thirst; *violent headache; livid complexion; oppression of the chest;* backache, *deep breathing and sleep;* or *great loquacity* (**Mar. v.**—during chill and heat, **Pod.**). Violent fever every evening, with loss of appetite and headache; internal chill, external heat; in the evening great febrile heat which lasted all night. Heat in the evening, with red spots on the cheeks. *Internal sensation of heat with cold feet.* Burning in the palms and soles, evening and night, *must be uncovered* (**Acon., Sec.**). Heat in ears, face, abdomen, pit of stomach, alternating with coldness, with shivering when lifting the bedclothes (**Nux v.**). Flushes of heat as from orgasm of the blood, with great sensitiveness of throat at night.

**Sweat.**—*Profuse sweat, which affords relief,* or light, warm, transient sweat. Perspiration *between* the paroxysms of fever; on the back which stains sulfur-yellow. *Strong-smelling* perspiration in axilla, *smelling like garlic* (*sweat in axilla, like onions*, **Bov.**). Sweat cold; *stains yellow;* or *bloody, staining red.*

**Tongue.**—*Trembles when protruded;* or *catches behind the teeth; mapped*, coated white, or dry, red tip and brown centre. Sour taste, everything turns sour (everything bitter, **Ipec.**).

**Pulse.**—Palpitation; *can bear no pressure on throat or chest.* Pulse weak and small, or full and small alternately, but accelerated; intermittent; unequal. The least movement causes feeling of suffocation around the heart.

**Apyrexia.**—Complete remission of all the symptoms; complexion livid, yellow, or ashy, often with vermillion redness of the cheeks; great weakness of the whole body, in the morning on rising, especially of the extremities.

"*Intermittent fever:* the paroxysms come on every spring, or after the suppression of the fever in the previous fall by Quinine; occur in the afternoon; are accompanied by violent pain in the small of the back and limbs, oppression of the chest, violent headache, with a red face and cold feet; during the hot stage continuous talking; face yellow or ash-colored."—LIPPE.

"*Lachesis* has proved efficient in relieving the excessive burning and rending pain, which is often experienced during a relapse into bilious intermittent fevers, the type of which had been violently suppressed by renewed doses of Quinine and Mercury."—C. J. HEMPEL.

## CLINICAL.

CASE I.—A girl, æt. 6, chills for six months in summer and fall of 1870, suppressed with "blue mass" and Quinine, returned May 15th, 1871. Convulsions during chill was most prominent symptom. Lach.$^7$, cured.—DR. WALKER, *Med. Inv.*,—Vol. VII.

CASE II.—A man, æt. 32, sanguine-nervous temperament, had intermittent fever for eight years, suppressed by large doses of Quinine in summer to return every spring. Complexion when fever was present a gray, ash-color. Prescribed on spring recurrence, Dunham's$^{200}$, one dose. No more chills for five years.—I. DEVER,—*Pr. Com.*

CASE III.—A lady, æt. 60, tall, dark, leathery skin; feeble, thin; nervo-bilious; fond of good living; had suffered from "sinking chills" *annually in August for nine years*. Had always been dosed heavily with Morphine, brandy and Quinine to prevent the "fatal third chill." Drenched in cold sweat for many days after each attack, it was the work of months to recuperate. The fever was always tertian, and this was her tenth year. Restlessness; pain in lumbar region, constipation; tongue coated thick, brown, furrowed and tending to dryness. Soreness across the bowels, and a short time before chill in attempting to walk became rapidly blind, giddy and hastened to couch. *Chill due at 2.30 P.M., and it is prompt. Body drawn up in a heap, tip of nose and ears cold and becoming icy; forehead cold; skin shrivelling and becoming livid; pulse filiform and dying away; rapid yawning and incessant sighing; dark areola around the eyes*, and *fast becoming darker as she sinks into stupor*. Lach.$^{30}$ in water. Almost instantly the yawning and sighing ceased, and in a few minutes a warm sweat broke out. In two days, rides out, and in two more superintending her usual household duties. No return.—C. P. JENNINGS, *Med. Inv.*, VII,—p. 314.

## LEDUM.

**Characteristic.**—Adapted to the rheumatic gouty diathesis; constitutions abused by alcohol.

Rheumatism and rheumatic gout; begins in lower limbs and ascends (descends, Kalmia); especially if brought to a low asthenic condition by abuse of Colchicum; joints become the seat of nodosities and "goutstones," which are painful.

Affects left shoulder and right hip-joint.

Emaciation of affected parts (Graph.).

Pains are sticking, tearing, throbbing, and pains in joints are aggravated by motion.

All symptoms except above are attended with general coldness and lack of vital heat.

**Aggravation.**—*Heat;* cannot bear heat of bed; becomes intolerable by midnight, compelling to throw off the bedclothes (rev. of Sil.).

Motion (joints only): misstep; alcohol.

**Amelioration.**—Uncovering, relieves the terrible burning at night in the gouty nodosities of joints.

**Type.**—Double quotidian.

**Time.**—9.45 A.M., 2.30 P.M., same day. Generally only a forenoon paroxysm.

**Cause.**—Exposure to cold. Diseases arising from cold and debility,

**Chill.**—*With thirst.* Chilliness *of single parts, as if cold water were poured over the parts* (chill over whole body as if dashed with cold water, **Rhus**). Chilliness mornings and forenoons; want of natural heat. Shaking all over, with little chilliness (**Eup. purp.**), without heat, but with thirst for cold water. *Shaking chill over the whole back, with hot cheeks and hot forehead, without redness of face or thirst, hands cold.* Shivering and chilliness with goose-flesh, without external coldness. Coldness of the back between the shoulders and in lumbar region. (See **Caps.**—sensation as if a piece of ice were lying on the back between the shoulders, followed by coldness over the whole body with gooseflesh; relieved by hot irons, **Lachn.**). General coldness with heat and redness of the face. Chill, *with colic every evening.*

"*Violent chills and horripilation with cold limbs.*"—HAHNEMANN.

**Heat.**—All over, *without thirst;* on waking up the body is covered with perspiration, accompanied by itching of the whole body. **The warmth of the bed is intolerable** *on account of the heat and burning of the limbs* (*external warmth is unbearable,* **Puls.**). *Heat in the hands and feet in the evening,* with much **distended veins of hands** (veins of face and neck distended, '**Bell., Cinch.**—veins in forearms and hands, **Puls.**).

**Sweat.**—*Perspires, and cannot bear the bed-covers* (must be uncovered as soon as sweat begins, **Acon.**). Slight sweat all over, with itching of the whole body, provoking scratching. Warm sweat on the hands and feet, long continuing. Sour, offensive sweat on the forehead if he perspires when walking.

"Intermittent fevers with malignant rheumatism or gouty complications."

"The fever consists almost entirely of coldness, shivering, here and there a little heat, of the cheeks or forehead, while the limbs are very cold, and a sour-smelling sweat especially on the forehead; the sweat is often interspersed with shivering."—DUNHAM.

## LOBELIA INFLATA.

**Characteristic.**—For asthmatic affections, with deranged digestion; weakness and oppression at epigastrium and simultaneous oppression at heart and chest.

Dyspnœa; aggravated by the slightest exertion, and increased by short exposure to cold to an asthmatic paroxysm. Extremely difficult breathing. Dyspnœa and asthma, with a sensation of lump or foreign body in supra-sternal fossæ.

Nausea in the morning, disappearing after a swallow of water.

Morning sickness, with profuse flow of saliva (after **Ant. t.** or **Ipec.** fail).

Faintness or weakness at pit of stomach, from excessive use of green tea or tobacco.

Chronic vomiting in paroxysms, with nausea, profuse perspiration, prostration of strength, with good appetite and brick-dust sediment in urine.

**Aggravation.**—Cold washing; cold bathing; cause dyspnœa and increase or return of pain (see **Ant. c.**).

**Amelioration.**—After drinking; evening.

**Type.**—Quotidian.

**Time.**—10.30, 11 A.M., 12 M.

**Prodrome.**—Thirst (**Caps., Cinch., Eup.**).

**Chill.**—*With thirst;* severe, shaking; coldness, increased after drinking (**Caps.**); down the back with heat in stomach; general shivering alternating with flushes of heat.

**Heat.**—With thirst; with sweat or inclination to sweat, particularly in the face; heat alternating with slight chilliness from noon till evening. Respiration short, anxious, laborious and wheezing, with tightness of the chest. Tickling in the throat-pit, with frequent hacking cough, severe headache extending round the forehead from one temple to the other. Great debility.

**Sweat.**—With heat, or after the heat has lasted some time; with sleep (**Pod.**); profuse, at night; cold.

**Tongue.**—White or coated on the right side, clean on the left. Loss of appetite.

**Pulse.**—Frequent, but small and weak in the evening.

**Apyrexia.**—Attended with great debility; dyspnœa and oppression at pit of stomach, with weakness and sensation as if stomach was too full, as from undigested food. Complete loss of appetite. Nausea relieved by drinking. The weak sensation in stomach may extend through whole chest or down to abdomen. The thirst is often found only during heat and prodrome and not in chill. The sweat resembles that of Podophyllum, coming on after the heat has continued for some time and is accompanied by sleep.

## LYCOPODIUM.

**Characteristic.**—Best suited to persons intellectually keen, but of weak muscular power; upper part of body wasted, lower part semi-dropsical; lean and predisposed to lung and hepatic affections (Phos., Sulf.).

Deep-seated, progressing chronic disease.

Pains, chiefly aching-pressure, drawing, right-sided.

Dread of men; of solitude; fear of being left alone (Bis., Kali c.).

Red sand in urine; on child's diaper (Phos.); child cries before urinating (Bor.); pain in back relieved by urinating.

Gastric affections: excessive accumulation of flatulence; constant sensation of satiety; good appetite, but a few mouthfuls fill up to the throat.

Complexion, pale, dirty, unhealthy; fan-like motion of alæ nasi (see Ant. t.).

Affects right side, or goes from right to left; throat, chest, abdomen, ovaries.

Complementary to Iodum.

Follows well after Lach., Calc., Puls.

**Aggravation.**—From 4 to 8 P.M.; after eating; cold food or drinks; oysters; salt food.

**Amelioration.**—On getting cold; uncovering; warm food and drinks.

**Type.**—Quotidian; tertian; double tertian; quartan; double quartan; every seventh day (**Cinch.**).

**Time.**—Morning paroxysm, 8 or 9 A.M. Afternoon paroxysm, 3 or 4 P.M.

Evening paroxysm (the most severe), **6 or 7 P.M.,** and continues until morning.

Evening fever without chill, every day, **or every other** day, *at same hour.*

This remedy is frequently rejected, when indicated, in intermittent fever, if the paroxysm does not occur at 4 P.M., and the *red, sandy* sediment is not present in the urine. The *sediment* rarely occurs in acute cases; and the most severe and most frequent paroxysm is the evening one at 6 or 7 P.M., which lasts all night (see Case I). The *sour eructations, sour taste, sour sweat,* **sour vomiting,** are much more reliable guides, because more often present. No single symptom, however guiding, is sufficient to warrant a prescription. If the totality corresponds, Lycopodium will cure, irrespective of time of paroxysm. The general symptoms of Lycopodium *are aggravated from 4 to 8 P.M.*, and if present, constitute an additional indication.

**Prodrome.**—Sometimes flushes of heat, and nausea and vomiting precede the chill, without thirst.

**Chill.**—Without thirst. First, she awoke *in the morning with chilliness,* followed by great heat. Violent chill at 8 A.M. lasting half an hour, and followed by little heat. Chilliness at 9 A.M. *over the whole body; she cannot get warm even by a stove.* Febrile paroxysm every afternoon at 3 o'clock, lasting till late in the evening; a constantly increasing chilliness, without subsequent heat or sweat (**Bov.**). Evening paroxysm; slight chill, followed immediately by violent, long-continuing heat, weariness, prostration, and pains in the limbs (**Ars.**). Alternating chill and heat, with great redness and heat of the cheeks (**Bell.**). *Chilliness at 4 P.M., goose-flesh over the whole body, with incessant yawning, nausea, inclination to vomit,* chilliness *starting from the* *back* and extending over the whole body (**Caps., Gels.**), with numbness and coldness of the hands and feet; *no sweat, no thirst; but heat,* which was confined to the face; the chill lasted two hours and a half, and ended with excessive weakness and weariness of the feet, inclination to sleep, and slight drawings in the wrists and fingers of both hands; she slept well through the night and woke well the next morning.

Chilliness over the whole body in the evening at 6 P.M., starting from the back, with a feeling as if water were spurted upon the back (**Ant. t., Led., Rhus**); chilliness with stupefying sleep, followed by uneasy sleep, with dreams; chilliness over whole body lasting two hours, with stupefaction of the head, sleepiness, tearing in the limbs, no thirst, and no sweat. At 7 P.M., *shaking chill, commencing in the back*, with *numb, icy-cold hands and feet* (**Ced., Sep.**); *she cannot get warm in bed for two hours,* the tearing in the limbs is worse, with uninterrupted yawning, nausea and inclination to vomit.

Febrile paroxysm at 7 P.M.; *shaking chill, with icy-coldness even in bed*, **as if she were lying on ice,** lasting two hours, with drawings in all the limbs, back and whole body; on waking from sleep full of dreams, *perspiration all over*, with **great thirst after the sweat.** During chill it seems as if the blood ceased to be warm and everything internal would come to a stand-still. **Chill on left side of the body (Caust., Carb. v.**—right side, **Bry.**). Nausea and vomiting, then chill, followed by sweat, without intervening heat (**Caust.**); **sour vomiting between chill and heat** (*bitter, bilious vomiting,* **Eup. perf., Ipec.**); *face and hands bloated* (**Apis, Ars.**). Shivering after drinking (**Ars., Caps., Eup. perf.**) and while eating.

The first chills are usually one-sided; most frequently on the left.

**Heat.**—With thirst. Flushes of heat over the whole body in the evening, with frequent drinking of small quantities at a time (**Ars., Cinch.**). *After eating, heat of the head and a red spot on the left cheek.* Frequent rising of heat from the abdomen to the head, with burning in the cheeks. Great heat and redness of the face, with irresistible inclination to sleep (**Apis., Ign.**). Face, cheeks, ears, eyes, fingers and palms of the hands hot and burning. *Nausea after cold drinks* (*nausea relieved by drinking, Lob.*); *warm drinks are grateful* (Casc., Cedr.). Constipation; increased urination, which relieves the backache. *Sour vomiting often occurs in* or lasts during *entire hot stage.* Must uncover (**Lach.**).

**Sweat.**—Perspiration in the night, or in the morning after a restless night. *Profuse sour-smelling perspiration on the body,* but not on the lower legs. Night-sweat on body, not on the limbs. Morning-sweat only of the joints. Morning-sweat *cold, sour, offensive, bloody,* or *smelling like onions.* May be general over whole body. **Perspiration immediately after the chill,** *without intervening heat* (**Caust.**). **Thirst after sweating stage.**

**Tongue.**—Clean, but dry; red, trembling, stiff; vesicles on tip, or brown, or cracked. Taste: *sour;* bitter; fatty; *eructations sour.* Desire for sweat (**Ipec.**); for oysters, which disagree. Aversion to boiled warm food; tobacco smoke (**Ign.**).

Canine hunger; head aches if he does not eat. Satiety, a few mouthfuls fill him up.

**Pulse.**—Sensation as if the circulation stood still; accelerated in evening or after eating.

**Apyrexia.**—Not pronounced; but the concomitants are often guiding symptoms. Constant sense of fulness in the stomach and abdomen as if they would burst. Repletion after eating ever so little. Rumbling in the bowels; obstinate constipation. Cough, with thick, yellow, salty expectoration. *Red, sandy sediment in the urine* (**Natr. m.**). Patient cannot bear to be left alone (wants to be alone, **Cinch.**, **Nux.**).

## CLINICAL.

In a recent epidemic:

"A number of cases had no chilly stage at all. During the heat the patient was generally thirsty and sleepy. The fever passed off after midnight with perspiration. The patient has had either a sour taste in the mouth or sour vomiting where Lyc. has been successful." —E. C. PRICE, *Med. Inv.,*—Vol. II., p. 322.

CASE I.—H. B.—My own child, æt. 8, of an amiable disposition —rather more so in sickness than in health—light hair, blue eyes, slender; first attack about 9 A.M.; next 7 A.M.; all others, with two exceptions, on awakening in the morning. Chill mostly felt in lumbar region, and lasting from thirty minutes to one hour. The *heat* lasted until 7 or 8 P.M., whether the paroxysm commenced on awaking or at 4 P.M. Some perspiration during the heat. Thirst predominated during chill, always called for water at commencement. Vomiting of water, mixed with food, of a greenish color, with two-thirds of the paroxysms, and always *between chill and heat.* The early appearance, with vomiting, between chill and heat, led me to give Eup. perf.; the

$^{200}$ for four days; then the tincture. It had no effect. Chill in the back induced me to give Caps., high and low. No response. Ign. and others were tried with similar results. Circumstances, which cannot be mentioned here, made it necessary to arrest them with Quinine. Two weeks after another chill at 4 P.M., lasting with the heat, until 8 P.M. No medicine was given. The following attack at 2 P.M. Both were accompanied by vomiting between chill and heat, which perplexed me, as Eup., the only remedy that I then knew that had this symptom, had no effect. The *time* of last attack led me to study Lyc., and in Lippe's Text-Book I found *sour vomiting between chill and fever*. The child now said the vomited matter was sour as vinegar. This settled the question. Three doses of Lyc.$^{41000}$ (Fincke); one slight attack after. I think this was a Lyc. case from the beginning, the same vomiting being present throughout.—C. BERNREUTER, *Med. Inv.*,—Vol. II., p. 150.

We may learn from this case the necessity of obtaining some of the finer characteristics of the drug and the patient. Here was vomiting *between chill and heat*, so characteristic of Eup. perf. and Lyc. The *kind of vomiting* distinguishes between them; the former *being bitter*, the latter *sour as vinegar*.

CASE II.—A large, fleshy man, about 30, was prostrated by chills and fever; chill every other day, about 4 P.M., for two hours, followed by more or less fever till late bed-time, when he would be comparatively well till morning. Both chill and fever were very severe, patient tossing, anxious, hot and restless. Urine heavily loaded with a pinkish, half-floating sediment, and a brick-dust sediment at bottom of vessel; severe pain in the renal region, which was aggravated by retention of urine after desire to urinate, and increasing in severity in proportion to time of retention; was relieved by urinating; belched much flatulence, which rumbled and pained him. Lyc. high, because it has proved useless in my hands in the cruder preparations. The relief was prompt, steady, continuous, and in less than a week was cured.—W. J. HAWKES, *Am. Hom.*,—III., p. 91.

CASE III.—A. L. W.; æt. 30, dark complexion, had a severe attack of intermittent fever, from which he was confined three weeks. Was treated by a colleague, and got out, but came down again in a week with a relapse. When he consulted me, chill appeared at 4 P.M. Chill predominated over the fever; constipation; sour, offensive sweat; complexion sallow; eyes dull and conjunctiva slightly yellow; urine scanty, somewhat turbid. Lyc.$^{200}$, without chill returning.—G. N. BRIGHAM, *Priv. Com.*

## MAGNESIA CARBONICA.

**Characteristic.**—Adapted to persons, especially children, of irritable disposition, nervous temperament (Chamom.).

The whole body feels tired and painful, especially the legs and feet.

Pains; neuralgic, lightning-like, worse left side (Col.); insupportable during repose, must get up and walk about.

Pain on vertex as if the hair were pulled.

All the symptoms are aggravated every third week (feels badly week before menstruation, Kali carb.).

Menses, preceded by sore throat, labor-like pains, cutting colic, backache, weakness, chilliness; flow only at night and in absence of uterine pains.

Diarrhœa; preceded by cutting colic; occurs regularly every three weeks; stools, green, frothy; green scum like that of a frog-pond; white, tallow-like masses are found floating in stool.

Complementary to Chamomilla,

**Aggravation.**—Cold; draught; change of temperature; contact; every third week; rest.

**Amelioration.**—Warm air, but worse in warmth of bed (**Ars., Mer.**).

**Type.**—Periodicity not marked. Quotidian generally.

Symptoms return periodically every three weeks.

**Time.**—9 A.M., and 5, 7, 8, 9 and 10 P.M.

**Chill.**—Chilliness in bed, *as if dashed with cold water* (**Ant. t., Led., Sab.**). Shaking chill beginning in the feet, going off in bed. Shaking chill at 9 P.M.; even in bed she was unable to get warm for an hour. Shivering at 10 P.M. in bed without subsequent heat, sweat or thirst (without subsequent heat or sweat, **Bov., Sulf.**). Coldness of feet, as though wading in cold water (as though standing in cold water up to the ankles, **Sep.**). *Chill running up the back; lessened by out-door exercise.*

**Heat.**—A feeling of warmth streams through her whole body (as if vapors rise up to the brain, **Sarac.**—as if hot water running through the veins, **Ars., Bry., Rhus**). *Great internal heat at night, could scarcely remain in bed, yet dreads the slightest exposure* (**Bar. c., Nux v.**). *Great aversion to uncovering* (**Bell.**—cannot move in the least or be uncovered without feeling chilly, **Nux v.**). Heat of the *head, face, hands*; one-sided (right), mostly in forenoon; *redness, burning* and *thirst* for half an hour; often with sweat on the head.

**Sweat.**—Profuse, with thirst; *from 12 P.M. till morning;* on slight motion; offensive night-sweat. *Sour-smelling, oily perspiration, difficult to wash off;* stains yellow.

**Tongue.**—Clean or white-coated; taste, sour, bitter. *Desire for meats, acid drinks.*

## MAGNESIA MURIATICA.

**Characteristic.**—Especially suitable to diseases of women; spasmodic and hysterical complaints complicated with uterine diseases.

Children; during difficult dentition are unable to digest milk, it causes pain in stomach and passes undigested.

General sensation of soreness, with great sensitiveness to noise.

Headache: every six weeks; in forehead and around the eyes; as if it would burst; worse from motion and in open air; better lying down, strong pressure, wrapping up. (See Sil.).

Tendency of head to sweat (Cal., Sil.).

Continual rising of white froth into the mouth.

Eructations; tasting like onions.

Constipation; stool large, hard; knotty, like sheeps' dung; difficult to pass; crumbling at verge of anus.

Urine; pale yellow; can only be passed by bearing down with abdominal muscles.

Menses: with great excitement at every period; flow black, clotted; spasms and pain extend into thighs; metrorrhagia, worse at night in bed, causing hysteria.

Leucorrhœa; after exercise; with every stool; with uterine spasm; followed by metrorrhagia.

Great tendency to foot-sweat (Sil.).

**Aggravation.**—At night; when riding on horseback; sea bathing (great weakness); cold.

**Amelioration.**—Warmth; in bed; exercise.

**Type.**—Quotidian. Same every day. Headache every six weeks.

**Time.**—4, 6, 7, 8 P.M.—4 to 8 P.M. worse (**Hep., Lyc., Sab.**—

pains commencing at 4 or 5 P.M., worse until midnight, diminishing after, and ceasing at daylight, **Syph.**).

**Chill.**—With shaking, not relieved by warmth of stove; lessened in the open air and in bed. Shivering over the whole body, with icy-cold feet. Chilliness, with goose-flesh, frequent yawning, cutting in abdomen and constant desire for stool. Chilliness in the evening, that disappears after lying down, followed before midnight by heat, and after midnight, sweat, with thirst lasting till morning.

**Heat.**—With thirst, in the evening; averse to uncovering. Flushes of heat, with vertigo. Heat of head, with redness of face, without external warmth, with internal shivering and desire for stool.

**Sweat.**—Without thirst, after midnight, till morning; averse to uncovering. Early morning with thirst and dryness of the mouth.

**Tongue.**—Coated white in morning, or tip and edges clean. Taste sour at night. Desire for sweets.

## MENYANTHES.

**Characteristic.**—Adapted to complaints from abuse of Cinchona and Quinine.

Fevers in which the cold stage predominates; coldness felt most acutely in abdomen and extremities (Verat.).

Anxiety about the heart, as if something evil were going to happen, precedes or attends many attacks.

Headache; a pressing in the head (vertex) from above downwards, as of a heavy weight (Cac.), worse ascending, better during hard pressure with the hand, and accompanied by icy-coldness of hands and feet. (Pressure upon the vertex with gastric pain or abdominal colic, relieved by pressure with the hand, Verat.)

**Aggravation.**—Evening; during rest; lying down.

**Amelioration.**—Motion; pressing on the affected part.

**Type.**—Quartan. Irregular.

**Time.**—Irregular time.

**Chill.**—Without thirst. *Chilliness, especially of the fingers and toes.* Chill over whole body, most severe in back, relieved by heat of stove; or chilliness, disappearing by warmth of stove and returning soon as he leaves the stove or remaining in the back only (not relieved by external warmth, **Verat.**—increased by external heat, **Ipec.**).

Chilliness and cold creepings externally, without internal chilliness. Horripilation over the back, as if the parts had long been exposed to cold air, without chilliness. **Coldness in the abdomen,** *especially on pressure with the hand;* on rising from bed in the morning, creeping coldness over abdomen, back and sides. *Coldness of the spine,* with shaking. **Feet cold as far up as the knees,** *as if they were in cold water* (coldness *as far up as the ankles,* **Mag. c., Sepia**). **Icy-coldness of the hands and feet, with warmth of the rest of the body.** *Coldness of the dorsal spine, with shaking* (see **Quinia**). Coldness of the feet lasting till night, could not get them warm in bed. *Shivering over the upper part of the body, with yawning,* immediately. Febrile shivering over the whole back as if he had been uncovered for a long time in the open air. *Veins of lower arms and hands distended, while the feet are icy-cold* (**Puls.**—of hands, **Led.**).

*Chill the predominant stage.*

**Heat.**—Without thirst, especially in the face, followed by chilly feeling. Great heat over the whole body, without sweat or thirst, with cold feet. Flushes of heat on trunk and back, with redness of face, mingled with sensation of coldness. *Flushes of heat,* with *hot ears and cheeks.* Increase of heat, with delirium.

**Sweat.**—From evening till morning. Sweat at night immediately after lying down, continuing all night.

**Tongue.**—Bitter-sweetish taste in the mouth. *Ravenous hunger;* **great desire for meat** (great aversion to meat, Arn.).

**Pulse.**—Slow during the cold stage (Dig.); only slightly accelerated during heat.

"It is a very efficient remedy in irregular intermittent fever, when paroxysm consists chiefly of cold stage, which is incompletely developed, the hands or ends of fingers, and the toes or feet, and the end of the nose, becoming very cold."—CARROLL DUNHAM, *U. S. M. & S. J.,* Jan., 1869.

"*Quartan Intermittents* were the pest of my life until I struck Menyanthes. The symptoms in 'Lippe' (No. 60 to 66, inclusive) and the *excessive coldness of legs* (not thighs) have been the leading symptoms. Lately, when I get a 'quartan,' *and it has not this excessive coldness of legs,* I give the solid extract of Menyanthes in two-grain doses, twice a day, otherwise in the $^{30}$; and it has *never* failed me, nor has a relapse occurred in any case."—A. L. FISHER, *Priv. Com*

"Intermittent fever, with chilliness in the abdomen, lasting six hours, then a disagreeable feeling of heat comes on, alternating or intermingled with chilliness, with cold feet and legs, and slow pulse."—J. S. DOUGLAS.

## MERCURIALIS.

**Time.**—Afternoon; 9 P.M.

**Chill.**—Chilliness over the whole body, with heat of the face; she could only get warm by lying down and covering herself up, then fell asleep, became warm, and afterwards perspired. *Chilliness over the whole body,* **commencing in the right arm and right side of chest** (left hand and left arm, **Carb. v.**—of the whole left side of body, **Caust.**), with shivering, great exhaustion, weakness, weariness, pains in the limbs, and constant desire to sleep; pain in stomach and abdomen aggravated by touch; dyspnœa; *cutis anserina on* **the cold right arm,** *which extends over the whole body;* after midnight *offensive perspiration on both sides, worse on arms.* Cold and chilly, with dark red cheeks. Chill in stomach at 9 P.M., which extends to *right arm, right side of chest, abdomen* and *right hip,* with difficulty of breathing; at 4 A.M., heat, thirst, and sweat of right side of body, with heat of face and redness of cheeks.

**Heat.**—With thirst; of head and dark redness of cheeks. Great heat of head and hands, face red, *veins of hands distended* (**Puls., Led.**), and feet hot. Violent and burning heat of head, face, hands and afterwards of feet, with *distended veins of hands.* Heat without preceding chill, rarely followed by perspiration.

**Sweat.**—Over the whole body from 3 A.M. till towards morning, after sleep. Great thirst.

## CLINICAL.

I once had a young man who came to me from the country; the chill began *on right arm and right side of the chest.* Had taken large quantities of Quinine. One package of Merc. peren. cured him.—E. C. PRICE, *Med. Inv.,*—II., p. 322.

## MERCURIUS.

**Characteristic.**—Indicated in bone diseases, pains worse at night; glandular swellings, with or without suppuration, but especially if suppuration be too profuse (**Hep.**).

Profuse perspiration attends nearly every complaint, but does not relieve and may even increase the suffering (profuse perspiration relieves, Natr. m., Verat.).

Ptyalism; profuse, fetid, metallic-tasting saliva.

Dysentery; stools slimy, bloody, colic, fainting; great tenesmus during and after, followed by chilliness, and a "cannot finish sensation." The more blood and pain the better indicated.

Morning sickness; profuse salivation wets the pillow in sleep.

Mammæ painful, as if they would ulcerate, at every menstrual period; milk in breasts instead of the menses.

Cough; dry, fatiguing, racking; in two paroxysms; worse nights; with utter impossibility of lying on right side.

Leucorrhœa; acrid, burning, itching, with rawness; always worse at night.

"Ulcers appear on the gums, tongue, throat, inside the cheek, with salivation; irregular in shape; undefined edges; have a dirty, unhealthy look; lardaceous base surrounded with a dark halo; apt to run together. The syphilitic ulcers are circular, attack the posterior parts of the mouth, have well-defined edges; surrounded with a coppery hue, and they do not extend from their primary seat."— Dunham.

Follows Hepar and Lachesis well, but should not be given before or after Silica.

**Aggravation.**—At night; wet, damp, cool air especially in evening; in autumn, warm days and cold, damp nights; uncovering, cold air coming in contact with exposed parts (Bar. c., Hep.); lying on the right side; perspiring; heat of bed.

**Amelioration.**—In open air; active motion, during work; rest in bed. Both Arsenic and Mercury have aggravation and amelioration in bed.

Mercury is aggravated by heat of bed, but relieved by rest in bed.
Arsenic is aggravated by rest in bed, but relieved by heat of bed.

**Type.**—Periodicity not marked. Tertian rarely; anticipating occasionally.

**Time.**—No certain hour. Midday; 12 M., 1 P.M.; evening; night.

**Cause.**—Rheumatic exposure. Warm autumn days and cold, damp nights.

**Chill.**—Without thirst; in the morning when rising; more generally in the evening after lying down, or in bed at night. Chilliness *on going into the open air*, (**Rhus**—reverse of, **Puls.**). Chilliness all over, with ice-cold hands; *as from cold water poured over one* (**Mag. c., Rhus**). More chilly in the open air than in the house, same temperature. Violent shaking chill in evening, in bed; she could not get warm. *Chilliness in the abdomen* (coldness of abdomen, **Meny.**). Chill; not relieved by warmth of stove; alternating with heat; of single parts only; internal with hot face. Sensation in soles of feet as if put in cold water, simultaneously with burning in them. *Hands and feet constantly cold.*

**Heat.**—With thirst. *Alternate sensation of heat and chilliness;* not perceptible to external touch. *Heat in bed; chilly when not in bed.* Heat alternating with chill, often of single parts. Aversion to uncover (**Mag. c.**). Heat and redness of face, and palms; then shaking chill far into the night, and thirst towards morning.

**Sweat.**—**Profuse on every motion** (**Bry., Samb.**). **Profuse sweat at night; same in the morning.** Unusually profuse sweat that is sour and offensive and makes the fingers look *softened, spongy, wrinkled, like a washerwoman's* (**Ant. c., Canch.**). *Profuse,* **fatty and oily perspiration at night** (**Thuja, Sab.**), makes linen yellow and stiff. *Profuse, offensive perspiration, soaking through the bed-clothes; the linen was stained saffron yellow and could not be removed by washing* (**Carb. an., Cinch., Bry.**). Sweat that causes a burning sensation in skin (**Caps.**). Profuse sweat on single parts not over six inches large, while other parts are dry. *Worse while sweating; weakness aggravated* (**Rhus**). *Sweat towards morning, with palpitation and nausea.*

**Apyrexia.**—Great weakness, trembling from least exertion; vertigo when sitting down; gums inflamed and painful; thick, salty saliva; throat sore, painful when swallowing.

## MEZEREUM.

**Characteristic.**—For the irresolute, of a phlegmatic temperament.

Hypochondriacal and despondent; indifferent to everything and everybody; angry at trifles and perfectly harmless things, but is soon sorry for it.

## MEZEREUM. 175

Violent headache, after slight vexation; it was painful on the slightest touch.

The head is covered with a thick, leather-like crust, under which thick and white pus collects here and there; hair is glued together; pus after a time is ichorous, becomes offensive, breeds vermin.

Ulcers covered with thick, whitish-yellow scabs, under which thick yellow pus collects.

Linen or charpie sticks to the ulcers, when it is torn away they bleed.

Vesicles appear around the ulcers, itch violently, burn like fire (see Hepar); fiery-red areola around, shining like fire.

Neuralgic burning pains, after Zona.

**Aggravation.**—Cold air; cold washing; night; contact, motion; one side (right) is usually affected; bad effects of mercury or alcohol.

**Time.**—8 to 9 A.M. Evening.

**Chill.**—With thirst, *with dry mouth posteriorly*, and *much saliva anteriorly*; predominates even in a warm room, with sleepiness; from upper arms extending to back and legs (Merc.). Chilliness out of bed; heat in bed (same during heat, **Merc.**). *Asthmatic constriction and oppression of chest* (oppression of chest as though patient would smother, **Apis**.) Chilliness, *of single parts, as if dashed with cold water*, especially over *arms, abdomen, hips, feet*, with yawning, while face and hands are warm (**Led.**). *Great chilliness over the whole body, hands and feet very cold*, with *blue nails*, with small hot spot on top of the head. *External coldness for 36 hours, with great thirst, without desire for warmth, or dread of open air, and without subsequent heat* (chill 24 hours, **Aranea**—12 hours, **Canth.**). Chill *lessened by heat* (**Ars.**, **Ign.**—lessened by drinking, **Ipec.**, **Caust.**). Very sensitive to cold air—less so in hot stage.

**Heat.**—Burning of internal parts with external chilliness. **Heat of left side of body** (of right side, **Meny.**). *Following the chill*, **intense heat with sleep, sweat breaking out during sleep** (deep sleep as chill passes off and breaks out with urticaria, **Apis**—falls asleep at climax of hot stage, and sweats profusely, **Pod.**).

**Sweat.**—Skin dripping with cold perspiration.

**Tongue.**—Thick, white coating on the tongue, with large, red, elevated papillæ (**Acon., Bell.**).

**Pulse.**—Full and hard; accelerated in the evening; intermittent at times; morning frequent, evening slow.

**Apyrexia.**—Headache; pale face; hardness and swelling of the spleen, with pressive pain in left hypochondrium; loss of appetite; sensitiveness to cold air. General weakness. Great tendency to run into remittent or typhoid, particularly the latter.

## NATRUM MURIATICUM.

**Characteristic.**—Great emaciation; losing flesh even while living well (Iod.); throat and neck of children emaciate rapidly during summer complaint.

Great liability to take cold.

Headache: of school-girls (Calc. phos.); from sunrise to sunset; with left-sided clavus; as if bursting; with red face, nausea and vomiting before, during, and after catamenia; as if beaten with little hammers, during fever, better after sweat begins.

Squirming in the nostril as of a small worm, in Hay asthma.

Lachrymation; tears stream down the face whenever he coughs.

Constipation: sensation as of contraction of anus, torn, bleeding, smarting afterwards; stool hard, difficult, crumbling; stitches in rectum (see Nitric acid); involuntary, knows not whether flatus or fæces escape (Aloe, Pod.).

Urine: involuntary, when walking, coughing, laughing; has to wait a long time if others are present.

Pressing and pushing toward genitals, every morning, must sit down to prevent prolapsus (Lil., Sep.).

The hair falls out when touched, in nursing women (after fevers, Lyc.).

For the bad effects: of anger (caused by offence); acid food; bread; Quinine; cauterizations with Arg. nitr. of all kinds.

Hangnails: skin around the nails dry and cracked; herpes about the anus (in bend of knees, see Hep.).

Dreams of robbers in the house, and on waking will not believe to the contrary till search is made (of robbers, danger, Psor.); of burning thirst.

## NATRUM MURIATICUM.    177

"Cannot often be repeated, in chronic cases, without an intercurrent."—Dunham.

Should not be given during paroxysm.

If vertigo and headache be very persistent or prostration prolonged, Nux vom. will relieve.

Complementary to Apis: acts well both before and after it.

**Aggravation.**—At 10 or 11 A.M.; heat of sun or stove; in summer; at sea shore or from sea air; exertion; talking, writing, reading; lying down.

**Amelioration.**—In open air (Puls.); cold washing; sitting up; fasting.

**Type.**—Every type of fever belongs to *Natrum Muriaticum:* vernal, midsummer, autumnal, midwinter; quotidian; tertian; quartan. Simple type. Anticipating tertian.

**Time.**—3, 4, 5, 6, 7, 8, 9 A.M.—**10 to 11 A.M.** Like *Nux v.* the characteristic paroxysm is in the morning or forenoon; the lesser paroxysm occurs in afternoon or evening. 4 to 7 P.M.; 6 to 7 P.M.; 5.30 to 7.30 P.M. Chilly all day, with fever all night.

*Fever without chill,* 10 *to* 11 *A.M.*

**Cause.**—Exposure to emanations from salt or fresh water; living on, or in the vicinity of water, margins of streams, or ponds; in damp regions or near recently turned up soil, especially freshly plowed fields of virgin soil. When Quinine has perverted and temporarily suppressed the original or regular paroxysm.

**Prodrome.**—**Patient dreads the chill.** *Languor, headache, thirst;* knows the paroxysm is coming because of headache and thirst; nausea and vomiting sometimes present; if vomiting, it is water recently drunk; tearing pains in hands, feet, and kidneys.

**Chill.**—*With thirst.* Paroxysm at 8 AM.; *violent chill till noon; then heat till evening;* without perspiration or thirst during the chill or heat; **unconscious, with violent headache**; sensation as if the head would fly into fragments, is stupefied, knows not where he is. Great chilliness every morning between 3 and 4 o'clock, with *languor, headache, great dyspnœa,* followed by great heat and thirst, and terminated by profuse perspiration. **Long and severe chill from 10 to 11 A.M., beginning in the feet, fingers, and toes,** or small of the back (**Gels.**), with blue lips and nails (**Nux v.**). *Thirst, drinking often and much at a time* (drinking often and large quantities, but it produces vomiting, **Eup. perf.**—drinks little and often, **Ars.**). **Bursting headache; nausea and vomiting; and sometimes complete unconsciousness.** Frequent creeping chills about 5.30 P.M., followed by heat and perspiration that lasted till 7.30. Violent chill, especially in a warm room, from 4.30 to 7 P.M.; relieved in the open air. Chilliness over the whole body between 6 and 7 P.M., with great sleepiness; was able to keep awake only by a great effort. Chill over the whole body in a warm room, between 4 and 7 P.M., with frequent yawning, though warm to the touch, except in the face.

Internal shivering from 4 to 7 P.M.; she is generally chilly; each night suffers excessively from rigors, followed by heat and profuse perspiration; as rigors come on, and during continuance, *excessive languor*, with *headache and dyspnœa " almost indescribable."* Chill predominates *mostly internal; hands and feet icy-cold; could not be warmed.* **Chilliness, great thirst, tearing in the bones, blue nails, chattering of the teeth, at 10 A.M.** Chilliness, with *increasing headache in the forehead every day from 9 A.M. till noon;* afterwards *heat with thirst*, and *gradual appearance of sweat;* the headache *decreasing gradually as the sweat increases* until 5 o'clock in the evening. Chill of right side (**Bry.**—left, **Caust., Carb. v.**).

" Icy-coldness about the heart (**Arn., Camph., Kali c., Olean., Petr.**), continuing after the paroxysm; blindness and unconsciousness during the chill, with great prostration, worse after chill; slight fever (**Ars.**)."—LIPPE.

" Chill predominates; chilliness internally, as from want of natural heat, with icy-coldness of hands and feet. Continuous chilliness from morning till noon."—LIPPE.

**Heat.**—With *increased thirst; intolerable hammering headache (as if beaten with thousands of little hammers),* with **stupefaction and unconsciousness (Bell., Cac., Opium)**, or obscuration of sight and fainting.

*Long, severe heat,* with *excessive weakness, which compels him to lie down* (weakness and prostration during chill, **Lyc.**—great prostration after paroxysm, **Ars.**). *Great thirst* for large quantities of water; drinks *much and often*, which refreshes (Bry.—drinks little and often, but it produces vomiting, **Ars.**). *Nausea and vomiting* (**Ipec.**).

" Fever blisters cover the lips like pearls."—RAUE. Hydroa, especially on upper lip (Rhus—see Ign., Nux v.).

"Continuous heat in the afternoon, with violent headache and unconsciousness; they are gradually relieved during the perspiration which follows."—LIPPE.

**Sweat.**—With thirst; *profuse, gradually relieving all pains*, except headache, which may continue during and after sweating stage (Samb., —headache is increased, **Eup. perf.**). *Profuse sweat breaks out easily during motion*, although he is very chilly (**Bry., Psor.**); over whole body at night and in the morning (over whole body, except legs, **Lyc.**); sour-smelling sweat.

**Tongue.**—Thin, yellowish-white coating on dry tongue; blisters on the mapped tongue or *looks like ringworm (herpes) on the sides* (**Lach., Tarax.**). Taste, water tastes putrid (water tastes bitter, **Ars.**); bitter, salt, sour; food has no taste at all. Longing for salt or bitter things. Aversion to bread.

**Pulse.**—*Irregular intermission when lying on left side*, at one time rapid and weak; at another full and slow; every third beat intermits. **The heart's pulsations shake the body.**

**Apyrexia.**—Never clear; *emaciation, languor, debility; livid, sallow complexion;* stitches about the liver and spleen; urine muddy, with *red, sandy sediment* (**Lyc.**); loss of appetite, loss of taste; *aversion to bread* (aversion to meat, **Arn.**); hiccup, after suppression by Quinine; *hydroa, like beads on the lips* (**Ign., Nux,** Rhus); *ulceration of labial commissures; sensation of fulness of the stomach after eating ever so little* (**Bry., Lyc.**); sexual desire diminished, or entirely lost, in men.

"Hard chill about 11 A.M., with great thirst, which continues through all stages; the heat is characterized by the most violent headache, relieved by perspiration."—RAUE.

## Arsenicum.

Advancing type.
Worse afternoon and night.
Headache commencing with fever, and continuing long after sweat.

Vomiting of *bile* with the chill; of water after drinking, in every stage.
Thirst, drinks little and often during chill and heat; large quantities during perspiration.

## Natrum mur.

Receding type.
Worse forenoon and daytime.
Headache commences in chill, increased in fever, partially relieved by profuse sweat.
Vomiting of bile between chill and fever (Eup. perf., Lyc.), or during heat.
Thirst in all stages; drinks large quantities and often, which refresh him.

| | |
|---|---|
| Hungry. | Loss of appetite. |
| Had been at seashore or summer watering-resorts during hot weather (Gels.). | Had been near freshly plowed or newly turned grounds, swamps, canals, or standing water, such as millponds, etc. |
| Lips pale, dry and cracked. | *Lips covered with hydroa, like strings of pearls.* |

"It is taught by every writer, that the chill must come on about 11 A.M., for Natrum muriaticum to be curative. This is all bosh and nonsense. I have cured many, many cases of chronic and acute intermittents where the chill has come on late in the afternoon. If the rest of the symptoms indicate this remedy, it makes no difference when the chill commences. And let me say here, that Natrum will cure more cases of intermittent fever, both acute and chronic, especially the latter, than any known remedy. With the *thirtieth dilution,* I have cured several hundred cases with this drug alone. It is the best friend a physician has in a malarious district."—BURT.

While it is true that time is but one element in a case, and that we must always obtain the totality or majority of symptoms, it is also true that the morning paroxysm predominates, especially at 11 A.M.

"During my travels in Hungary, in the malarious plains of the Theiss and Maros, as well as during a prolonged residence among the Guarosi Indians, of South America, I used a cheap remedy which radically cures every case of ague in twenty-four hours by taking one or, at the utmost, two doses of it. I order a good handful of fine, clean kitchen Salt to be thoroughly roasted—if possible, in a new pan, or at least, in one thoroughly cleansed—over a slow fire, till it takes on a brown color, similar to that of lightly roasted coffee. From this roasted Salt, a grown up man takes a full tablespoonful, rather more than less, dissolved in a glass of hot water, at once, on the morning following the paroxysm, on an empty stomach, and in quotidian fevers a few hours after the paroxysm is over. As the remedy is only sure of its action on an empty stomach, neither food nor drink must be taken. Though great thirst follow, the patient must only sip a little water through straws; and, when the patient becomes hungry, forty-eight hours after taking the Salt, he might take a little chicken-broth, or a little beef-tea. Strict diet and great care not to catch cold, are of the utmost importance. I have used this remedy for the last eighteen years, and it has never failed in a single case when rightly applied. Hundreds of cases in Hungary were cured by it; and, during my voyage to Buenos Ayres, the mate of the steamer Ibis was cured by a single dose in twenty-four hours from an ague which had troubled him periodically for years, and the cure remained permanent. In the tropics of America every European immigrant, as soon as he goes inland, is attacked by intermittent fever, which, if neglected, is too frequently fatal. Thus, four hundred English people succumbed to it in the most paludal forests of Stape, in spite of the immense doses of Quinine and brandy taken; whereas the equally suffering German colony in the adjacent department of Haqua and Paraguay took their roasted Salt, and no death occurred among them."—Dr. Brooke, in *N. A. J.*, 1878.

There is, probably, no remedy in our Materia Medica (Arsenic alone excepted) so often indicated in severe cases—acute or chronic, even those maltreated by Arsenic and Quinine—as Natrum mur. It will cure promptly when indicated; and much quicker and more permanently in the attenuations *above* than *below* the thirtieth. Like Lyc., Cal. c., Sep., Sulph., and some of the metals, it is comparatively inert in the crude form. Hydroa on the lips is a guiding symptom, although Ign., Nux and Rhus all have it. If hydroa be present in first onset of the fever, although after frequent suppression by Quinine, it may not be present in old cases, Natr. mur. should be thought of. In nursing children, hydroa on the lips, and later the ulcers which succeed them with forenoon attack, are guiding.

## CLINICAL.

Case I.—A young girl, æt. 8, brown hair and blue eyes, had a hard chill daily, at 9 or 10 a.m., with no thirst; *heat*, with great thirst, followed by copious sweating; drinking and sweating giving much relief; frontal headache, increasing with fever, diminishing with sweat. Twelve powders Natr. m.$^{200}$ cured.—T. D. Stowe.

Case II.—Mrs. P., æt. 30, has chill every eleventh day. Has taken Quinine. The symptoms now were: Chill beginning at about 10 a.m., first felt in the toes and ends of the fingers, extending thence over whole body. Drawing pains in the limbs during the chill, and violent headache, increased during the hot stage; great sensitiveness to cold air, even after chill has passed off. During the heat, simply raising the bed covering seemed to her like the application of cakes of ice to the body. The fever stage was ushered in by vomiting, and attended by delirium; great heat of the head; the headache, which commences with the chill, continues unabated during the fever, and is greatly aggravated by raising the head and coughing; ringing in the head and ears during and after the headache has passed away, with dizziness and loss of sight when turning the head and when rising from stooping. Very obstinate constipation, which has been present ever since an attack of diphtheria, bowels moved only about every tenth or eleventh day, except by the employment of strong purgatives. Appetite very poor. Now, in this case, the appearance of the chill at about 10 A.M., beginning in the toes and fingers, with drawing pains in the limbs, led me to give Natr. m.$^{5m}$, two powders, to be taken twenty-four hours apart, and followed by Sac. lac. Cured.—WM. E. PAYNE, *H. M.,*—1871, p. 354.

CASE III.—Mr. T., æt. 65. Six years ago had ague sixteen months in spite of Quinine. Change of residence to upland country (Wabash valley to hills of central New York) re-developed disease for five months under Quinine, when he returned home. For four years suffered from Quinine cachexia, and all its attendant evils. Another return to upland country, with return of tertian ague. Orthodox treatment again of no avail. Present symptoms: *Chill,* beginning every other day at 10 A.M., continuing one and a half hours, with severe shaking; *heat,* all the afternoon; profuse and offensive sweat at night. Severe aching in knees and legs during chill; during heat, much thirst, terrible headache and delirium. During sweat, complete relief of all the symptoms. Natr. m.$^{200}$, one dose cured.—H. V. MILLER, *H. M.,* —1872, p. 404.

CASE IV.—A working man, an Italian by birth, about 25 years old, dark complexion, and of a previous robust habit. He was suffering from a well-developed intermittent, with chill coming on about 10 A.M. Paroxysm very pronounced; no appetite; fever had produced rapid emaciation, with great loss of strength. He trembled excessively from muscular weakness, and was only able to be about on his well day, the fever occurring every other day. Had been in charge of a homœopathic physician for a week, with no improvement. I gave him four powders of Natr. m.$^{10m}$ and he had no more chills.—G. N. BRIGHAM, *Am. Hom.,*—III, p. 135.

CASE V.—Mr. L. has suffered from chills and fever over three months. Treated heroically seven weeks by crude doses of Cinchona in various forms, without benefit; then homœopathic medicine for a time, when he removed to this city and decided to "let the chills get well without medicine." Paroxysm *every other day at* 11 A.M., with *severe pain in the limbs* and *small of the back;* chill lasted nearly two hours, with no thirst during chill. Fever all the afternoon, with *bursting headache* and *intense thirst for large quantities of cold water.* Little or no perspiration, eats and sleeps well, and next day resumes his occupation. Natr. m., 30th trit., every four hours during apyrexia. Next chill light, and no return to date.—H. C. ALLEN, *Am. Hom.,*—III, p 206.

Case VI.—Patient was a medical student, from Minnesota, about 35 years old, strong and well. Slight but increasing chill, every alternate morning for ten days. Chill very prompt, at 10 A.M., followed by severe headache which lasted till noon, when violent symptoms gradually disappeared. The *heat and headache were disproportionately severe.* The patient being a medical student, I told him the remedy, and why. He said he had been taking Natr. m.⁶ several days, without benefit, fever increasing in severity all the time. I replied, as I believe, that he might as well take a pinch from the salt barrel. I gave him four powders of a high attenuation, which ended the fever.—W. J. Hawkes, *Homœop.*,—III, p. 93.

Case VII.—Violent chilliness in the evening with chattering of the teeth, for three hours; followed by mere increase of temperature. Violent headache, lasting four or five hours, as if the head would burst; little thirst or appetite. Hard, intermittent stool. Eruption on the lips. Natr. m.³⁰ cured.—*Ann.*,—II, p. 342.

Case VIII.—Violent chill, with thirst, every fourth afternoon; blueness of the lips and nails, and spasmodic tightness of breathing. One hour after, the heat set in, lasting until night. Sweat after midnight. During the apyrexia, pressure in the region of the liver, sometimes alternating with pain in the spleen. Labor-like drawing in the abdomen, in the intestinal canal. Sensation of pressure in the chest. Weakness and appearance as if worn out. Natr. m. cured.—*Hom. Clinique,*—Pr. C., p. 49.

Case IX.—Mr. S., æt. 50, bilious temperament, hard-working farmer, living in an aguish locality, where many of his neighbors were suffering from chills. Had hard chills on morning of November 30th and December 2d, each lasting two hours, *preceded by thirst and bilious vomiting*, heat with thirst, and perspiration at night; yellow complexion, headache and general debility. Had no confidence in homœopathy; had never tried it. One powder Natr. m.²⁰⁰ at 11 A.M. and another to be taken evening before next paroxysm; Sac. lac. every three hours for two days, then to report. He came six miles in a cold wind to tell me " he was convinced there was something in the sugar." Not the slightest indication of any more chills, fever, or headache.—C. Pearson, *Med. Inv.*,—VIII, p. 152.

Case X.— April 21st, 1878, John H., æt. 29, seaman, had fever and ague two or three times a day, with watery vomiting, in Calcutta, in September, 1877. Was in the Calcutta Hospital three weeks for it, then took emetics, Quinine and tonics. Left at the end of three weeks cured; but before he was out of port the ague returned, or he got another and he had a five months' voyage home to the port of Liverpool. During the first three months of this homeward voyage he had two, three, four, five attacks a week, and took a great deal of a powder from the captain, which, from his description was probably Cinchona bark; then the fever left him and the following conditions supervened, viz.:

"Pain in right side under ribs; cannot lie on right side; both calves very painful to touch, are hard and stiff; left leg semi-flexed; he cannot stretch it." He was in this condition two months at sea and two weeks ashore, and in this condition he comes to me hobbling with the aid of a stick, and in great pain from the moving. Urine muddy and red; bowels regular; skin tawny; conjunctivæ yellow. Drinks about three pints of beer daily.

Here we have evidently to do with an ague suppressed with Cinchona. Therefore ordered Natr. mur. 6x trit., six grains in water, every four hours. April 27th.—Pain in side and leg went away entirely in three days, and the water cleared at once; but the pain returned on the forth day in the left calf only, which to-day is red, painful, swelled and pits. He walks without a stick. Continue medicine. May 4th.—Almost well; feels only a very little pain in left calf when walking. Looks and feels quite well, and walked into room with ease without any stick. Continue medicine. May 11th.—Quite well; no medicine. July 20th.—Continues well.—J. C. BURNETT.

## NITRIC ACID.

Suitable especially to lean persons of rigid fibre, dark complexion, black hair and eyes—the brunette rather than blonde—nervous temperament.

Persons suffering with chronic disease who take cold easily; are disposed to diarrhœa; very seldom to those who suffer with constipation.

Old people, diarrhœa and great weakness.

Excessive physical irritability.

Pains: sticking, pricking, as from splinters; suddenly appearing and disappearing; on change of temperature or weather; during sleep; gnawing here and there, as from ulcers forming.

Diseases which depend on some virulent poison; mercury, syphilis, scrofula; in broken-down, cachectic constitutions; hateful and vindictive.

Often anxious about his own illness; constantly thinking about his past troubles; mind weakened and wanders.

Ozena: green casts from the nose every morning.

Diarrhœa: great straining but little passes; as if stayed in rectum and could not be expelled (Alum.); pain as if rectum and anus were torn or fissured; violent cutting pain after stool, lasting for hours.

Urine: scanty, dark brown, strong-smelling, like horses' urine; cold when it passes; turbid, looks like remains of a cider barrel.

Ulcers: easily bleeding, pricking pains especially on contact; zigzag, irregular edges; base looks like raw flesh; exuberant granulations; after mercury or syphilis or both, engrafted on a scrofulous base.

Hemorrhage: from bowels in typhoid; after miscarriage or postpartum; from overexertion of body.

Complementary to Caladium.

Follows well after Calcarea, Hepar, or Thuja, but is most effective after Kali carbonicum.

Should not be used before or after Lachesis.

**Aggravation.**—Evening and at night; contact; change of temperature or weather; on waking; while walking; rising from a seat.

**Amelioration.**—While riding in a carriage (the reverse of **Coc.**); from eructations.

**Type.**—Quotidian; tertian.

**Time.**—Afternoon and evening.

**Chill.**—*Continuous chilliness in the evening, before going to bed and after lying down; in bed, worse from uncovering or moving* (**Nux v.**). Chill in the afternoon while in the open air, for an hour and a half; afterwards dry heat in bed, with delirium and a sort of half-waking, dreamy state; *sweat and sleep towards evening.* Chilliness in the afternoon, for an hour; then heat over the whole body, for a quarter of an hour; afterwards profuse perspiration over the whole body for two hours; there is no thirst in either cold or hot stages. Cold hands, with *extreme ill-humor.* *Constant coldness of the feet* as far up as the calves. *Icy-coldness of soles of feet,* preventing sleep at night.

**Heat.**—Dry, internal at night; *desire to uncover* (**Acon.**); pricking all over, as from needles. Dry heat of hands and face in flushes, with sweat of hands. **Constant paroxysms of flushes of heat, of single parts, or over entire body** (**Ferr., Sep.**). *The blood seemed hot at night, especially in the hands,* preventing sleep. Great heat in the face and hands; or heat in face, with icy-cold hands. *Dryness of the throat.*

**Sweat.**—*All over the entire body after eating* (**Carb. an.**). **Sweat, with cold hands and blue nails. Sweat sour, offensive,**

like horse's urine. Night-sweat, *on covering up in bed* (on being covered sweats profusely all over, **Cinch.**). *Night-sweat, only on the parts on which he is lying* (**Acon., Bry.**—on the part not lain upon, **Benz.**). Profuse night-sweat, *every other night. Offensive axillary sweat* (**Bov.**). Profuse sweat on the soles, causing soreness of the toes and balls of the feet, with sticking pain as if he were walking on pins. Perspiration in the morning.

**Tongue.**—Coated white or lemon-color; dry in the morning; saliva profuse, fetid, acrid; corners of mouth sore and ulcerated; cadaverous odor. Taste, bitter after eating (**Puls.**); aversion to meat and bread; longing for fat (reverse of **Puls.**). Corners of mouth ulcerated. Cracking in the maxillary articulation when chewing or eating.

**Pulse.**—During heat full, hard and tense. In old cases irregular; fourth beat intermits; one normal beat is often followed by two rapid beats.

"In India eighty cases were cured out of ninety treated, seventy-five quotidian and fifteen tertian type. In sixty-three cases in this country, there was a like degree of success. Acts better in long-lasting chronic cases, where the liver is involved and the patient anæmic, with a general cachectic condition."

## NUX MOSCHATA.

**Characteristic.**—Adapted especially to women and children of a nervous, hysterical temperament; to people with a dry skin who rarely perspire.

All the ailments are accompanied by drowsiness, sleepiness, or an inclination to faint: complaints cause sleepiness.

Absence of mind, cannot think; great indifference to everything.

Changeable humor; one moment laughing, the next crying (**Ign.**).

"Sudden change from grave to gay, from lively to serene."

Great dryness of the mouth; tongue so dry it adheres to mouth; saliva seemed like cotton; throat dry, stiffened, no thirst.

Sensation of great dryness; without real thirst and without dryness of the tongue.

Abdomen enormously distended after every meal.

Diarrhœa: from cold drinks; boiled milk; dentition; during pregnancy; with sleepiness and fainting.

At every menstrual nisus, mouth, throat, and tongue become intolerably dry, especially when sleeping.

Leucorrhœa, in place of menses; awakens with dry tongue.

Pain, nausea and vomiting, caused by pessaries, relieved by Nux moschata.

Sudden hoarseness from walking against the wind (Euph., Hep.).

Cough, caused by: getting warm in bed; overheated; during pregnancy (Con.); bathing; standing in water; living in cold, dark places; loose after eating, dry after drinking.

Soreness of all parts on which one lies (Bapt.).

Fatigued, must lie down after least exertion.

**Aggravation.**—Cold, wet, windy weather; cold food; water and washing; riding in a carriage (**Coc.**); motion; lying on painful side.

**Amelioration.**—Rest; dry weather; warm room; wrapping up warmly.

**Type.**—Tertian; double tertian; quartan; double quartan.

**Time.**—7 A.M., 1, 5, 6, 9 P.M.

**Chill.**—Without thirst. *Skin cold and blue over the whole body*, at 5.30 P.M. Became cold, chilly and pale on going into open, especially damp, cold air, disappeared at once in a warm room (worse in a warm room, **Apis**). Coldness *commencing in left arm and lower limbs* (in left hand and arm, **Carb. v.**), in frequent attacks, and clear intermissions between, *with desire to sleep between attacks*. Chill from uncovering (**Nux v.**); hands and feet icy-cold and as if numb from coldness (**Rhus**). As chill progressed became very drowsy, and at close of chill fell asleep (**Apis, Nux v.**); continued through heat, which was very light.

**Heat.**—With slight thirst, with redness of face and hot hands. Great heat, with prostration, hypochondriac mood; *mouth and throat dry; drowsiness and deep sleep* (**Apis, Opium**—falls asleep at climax of heat and breaks out with sweat, **Pod.**).

**Sweat.**—Drowsiness during sweat (**Pod.**); cannot bear to be uncovered (**Bar. c., Hepar, Nux v.**). Sweat light, or wanting altogether; sweat red or bloody (**Lach.**).

"Double tertian intermittent fevers, with sleepiness, white tongue, rattling breathing, bloody expectoration, and very little thirst only during the hot stage."—LIPPE.

"Fever, not paludal, purely nervous; its periodicity places it here. At seven o'clock every morming the chills set in and increase, but, in the midst of this progression of chills, the patient becomes drowsy, and, when the chills cease, is fast asleep. The hot stage is very slightly pronounced, the patient continues to sleep; on awakening great dryness of throat; fever, with colliquative diarrhœa."—A. CHARGE.

**Tongue.**—Coated white, dotted with red papillæ. "Cotton" saliva, *sticky dry lips*, and *tongue adhering to roof of mouth*, without any actual dryness or real thirst. Can only digest highly seasoned food.

## NUX VOMICA.

**Characteristic.**—Adapted to thin, irritable, choleric persons, with dark hair and bilious or sanguine temperament, disposed to be quarrelsome and malicious.

Debauchers of a thin, irritable, nervous disposition.

"Nux vomica is chiefly successful with persons of an ardent character; of an irritable, impatient temperament, disposed to anger, spite, or deception."—Hahnemann.

Oversensitive: to external impressions; noise; odors; light or music; trifling ailments are unbearable; every harmless word offends.

Persons who are very particular, careful, zealous, inclined to become excited or angry.

Bad effects: of coffee, tobacco, alcoholic stimulants; highly seasoned food; overeating; over-mental exertion; sedentary habits; loss of sleep; aromatic or patent medicines; sitting on cold stones.

One of the best remedies with which to commence the treatment of cases that have been drugged by mixtures, bitters, vegetable pills, nostrums and quack remedies, especially aromatic or "hot medicines."

Pains are tingling, sticking, hard, aching, worse from motion and contact.

Cannot keep from falling asleep in the evening, while sitting, hours before bedtime, and wakes at 3 or 4 A.M.; falls into a dreamy sleep at daybreak, from which he is hard to arouse, and then feels tired and weak (with many complaints).

Eructations: sour, bitter; nausea and vomiting every morning, with depression of spirits; after eating.

Constipation: frequent unsuccessful desire, passing small quantities of fæces, sensation as if not finished.

Should be given on retiring, or what is better, several hours before going to bed.

Complementary to Sulphur.

Is often indicated after Ipecacuanha, which it follows well.

**Aggravation.**—Morning; mental exertion; after eating; contact; noise; anger; overeating; spices; narcotics; dry weather.

**Amelioration.**—Evening; rest; lying down, and in damp, wet weather (**Caust.**).

**Type.**—Fevers of every type. Simple; quotidian; tertian; quartan; but like Natr. mur. it is more frequently called for in the morning paroxysm and in the tertian type, than perhaps in any other. Every spring (**Lach., Sulf.**). Anticipating; congestive; monthly; after the menses; apoplectic intermittents.

Irregular in paroxysm; may come on at any hour of the day, and return at the same hour, or earlier, or later.

Irregular in stage; may consist of heat, then chill, then sweat; or sweat, then chill, then sweat again; or external heat and internal chill or *vice versa*.

**Time.**—Night or early morning, 6 to 7 A.M., 11 A.M., 12 M., 4, 5, 6 P.M.; 7 to 9 P.M. Evening paroxysm usually lasts all night (**Lyc., Polyp., Puls., Rhus**).

Fever, without chill, at 6 or 7 P.M.

**Cause.**—Typical cases are apt to occur in men of active, "rushing," business habits, nervous, dyspeptic from worry, care, too much mental and too little physical exertion. Irregular, unseasonable, rapid eating; too much coffee, tobacco, stimulants; late suppers, late hours.

**Prodrome.**—Intolerable drawing pain through the thighs and legs, *that obliged him to draw them up and stretch them out.* Prostration. Sensation of paralytic weakness, especially in the limbs. *Often heat,* and sometimes *sweat* before the chill.

**Chill.**—Without thirst. Chilliness every morning after rising. *Violent, shaking chill, lasting three-quarters of an hour,* **with bluish cold face and hands,** followed by *violent heat* and moist skin.

**Anticipating morning fever;** chill with gaping, and *aching in the limbs* (sore, bruised pain in limbs, as if in periosteum, **Arn.**); **blue nails;** no thirst; then *long-lasting heat with thirst* (**Natr. m.**), and stitches in the temples; *sensation of chilliness on the back* and *limbs*, followed by light sweat, *in the morning*, with *painfulness of the skin, as if it had been frozen*, and *numbness of limbs, as if gone to sleep*, as they do in cold weather.

**Afternoon paroxysm: Chilliness and coldness, with blue nails, for four hours,** *followed by general heat and burning of the hands, with thirst at first for water, afterwards for beer*, without subsequent sweat. Shivering and chilliness *after drinking* (chill after every drink, **Caps., Eup. perf.**). Drinking increases and hastens chill, and causes vomiting (**Eup. perf.**—drinking relieves the chill, **Caust.**). *Coldness of the whole body*, **with blue hands and blueness of the skin. Great coldness, relieved neither by warmth of the stove, nor by covering in bed** (worse from uncovering, **Phos.**—worse in a warm room or near the stove, **Apis**—chill increased by external heat, **Ipec.**). Shivering and chilliness for an hour, *from the slightest contact with the open air* (excessively sensitive to cold air, **Camph.**—coldness and chills as soon as she attempted to rise or put one limb out of bed, **Canth.**). Violent chill, and sleep for an hour in the evening after lying down, followed by heat, with headache and roaring in the ears. Chill evening and night in bed, *lasting till morning, worse when moving.* **Pain in sacrum** during chill (**pain in dorsal vertebræ, Chin. s.**). **Congestive chill,** with vertigo, headache, anguish, delirium, terrible coldness of body, with blue face, nails, and hands, accompanied by vivid visions, distention of the stomach, stitches in the sides and abdomen; worse from the slightest attempt to uncover or move in bed. *Sleep after chill* (**Nux m., Pod.**—  —sleep during heat, **Apis.**).

**Heat.** — *With thirst. Violent, long-lasting heat, with great thirst.* Flushing redness and heat of the cheeks on the slightest motion or exertion (heat relieved by moving about, **Caps.**); worse in the open air; averse to uncovering when in bed, day or night; desire to uncover, but chilled when uncovering (**Acon.**—averse to uncovering, **Bell.**—cold and chilly on putting hands out from under bedclothes, **Bar. c.** —**cannot move or uncover in the least without feeling chilly, Arn.**); heat of hands and feet, which must be covered, *because cold causes intolerable pain* (**Stram.**). *Great heat; whole body burning hot,* **yet patient must be covered up** (must be uncovered, **Sec.**). Heat and redness of face, cheeks, hands, with stitching headache, especially in the sinciput; anguish, vertigo, and delirium, with redness of the face (**Bell.**); roaring in the ears; pain in chest, sides, abdomen; feet cold and shivering.

"During the fever a round spot at the pit of the stomach of two inches in diameter, *feels hot to the patient*, but *is cold to the touch*. Cured by Nux vom."—C. LIPPE.

**Sweat.**—*Without thirst* (with great thirst, **Ars., Cinch.**). Usually, *sweating stage light*, **with chilliness from motion or allowing the air to strike him.** *Sweat relieves pains in limbs* (**Eup. perf., Lyc., Natr. m.**). *Sweat alternating* with chill (**Ant. c.**—chill alternating with sweat, always either chilly or in a sweat, **Caust.**). Sweat *one-sided* (right), or only on upper part of the body (**Acon., Cinch., Nitr. ac., Puls.**—sweat on trunk, but not on legs, **Lyc.**); cold on face; sour, clammy, offensive.

**Profuse perspiration,** *after the severest paroxysms*, or *attending the congestive chill* (**reverse of Eup.,** which has **light chill** and **profuse sweat**; or **hard, shaking chill** and *light, scanty sweat*); *only on right side*.

**Tongue.**—Heavily coated, white or yellow. Taste so *bitter, sour, putrid;* **must rinse the mouth** (**Thuja**). Canine hunger; with *aversion to bread, water, coffee, tobacco*. Longing for brandy, beer, fat food (see **Puls.**).

**Apyrexia.**—Gastric and bilious symptoms are always present. Legs feel weak and paralytic; head heavy, dull, with vertigo and severe frontal headache, especially in morning, pains are pressive, pulsating, sticking, worse in temples and sinciput; face pale and waxy, as in chlorosis; debility; soreness of liver and spleen, which are sensitive to least pressure; loss of appetite and obstinate constipation, with frequent but ineffectual inclination (rarely canine hunger and diarrhœa); great sensitiveness in and distension of the epigastrium. Vomiting of food or bitter fluids and sour mucus; emaciation; anxiety; and great weakness of the whole body. Chilly on the least movement, repugnance to cold, or cold air. Nightly paroxysms of dry cough. Many of the symptoms, after continuing with greater or less intensity, gradually pass into the succeeding prodrome.

## Natrum mur.

**Time.**—5 to 8 A.M., 10 to 11 A.M., and 4 to 7 P.M.
Fever, without chill, 10 or 11 A.M.
**Type.**—Anticipating, every other day. Every day paroxysm, regular.
**Prodrome.**—*Dreads the chill.* Languor, headache, thirst, nausea and vomiting.
**Chill.**—With thirst, drinking often and much at a time, with blue lips and nails, and bursting headache; tearing in bones and chattering of teeth.

**Heat.**—With thirst; increased headache, unconsciousness and excessive weakness.
**Sweat.**—With thirst, gradually relieving all pains except headache, which is not so severe. Profuse sweat breaks out easily on motion. Sour-smelling.
**Tongue.**—Mapped tongue, like herpes, on the side; yellow coat; salt taste.

## Nux vomica.

**Time.**—6 to 7 A.M., 11 A.M., or 12 M.; and 5 to 9 P.M., lasting all night.
Fever, without chill, 6 or 7 P.M.
**Type.** — Anticipating. Paroxysm and stages usually irregular.
**Prodrome.**—Drawing pain in limbs; weak and paralyzed. Heat and sweat sometimes before the chill.
**Chill.** — Without thirst, shaking, with blue face and hands; pain and numbness of limbs, as if gone to sleep; relieved neither by warmth of stove nor covering in bed.
**Heat.**—With great thirst, violent and long-lasting. *Cannot move or uncover in the least without feeling chilly.*
**Sweat.**—Without thirst; with chilliness from motion or allowing the air to touch him. Sweat on one side (right) or upper part of body. Relieves pains in limbs.
**Tongue.**—Heavily coated white or yellow; putrid taste; must rinse the mouth.

"Children's intermittents; *shaking chill,* with *blue-mottled skin, especially on covered parts.* Morning chill, very severe, with *skin blue-mottled;* thirst very great during chill and fever; great tendency to spasms (and even convulsions), as *the chill went off* and *sweat came on.* Bowels constipated, with the ineffectual urging to stool, especially in nursing children; appetite poor, urine red and fetid, and generally a dry, hacking cough (Crotalus, if right side was *most mottled*)."—DR. HIGGINS, *N. A. J.*, p. 182.

*The anticipating chill always denotes increasing severity of the fever,* and the remedies which correspond to it are among the most prominent and frequently called for, viz., Arsenic., Bryonia, Cinchona, Chininum s., Natrum mur., and Nux vomica. Ipecacuanha may anticipate. Ignatia anticipates and postpones.

By many professing homœopaths Nux vomica is used in alternation with Ipecacuanha, and they boast of their success in the treatment of ague. However successful such treatment may be, it is routine practice, and, like the empiricism which leads the other school to the indiscriminate abuse of Quinia, must often fail. Nux vomica deserves, and will repay, a careful individualization.

## CLINICAL.

Case I.—Alternate chilliness and heat, more or less violent, every other day; accompanied with complete loss of strength. Violent beating pain in the sinciput, especially when stooping and during exercise in the open air. Bitter taste and eructations. Want of appetite. Costiveness. Yellowish complexion. Tongue coated white. A good deal of thirst during and after the hot stage. Nux v. three doses, one every night; cured.—*A. H. Z.*,—I, p. 105.

Case II.—Violent chilliness every other day, with shaking and chattering of the teeth, with thirst; but drinking increased the coldness. Chilliness when moving about in the bed. Blueness of the face and hands during the cold stage. Heat after the lapse of two hours, and soon after, sweat. Ugly taste in the mouth; sour eructations; loss of appetite; retention of stool; pain of the abdominal integuments. Heaviness of the head, especially when stooping. General debility after exercise in the open air. Ill humor. Nux v.$^{15}$, one drop; two more paroxysms, each lighter. Cured.—*Ann.*,—IV, p. 445.

Case III.—Miss T., æt. 15—at seashore—been sick with chills and fever five weeks. Her daily medication had been: Quinine pill three times a day; a black-looking syrup twice a day, a teaspoonful; a cathartic pill at night. Symptoms: *Chill* every evening, commencing at 7 *P.M.*, *with coldness all over*, but especially *hands and feet, with blue nails*, continues five to ten minutes. *Violent dry heat all night*. *Towards morning*, warm, *profuse perspiration*. During *the heat, thirst*, worse towards morning. Constipation; no appetite. Nux v.$^{mm}$, one dose; Sac lac, two doses to be taken seven days apart. On the fourteenth day all that was left was *sweat toward morning as if mixed with oil*. Circh., high, one dose removed. Entirely well. Eats well; complains of nothing. She had been continually in bed for a week when I first saw her. In three days she was hungry and wanted to go out doors, which she did on the fifth day. Her bowels moved regularly since the third day.—Samuel Swan.

## OPIUM.

**Characteristic.**—Suitable especially to children and old people (Bar. c., Mill.).

Diseases: of first and second childhood; from fright, bad effects of, the fear still remaining (Acon., Hyos.); from charcoal vapors; of drunkards.

All complaints: with great sopor; painless, complains of nothing, wants nothing.

Screaming, before or during the spasm (Apis, Hell.).

Sleep: heavy, stupid; with stertorous breathing, red face, eyes half-closed; after the spasm.

Sleepy, but cannot sleep; sleeplessness with acuteness of hearing; clock striking and cocks crowing at a great distance keep her awake.

Bed feels so hot she cannot lie on it; moves often in search of a cool place; must be uncovered (see Arn., Bapt.).

Want of susceptibility to remedies; lack of vital reaction (Carb. veg.).

Digestive organs inactive: peristaltic motion reversed or paralyzed; bowels seem closed.

Constipation: of children; corpulent, good-natured women (Graph.), from inaction or paresis; from lead; stool, hard, round black balls (Chel., Plumb., Thuja). Involuntary, especially after fright (Gels.).

Urine: retained, bladder full; post-partum; nursing children after passion of nurse; in fever or acute illness.

(In Stramonium we have suppression; while in Opium the secretion is not diminished, the bladder is full, but fulness is unrecognized.)

"Opium renders the intestines so sluggish, that the most active purgatives lose their power."—Hering.

"Persistent diarrhœa in those treated with large doses of the drug."—Lippe.

**Aggravation.**—Warmth; during rest; while perspiring; from stimulants; night and morning.

**Amelioration.**—From cold; motion; during day and evening.

**Type.**—Congestive. Epileptiform. Regular paroxysms; irregular stages. Sleepy.

**Time.**—11 A.M. Afternoon; night; after midnight.

**Chill.**—Without thirst. *Shaking chill at* 11 A.M.; *body cold*, or *coldness only of the limbs, abdomen, back, hands and feet*. Shaking chill, followed by heat, *with deep soporous sleep*, during which she *sweats profusely*. Chill with pains in limbs, **hot head and deep sleep**. Chilliness on going to bed; **sleep, with profuse sweat about the head**.

**Heat.**—Over *whole body, burning even when bathed in sweat*, with red face. **Soporous, snoring sleep,** with *open mouth,* twitching of the limbs. Spasmodic contraction of the muscles of the face; sardonic smile; unconsciousness, and *desire to uncover* (must be uncovered, **Apis, Puls.**). Headache, great prostration and often fainting when waking from sleep.

**Sweat.**—Over entire body, which is burning hot; *deep sleep, with stertorous breathing and open mouth.* *Hot, profuse morning-sweat, wants to be uncovered.* Sweat on the upper part of the body, lower part hot and dry; heat and sweat intermingled. Cold sweat on forehead. *Worse during sweat* (**Ipec.**—better after sweat, **Bell.**).

**Tongue.**—Coated dirty yellow, *quivering.* Loss of appetite; aversion to food. Longing for spirituous liquors.

**Pulse.**—Full and hard; or weak, slow, scarcely perceptible.

**Apyrexia.**—Symptoms of *cerebral congestion,* with profound stupor; entire nervous system insusceptible; complete indifference; the patient makes no audible complaint. Intermittents of old persons and children.

## CLINICAL.

CASE I.—May 16th, Ch. R., æt. 12. Chills last season, suppressed by Quinine, have returned this year. Chill latter part of night, accompanied with thirst, pain in limbs, heat in head, and sleepiness. Fever soon after chill; during fever, sleep, headache, pale face, loss of appetite and vomiting of bile; urine dark and increased in quantity; then sweat mostly in legs; sleepy, with headache. Ars.$^{200}$ in water every three hours. May 18th, another chill; deep and heavy sleep, with snoring. Opium$^{200}$ (Tafel) in water every three hours. No more medicine. No return of chill.—A. L. FISHER, *A. J. H. M. M.,*—IV, p. 18.

[This case was evidently an Opium one from the commencement. Ars. could not cure it.—H. C. A.]

CASE II.—C. S., a little boy, æt. 9, suffered for six weeks with intermittent fever; three weeks at first, every other day; last three weeks, daily, at midnight. Chill, then profound sleep, which lasted one hour, with heat and sweat following. Waking up he complained of headache and general debility. Gave him Opium. Next day attack absent; but second day fever returned as before. Opium$^{10}$ repeated, two doses in two days, and fever returned no more.—DR. SEEDEL, *Hom. Clinique.*

## PETROLEUM.

**Characteristic.**—Adapted to persons of light hair and skin; irritable, quarrelsome disposition (see Nux v.); offended at trifles; vexed at everything.

Symptoms appear and disappear rapidly.

During sleep or delirium: imagines that one leg is double; that another person lies alongside of him in the same bed; that there are two babies in the bed.

Vertigo on rising; in occiput; as if intoxicated; like seasickness.

Headache; in occiput, which is as heavy as lead; pressing pulsating pain; as if everything in the head were alive, numb, bruised, as if made of wood.

Gastralgia: of pregnancy; with pressing, drawing pains; whenever the stomach is empty; relieved by constant eating (Chel., Sep.).

Complaints; from riding in a carriage, railroad car, or in a ship (Cocc.).

Sweat and moisture of external genitals, of both sexes; fetid, of axillæ and feet.

Tips of fingers rough, cracked, fissured; skin of hands rough and cracked; of whole body, sore and painful.

**Aggravation.**—Carriage riding; during a thunder-storm; in winter (skin symptoms).

**Amelioration.**—Warmth; warm air.

**Type.**—Quotidian. Cold stage predominates.

**Time.**—10 *A.M.*, 3, 4, 6, 7 and 10 P.M. *Evening paroxysm predominant.*

Fever without chill, 5 to 6 P.M.

**Chill.**—Without thirst at 10 A.M. for half an hour, with coldness of the hands and face. Chilliness lasting two hours, every afternoon, at 3 or 4 o'clock, with cold hands and *dryness of the mouth.* Shaking chill at 7 P.M., with sweat over whole body, except lower extremities, wh ch were quite cold. Violent internal shaking chill at 10 P.M. *Shaking chill every evening. Chilliness with trembling, face cold, cheeks, fingers and nails blue. Chilliness at 6 P.M., with blue nails. Chilliness in the open air.* Chilliness in evening, with flushes of heat in the face. *Frequent chilliness through the whole body,* **followed by violent itching of the skin** (pricking of the skin, **Nitr. ac.**).

**Heat.**—And chill at same time, at 10 P.M. Heat at night, *bedclothes were intolerable, and was obliged to uncover* (external warmth is intolerable, **Puls.**). *Flushes of heat over whole body. Heat of head; redness of the face; burning pain in the mouth, and dryness of the trachea.* Heat in the evening after the chill.

**Sweat.**— *Of single parts at different times, as hands, palms, head, back, chest, axilla, arms, legs, feet* (Thuja). *Profuse perspiration of the forearms, lower legs, feet;* on the soles. Sweat; with partial chills; or immediately after the chill. No heat intervening.

**Tongue.**—Coated white in the centre, with a dark streak along the sides (white, with red edges, or red and white in alternate streaks, **Ant. t.**); offensive saliva. Taste, slimy, pappy, putrid; *aversion to fat, meat, and all warm cooked food.* Ravenous hunger, or loss of appetite.

**Pulse.**—Full; accelerated by every motion; becomes slow again during rest. Cold feeling about the heart (Natr. m.).

## CLINICAL.

Paroxysm occurring every day. Pain from the occiput over the head to the front and eyes, with transitory blindness; he gets stiff, loses consciousness, and gets blind. Spleen enlarged and painful; belching; nausea, and constipation. Petrol.[12], in repeated doses, in a short time cured, notwithstanding previous allopathic treatment for four months. —STENS, SR., *A. H. Z.*, 83–135.

## PHOSPHORIC ACID.

**Characteristic.**—Adapted to persons of originally strong constitutions, who have become debilitated by loss of animal fluids; sexual excesses (Chinch.); violent acute diseases; chagrin; a long succession of moral emotions, as grief, care, disappointed affections.

Is very weak, apathetic; indifferent to the affairs of life; to those things that used to be of most interest.

In children and young people who grow too rapidly (Cal.); pains in back and limbs as if beaten.

Patient trembles, legs weak, stumbles easily, or makes missteps.

Interstitial inflammation of bones; scrofulous, syphilitic, mercurial; periosteum inflamed, pains burning, tearing, as if scraped with a knife (Rhus); caries, rachitis, but not necrosis.

Urine; looks like milk mixed with jelly-like, bloody pieces; decomposes rapidly; profuse urination at night, of clear watery urine which forms a white cloud at once.

Onanism; when patient is greatly distressed by the culpability of the act.

**Aggravation.**—At rest; at night; cold, dry weather.

**Amelioraton.**—Motion; warmth; wet weather.

**Type.**—Periodicity not marked. Apt to become remittent or typhoid, with cerebral symptoms predominant.

**Time.**—9 to 10 A.M.; 4, 6, 7, 8, 9, 10; afternoon till 10 P.M.

**Chill.**—Without thirst. Shaking chill, with blue nails, coldness in tips of fingers, in abdomen, tearing in wrists, and paralytic weakness of the arms. Chilliness and palpitation (palpitation during sweat, **Mer.** —see **Bar. c.**). Violent shaking chill from afternoon till 10 P.M., *followed by such great heat that he almost lost consciousness.* Chilliness for an hour towards evening, without subsequent heat (**Sulf.**). Chill and heat, alternate, frequently. Shaking chill over whole body, with ice-cold fingers (**Ced., Sep.**). *The evening chill predominates.*

**Heat.**—Without thirst; *excessive, depriving one almost of consciousness;* internal, without being hot to the touch. Hot face, on the side on which he is not lying. Heat, yet cannot be uncovered (**Bell.**—must be uncovered, **Ign., Puls.**).

**Sweat.**—*Thirst only during sweat* (**Cinch.**—drinks often and in large quantities, **Ars.**—thirst after sweating stage, **Lyc.**). Perspiration, with heavy dreams of dead people and of being pursued. *Profuse morning-sweat; clammy; exhausting.*

**Tongue.**—Red streak in the middle of the tongue. *Craves refreshing, juicy food.*

**Pulse.**—Weak, small, frequent; irregular; intermitting one or two beats.

## PHOSPHORUS.

**Characteristic.**—Adapted to tall, slender persons of sanguine temperament, fair skin, blonde or red hair, quick, lively perceptions and sensitive nature.

Young people, who grow too rapidly, are inclined to stoop (walk stooping, Sulf.); chlorosis; anæmia.

## PHOSPHORUS.

Apathetic; unwilling to talk; answers slowly; moves sluggishly.
Weary of life; full of gloomy forebodings.
Great nervous debility; trembling.
Weakness and prostration; of whole body; weariness, from loss of vital fluids.
Sensation of weakness and emptiness in stomach and abdomen.
As soon as water becomes warm in stomach it is thrown up.
Constipation; fæces slender, long, dry, tough and hard like a dog's; voided with difficulty (see Caust., Prunus).
Diarrhœa: as soon as anything enters the rectum; profuse, pouring away as from a hydrant; watery with sago-like particles; the anus remaining open (Apis); involuntary; during cholera time.
During pregnancy; unable to drink water; sight of it causes vomiting; must close her eyes while bathing (see Hydroph.).
Hemorrhagic diathesis; slight wounds bleed profusely (Lach.).
Hemorrhage: frequent and profuse, pouring out freely and then ceasing for a time; hæmoptysis; metrorrhagia, cancer; vicarious, from nose, stomach, anus, urethra in amenorrhœa.
Cannot talk, the larynx is so painful; cough, going from warm to cold air (rev. of Bry.), laughing, talking, reading, eating, lying on left side.
Pain; acute, especially in right chest, worse from pressure (even slight) in intercostal spaces, and lying on left side.
Acts most beneficially when patients suffer from chronic diarrhœa.
Complementary to Arsenic, with which it is also in isomorphic relation.
Follows well after Cinchona or Calcarea.

**Aggravation.**—Evening before midnight; when alone; lying on left side or back; from light; during a thunder-storm; change of weather; eating something warm.

**Amelioration.**—In the dark; lying on right side; after sleep; eating something cold; rubbing.

Cold air relieves the head and face symptoms, but aggravates those of the chest, throat and neck.

**Type.**—Quotidian.

**Time.**—1, 6, 5 to 6, 7 P.M. Afternoon and evening. *Same hour every day.*

**Chill.**—Without thirst. Towards evening, *not relieved by heat of stove* (**Meny., Nux v.**). Chills at 1, lasting till 5 P.M. Chilliness over whole trunk, as if in cold water, *not relieved by external covering* (**Nux v.**). Chilliness in the evening on falling asleep; from 6 P.M. till midnight, falling asleep from weakness. **Chilliness every evening, with shivering,** *with aversion to uncovering.* Violent shaking chill at night, with diarrhœa, followed by heat and perspiration. *Chill alternating with heat* (**Ars.**)*; veins of hands swollen;* yawning; gooseflesh. *Chill descends; heat ascends,* the back (**Ver. a.**). **Coldness in the knees at night, in bed** (**Carb. v.**). *Coldness of the limbs;* **icy-coldness of the hands and feet, even in bed.**

**Heat.**—With thirst. Violent chill; he could not get warm at 5 to 6 P.M., followed by heat and internal chilliness; then heat and perspiration all night. Heat at night, beginning in stomach; faint and hungry; then chill followed by internal heat, especially in the hands, the cold continuing externally. **Heat and sweat at night, with ravenous hunger,** *that could not be appeased* (hunger in every stage, **Cina**—hunger after paroxysm, **Eup.**—hunger before chill, **Cinch.**). Hot flushes over whole body, beginning in the hands. Heat, anxiety, and burning in face and hands, both afternoon and evening; cold externally. Urine turbid, whitish, brick-dust sediment.

**Sweat.**—**Profuse over whole body and on slight exertion.** *Morning-sweat, most profuse during sleep* (**Cinch.**). *Profuse, exhausting morning-sweat,* sometimes clammy. Sweat on head, hands, feet, fore part of body, alternating with chilliness; urine turbid and milky.

**Tongue.**—Coated with a thick fur, white or brown, dark centre and red edges; or coated only in the middle.

Hunger, must eat during chill and heat, before he can get up; feels faint; wants cold food, ice water, ice cream. Regurgitation of food, in mouthfuls, without nausea. Food scarcely swallowed, comes up again.

"Intermittent fever; heat and perspiration at night, with faintness and ravenous hunger, which could not be satisfied by eating; afterwards chilliness, with chattering of teeth and external coldness; chilliness succeeded by internal heat, especially in hands, the external coldness continues."—LIPPE,

Apt to become remittent or typhoid; or a remittent fever takes on after a time—or after partial or complete suppression—an intermittent type, usually the quotidian.

## PLANTAGO.

**Characteristic.**—Suitable to chronic cases with regular type, which Quinine will neither change nor suppress.

Persons of irritable, morose disposition; impatient, restless mood, with dull stupid feeling in the brain.

Great mental prostration, increased by mental exertion, which also causes rapid respiration and a feeling of great anxiety.

Teeth (left side) elongated, sore; pain unbearably severe, boring, digging in sound teeth; worse from contact and extremes of heat and cold.

Bad effects of excessive use of tobacco, especially the mental anxiety; digging toothache and frequent attacks of sudden sneezing with profuse, watery, bland coryza.

Nocturnal enuresis; profuse colorless urine, depositing a white sediment; occurs from midnight to morning.

**Type.**—Every type. Quotidian, tertian, quartan. Every seven, or every fourteen days.

**Time.**—2 P.M. Any time during the day.

**Prodrome.**—Erratic pains in chest, dulness in head and stretching of limbs.

**Chill.**—Without thirst. Cold chills with goose-flesh at 2 P.M., running over the body, worse when moving about; fingers cold. Coldness of body with shivering; head feels irritable; feet and legs cold; hands cold even in a warm room.

**Heat.**—With thirst; great excitability, anxiety, mental agony, restlessness; room seems hot and close; oppression of chest, rapid respiration; breathing difficult, as if there was no air in the room (anxious, oppressed breathing, **Ipec.**—air of room intolerable, **Apis**). Burning heat of head, face, hands and feet; head feels hot, painful, dull and stupid. Hands hot and clammy.

**Sweat.**—Cold over lumbar and sacral region. Heat of room was unbearable, producing perspiration.

**Tongue.**—White coated; breath putrid, offensive. Taste dirty, putrid. Food tasteless. Eructations tasting of sulphur, last all day.

### CLINICAL.

Fever which runs its course for many weeks or months, either in daily paroxysms or repeated every 2, 3, 4, 7 or 14 days. Cases which have proved intractable to Quinine and all the popular remedies or febrifuges. Characteristics, recurrence of paroxysm in daytime, with a relaxation of sphincter vesicæ.

## PODOPHYLLUM.

**Characteristic.**—Adapted to persons of bilious temperament, who suffer from gastro-intestinal derangement, especially after abuse of Mercury.

Pains: sudden attacks of jerking pain.

Depression of spirits; imagines he is going to die or be very ill (Ars.).

Headache, alternating with diarrhœa (Aloe).

Painless cholera morbus; violent cramps in feet, calves, thighs; watery, painless stools.

Difficult dentition; moaning; grinding the teeth at night; head hot and rolling from side to side.

Diarrhœa of children; during teething; after eating; while being washed, dirty water soaking napkin through.

Diarrhœa; early in morning, continues through forenoon, followed by natural stool in evening (Aloe), and accompanied by sensation of sinking or weakness in abdomen and rectum.

Stool; green, watery, fetid, profuse (Cal. c.); gushing out (Jatro., Phos.); chalk-like, jelly-like (Aloe); undigested (Cinch., Ferr.); yellow, meal-like sediment; prolapse of rectum, before or with stool.

Prolapsus uteri: from overlifting or straining; after parturition. In early months of pregnancy, can lie comfortably only on stomach.

Affects right throat, right ovary, right hypochondrium (Lyc.).

**Aggravation.**—In early morning (**Nux v., Sulf.**); hot weather (diarrhœa).

**Amelioration.**—Evening; external warmth; pressure.

**Type.**—Quotidian; tertian; quartan. Periodicity marked. Morning paroxysm predominates. Intermittent may become remittent.

**Time.**—7 A.M., characteristic. Light paroxysm may occur in evening.

**Prodrome.**—Backache; *severe* in lumbar region. *Gastric and bilious symptoms are marked, sometimes for days before the paroxysm.*

**Chill.**—Without thirst, *with pressing pains* in *both hypochondria,* and dull aching in *knees, ankles, elbows* and *wrists.* Feverish during the afternoon, with occasional chilliness, which *was not re'ieved by the heat of stove,* but *was relieved by covering up warmly in bed.* **Great loquacity;** consciousness, but cannot talk, because he forgets the words; or tries to talk continually, but he forgets the words he wishes to employ (**Marum v.**). Chilly on first lying down in evening, with incoherent talking during the imperfect semi-sleep.

**Heat.**—*With thirst.* The heat begins *during the chill,* or *while he is yet chilly.* The shaking and sensation of coldness continue for some time *after the heat commences.* **Violent pain in the head, with excessive thirst.** Chilliness while moving about and in act of lying down; with sweat at once. **Great loquacity,** *constantly talking* (**Carb. v., Lach.**), *which continues with delirium until fever* reaches its climax, when **he falls asleep** *and transpires profusely,* with forgetfulness of all he had said (falls asleep during evening fever, and wakes when it stops, **Calad.**—see **Apis, Nux m.**).

**Sweat.**—Profuse sweating, so that it dropped off the finger-ends. **Sleep during perspiration;** relieves headache. Bathed in cold perspiration.

**Tongue.**—Coated white, moist, dirty, pappy, pasty, shows imprint of teeth (**Mer.**); dry, yellow. Offensive odor of breath, *which disgusts him* (offensive odor from mouth, *not perceptible to himself,* **Puls.**). Taste foul; total loss of taste, or everything tastes sour. **Gastric symptoms predominate.**

**Apyrexia.**—Total loss of appetite; even the smell of food produces loathing (**Colch.**); offensive breath; foul taste; profuse salivation; eructations smelling like rotten eggs. Constipation or diarrhœa.

The loquacity *during chill* and *far into heat,* with complete forgetfulness afterwards of all that had passed, is characteristic. *Falls asleep at climax of heat, and sleeps during perspiration* resembles Apis, but the urticaria is wanting, and the perspiration is more profuse.

## CLINICAL.

A gentleman, æt. 76, never had a severe illness of any kind in his life, was attacked in July last with chills and fever, paroxysm daily at 7 A.M., with aching pain in right hypochondrium, which is sensitive to pressure. Severe pain in back *before,* but not during chill. Chill not very severe, but heat begins before the shivering and coldness ceases. Some thirst during chill; excessive during heat. Violent headache and slight delirium during fever; falls asleep in heat, and breaks into profuse perspiration; tries to talk, but cannot find the right words. Dirty, pappy, pasty tongue, with foul taste and complete loss of appetite, even the smell of food produces loathing. The pain in limbs and back, time 7 A.M., indicated Eup. perf., which was given without benefit; but a closer comparison revealed Pod. to be the similimum, which he received in 30th trit. every four hours. Next chill much lighter, felt better every way, and a few powders of 200th completed the cure.—H. C. ALLEN, *Am. Hom.*,—III, p. 208.

## POLYPORUS OFFICINALIS.

**Type.**—Quotidian; tertian. Sporadic or endemic, of spring, summer, winter. Rarely called for in autumn.

**Time.**—5, 10 and 11 A.M.,—1, 3, 4, 3 to 4 and 9 P.M.

**Prodrome.**—Great languor and aching in the large joints.

**Chill.**—Chills, with slight thirst, alternate with heat several times a day. Chilliness with disposition to yawn and stretch. *Frequent creeping chills along the spine between the shoulder-blades, up the back to nape of neck*, intermingled with hot flushes (chills along the spine, running up the back in successive waves, **Gels.**). **Chills commencing in the back between the shoulder-blades** (**Caps.**). *Coldness of nose, hands and feet. Great languor, with severe aching pains in back, large joints, and bones of legs* (**Eup., Pod.**); *yawns and stretches.* Severe chills, lasting two hours, followed by heat and perspiration. *Unusual chilliness when the open air is encountered, with icy-coldness of the nose.*

**Heat.**—With thirst; constant, lasting all night (after evening chill, **Lyc., Puls., Rhus**). Skin extremely hot and dry. *Face hot and flushed*, with prickly sensation (**Nitr. ac.**); *hands, palms, feet hot and dry.* Thirst not excessive, nausea and vomiting often occur during heat.

**Sweat.**—*Profuse after midnight;* sweat all night; mild in recent cases; profuse in old, chronic.

**Tongue.**—Coated white; or yellow thick coat, with red tip. Taste, bitter, coppery. Loss of appetite. Desire for sour things, which always relieved symptom.

**Apyrexia.**—Pain in liver, with jaundice of the skin and great lassitude. Pain in abdomen between stomach and navel; loud rumbling in the bowels. Constipation, dull headache and great languor; or congestion of blood to the head with vertigo. Intermission very short; fever almost continuous in severe cases, and apt to become remittent.

Best adapted to old, long-standing cases that have been saturated with Quinine, and remained proof against all febrifuges.

## PSORINUM.

**Characteristic.**—Especially adapted to psoric constitutions; lack of reaction after severe acute diseases, appetite will not return.

Extremely scrofulous patients; nervous, restless, easily startled, sleepless from intolerable itching or frightful dreams of robbers, danger, etc.

In chronic cases, when well-selected remedies fail to permanently improve (in acute diseases, Sulf.); when Sulf. is indicated and fails to act.

Children are pale, delicate, sickly; sick babies will not sleep day or night, but worry, fret, cry (Jalapa); child good, plays all day; restless, troublesome, screaming all night.

Great weakness and debility; from loss of fluids; remaining after acute diseases; without any organic lesion.

Despairs of recovery; hopeless, thinks he will die, especially after fevers.

Religious melancholy.

Body has a filthy smell, even after bathing.

Headache, chronic: at every change of weather; awakened from sleep with pain; hungry during headache; relieved by washing, by nosebleed.

Great sensitiveness to cold air or change of weather; wears a fur cap, overcoat or shawl, even in hottest summer weather. Stormy weather affects him; feels restless for days before, and during a thunder-storm (see Phos.).

Cough returns every winter.

All excretions; diarrhœa, leucorrhœa, menstrual flow, perspiration have a carrion-like odor.

Hungry in the middle of the night; must have something to eat.

Eructations tasting of rotten eggs (in A.M., Arn.—at night, Ant. t.—in A.M. only, disappearing after rinsing the mouth, Graph).

Diarrhœa; stool watery, dark brown, fetid, carrion-like odor.

Leucorrhœa; clotted, large lumps, of an unbearable odor.

Vomiting of pregnancy, obstinate cases when the best selected remedy fails.

Asthma; worse sitting up, better lying down and keeping arms spread wide apart.

**Aggravation.**—Evening, before midnight; in open air; stormy weather, thunder-storm; sitting.

**Amelioration.**—Lying down; in the room; moving.

**Type.**—Periodicity of fever paroxysm not marked. Attacks (of other diseases) at same hour every day. Every alternate day; headache, thirst, cold.

**Time.**—Evening.

**Chill.**—With thirst, especially in the evening, *on the upper arms and thighs*, with horripilations, hot flashes, creeping chills, great weakness, debility, sleepiness. *Internal shivering, creeping chills*, and *icy-cold feet*. **Drinking causes cough** (causes cough and gagging, **Cimex.**).

**Heat.**—And sweat on the face in the evening; *when riding in a carriage* (better when riding in a carriage, **Nitr. ac.**). *Evening heat with delirium, great thirst*, followed by *profuse sweat*. Heat, sweat, thirst, during both chill and heat (**Cal. c., Sulf.**).

**Sweat.**—**Profusely and freely when walking, with consequent debility** (**Bry., Cinch., Carb. an.**). **Takes cold easily** (**Cal. c., Bar. c.**). *Copious perspiration* on *face, palms of hands* and *perinæum*, **when moving about** (profuse from *walking, reading, riding, talking*, **Sepia, Sulf.**).

**Tongue.**—Coated white or yellowish-white; tip dry and feels burnt as far as the middle (red, triangular tip, **Rhus**). Taste bitter, goes off after eating or drinking (reverse of **Nitr. ac., Puls.**); foul taste. Great hunger, without appetite.

Psorinum will often clear up a case, where there is lack of vital reaction after severe attacks, and other remedies, although well chosen, fail to relieve or permanently improve. The constitutional symptoms are the guiding ones; the chief symptoms do not come to the surface during the paroxysm. It has cleared up many a case for me in psoric constitutions after Sulfur failed. More frequently indicated than used (reverse of Quinine).

## PULSATILLA.

**Characteristic.**—Adapted to persons of indecisive, slow, phlegmatic temperament; sandy hair, blue eyes, pale face, easily moved to laughter or tears; affectionate, mild, gentle, timid, yielding disposition.

Weeps easily; almost impossible to detail her ailments without weeping.

Pains: drawing, tearing, erratic, rapidly shifting from one part to another (Kali b.); are accompanied with constant chilliness, and the more severe the pain the harder the chill; appear suddenly, leave gradually, or tension, which increases until very acute, and then "lets up with a snap" (toothache, neuralgia).

Symptoms ever changing; no two chills, no two stools, no two attacks alike; very well one hour, very miserable the next.

Thirstlessness with nearly all complaints.

Gastric difficulties from eating rich food, cake, pastry, especially fat pork or sausage; the sight or even thought of pork causes disgust.

Derangements at puberty; catamenia, suppressed from getting the feet wet; too late, scanty, slimy, intermitting flow, with evening chilliness.

Sleep: wide awake in the evening, does not want to go to bed; first sleep restless, sound asleep when it is time to get up; wakes languid and unrefreshed (rev. of Nux v.).

Styes, especially on upper lid (Lyc.—lower, Staph.) from eating fat, greasy, rich food or pork.

Threatened abortion; flow ceases and then returns with increased force; pains spasmodic, excite suffocation and fainting; must have fresh air; during chill.

After abuse of Chamomilla, Quinine, Mercury, Sulfur.

Complementary to Lycopodium, Sulphuric acid. Follows well after Kali b., Sepia, Sulfur.

**Aggravation.**—In warm, close room; evening; in twilight; lying on the left or painless side; indigestible food, fats, pork, ice cream, etc.

**Amelioration.**—In open air; lying on painful side (Bry.); cold room; eating cold things.

**Type.**—Every type. Simple and double. Quotidian; tertian; quartan. Monthly (Nux v., Sep.); every fourteen days (Ars., Cinch., Plan.). Irregular type; irregular stages; *long chill, little heat, no thirst* (short chill, long heat, no thirst, Ipec.); not marked and apt to run into each other (Ars., Nux v., Pod.).

**Time.**—1, 8 and 11 A.M. 1 and **4 P.M.** Afternoon and evening. The 4 o'clock paroxysm predominates. Evening paroxysm lasts all night (Lyc., Nux v., Rhus).

**Cause.**—Dietetic irregularities. Eating rich, fat food, pastries, pork, often originates an attack, or during convalescence produces a relapse (see Ant. c., Ipec.).

**Prodrome.**—Thirst; drowsy and sleepy all day, with mucous diarrhœa; nausea or vomiting of mucus. If morning chill, *diarrhœa previous night without thirst.*

**Chill.**— *Cold chills all over; chilliness all the time; feels cold even in a warm room, in the evening.* Chilliness the whole evening before bedtime, even while walking. *Chilliness; on going from a warm room into the cold* air; *with pains in the evening.* **Chill at 4 P.M.,** *no thirst;* vomiting of mucus when the chill comes on; anxiety; dyspnœa; flitting chilliness; in spots, now here, now there; worse in the evening. *One-sided coldness,* with numbness (**Bry., Natr. m.**—right side; Caust., **Carb. v.** and **Lach.**—the left). *Chilliness over the abdomen extending around the sacrum and back.* Shivering on the back extending into the hypochondria, especially into the anterior portion of the *arms* and *thighs*, with a coldness of the limbs, and a feeling as if they would fall asleep about 4 P.M. Shivering running up the back all day; creeping-shivering over the arms, with heat of the cheeks; *the air of the room seems too hot.* Cold hands and feet, they seem dead (**Lyc., Sepia**—whole body numb, **Ced.**). Hand and foot of one side cold and red; the other side hot, in the evening. The morning paroxysm at 8 A.M. has nausea, vomiting, headache and vertigo; chilliness, heat and sweat intermingled, or simultaneous (Ars.), and usually much thirst during entire attack. Evening paroxysm; violent chill, with external coldness, without shivering or thirst; in the morning sensation of heat, as if sweat would break out, without thirst or external heat, though with hot hands and aversion to uncovering.

**Heat.**—With thirst; with *red face,* or *one cheek red* and *one pale* (**Acon., Cham.**). *Heat of right side* (left side and left arm, Rhus), *or on upper part of body,* lessened by motion or washing (**Caps.**—increased by motion, **Nux v.**); heat of face, or of one hand, with coldness of the other; body hot, limbs cold (**Bell., Carb. v.**). Anxious heat, *as if dashed with hot water* (**Rhus**). Intolerable burning heat at night in bed with uneasiness. Dry heat of the body in the evening, with distended veins and burning hands, that seek out cool places (**Opium**). He is hot, wishes to be uncovered (**Apis., Camph., Sec.**). Moans and groans, licks the lips, but does not drink. Heat of the whole body, except the hands, which are cool, with pressive headache above the orbits. Internal dry heat with thirst; flushes of heat; with clothes on was too warm, on taking them off was chilly. External warmth is intolerable (heat of room is intolerable, **Apis**); the veins are enlarged (**Bell., Cinch.**). Fever; thirst at 2 P.M., followed by chill at 4 P.M., without thirst, with coldness of the face and hands; anxiety and oppression of the chest; afterward, when lying down, drawing pains in the back, extending to the occiput, and thence into the temples and vertex; after three hours, heat of the body, without thirst; the skin was burning hot, but there was sweat only on the face, trickling down in large drops like pearls, sleepiness without sleep, and restlessness; next morning sweat over whole body.

"The intermittent fever that Pulsatilla is able to excite has thirst only during heat (not during chill), seldom after the heat or before the chill. When there is only a sensation of heat, without externally perceptible heat, the thirst is wanting."—HAHNEMANN.

"When heat follows the chilliness, if it be only a sensation of heat with no objective warmth, there is no thirst; but if the heat be, as it sometimes is, both objective and subjective, it is then attended by thirst. Remember this, because absence of thirst is said to be a characteristic of Pulsatilla, and presence of thirst, therefore, to contra-indicate. This is true with the limitation stated."—DUNHAM.

**Sweat.**—One-sided; only on the left, or *only on the right side* of the body; sweat on the *right side of the face* (sweat on the side on which he lies, **Acon., Chin. s.**—on the side not lain upon, **Benz.**—on single parts only, **Bry.**); sweat worse at night or in the morning, *ceases when waking* (see **Samb.**). Perspiration on the head, face, and scalp. Sweat all night, with **loquacity during stupefied slumber** (loquacity during chill, **Pod.**—during heat, **Lach.** and **Pod.**). Pains continue during sweat (**Eup. perf., Lach., Natr. m., Nux v.**—worse during sweat, Ipec.).

**Tongue.**—Coated *white* or *yellow*, and covered with *a tenacious mucus;* too large, too broad. *Taste foul, of putrid meat; disgusting; bitter, slimy,* bilious taste after eating, drinking and smoking. Desire for beer, alcohol, stimulants, sour, refreshing things. *Aversion to fat pork,* milk, bread.

**Pulse.**—Weak, small, but accelerated. Pulsations through the whole body; in violent paroxysms; from chagrin, fright, joy; with anæmia, chlorosis; great anxiety, was obliged to throw off his clothes.

**Apyrexia.**—Spleen enlarged and sensitive. *Constant chilliness during apyrexia.* Headache, moist cough, painful oppression of the chest, somnolence, loss of appetite, bitterness of the mouth, sour eructations, nausea and vomiting of mucus, diarrhœa of glairy, watery stools, with prevalence of gastric and bilious symptoms.

After abuse of Quinine, with bitter taste of food and clean tongue. Suppression of menses, or irregular menses (**Sepia**). Slightest derangement of the stomach will cause a relapse (**Ipec.**). *Mild, tearful disposition* of women and children often becomes converted into a peevish, irritable, fretful mood; symptoms of threatened abortion during paroxysm in early months of pregnancy. **Paroxysm of increasing severity and ever changing symptoms; no two attacks alike.**

## CLINICAL.

CASE I.—Patient with red hair, light skin, freckles easily. First attack at 3 P.M., later ones at 1 A.M. *During the chill,* great coldness with shuddering; chills up and down the back, with aching and drawing pains in the bones and muscles of the hips; chilliness lasting three-quarters of an hour. *Fever high, with faintness and restlessness from want of air and heat of room.* Considerable perspiration after fever, but easily chilled. *Cannot remain in the warm room.* Pulse small and quite full; tongue moist and dirty-white. *No thirst.* Puls.$^{200}$. Cured promptly.—T. D. STOW, *H. M.,*—V, p. 237.

CASE II.—Mrs. S. E., æt. 65. Chill followed by fever and sweat nearly every day, *coming on towards evening;* no thirst in any of the *stages;* aversion to fat or rich food, and but very little appetite for anything; what little she did eat distressed her, and she had to live quite abstemiously. She had at same time a severe pain in left chest, with a troublesome cough, *worse on lying down.* Puls.$^{51m}$ (Fincke) cured, with but one more chill next afternoon, and none thereafter. In four weeks she reported herself better than for fifteen years.—S. H. COLBURN, *A. J. H. M. M.*,—IV, p. 86.

CASE III.—Mr. D., æt. 35; dark complexion; contracted while in the army in the Savannah marshes, fever, for which he took Quinine and whiskey. Has now no regular chills, but is troubled with great debility; very nervous and fidgety; night-sweats, awakes to find himself wet with sweat, and cold. This is repeated through the night; no appetite; before sitting down to the table thinks he can eat, but after tasting of food his appetite leaves him; *better in the open air;* soreness of the abdomen extending around to the back, feels sore and lame after his day's work. While in army he had diarrhœa, which any overexertion now brings on. Puls.$^{40m}$, one powder in water, teaspoonful before each meal. Cured in six weeks.—T. L. BRADFORD, *Am. Obs.*, —1875, p. 425.

CASE IV.—A married lady, æt. 28, nursing an infant six months old, had been much exposed for five weeks, while traveling in Missouri, sleeping in a wagon at night. Had suppressed *the chills* for ten days with Quinine, returned again every other night before midnight; not amounting to a shake, but a chilly, cold feeling, lasting from one to two hours, followed by high fever which lasted fully eighteen hours, ending in slight sweat. There was very little thirst at any time, a good deal of headache during the fever, and nausea before the chill; a pretty good picture of Pulsatilla, one powder of the 200th in the morning after the chill. One slight return of fever thereafter. Three powders in all were taken. Cured.—C. PEARSON, *Med. Inv.*,—VIII, p. 152.

CASE V.—" While visiting the office of a ' Doubting Thomas,' in July, 1881, I was challenged to prescribe for a case of intermittent fever, which had for nearly six months resisted his best efforts both with homœopathic remedies and Quinine. The patient, a large, blue-eyed, good-natured man, after attempting to minutely describe an attack, finally exclaimed : ' It's no use, doctor, no two of the paroxysms are alike.' One prescription of *Pulsatilla*, 3x, completely cured."—W. P. POLHEMUS.

## RHUS TOXICODENDRON.

**Characteristic.**—Adapted to persons of a rheumatic diathesis. Bad effects of getting wet, especially after being heated.

Ailments from spraining or straining a single part, muscle or tendon; overlifting, particularly from stretching arms high up to reach things; lying on damp ground.

Affects the fibrous tissue especially (the serous, Bry.); right side more than left.

Pains: as if sprained; as if a muscle or tendon was torn from its attachment; as if bones were scraped with a knife; worse after midnight; in wet weather.

Great restlessness, anxiety, apprehension; cannot remain in bed; must change position often to obtain relief from pain (restlessness from mental anxiety, Ars.).

Muscular rheumatism, sciatica, left side (Col.); aching in left arm, with heart disease.

Great sensitiveness to open air; putting the hand from under the bed-cover brings on the cough (Bar., Hep.).

Vertigo when standing or walking, is worse when lying down (better when lying down, Apis).

Dreams of great exertion; rowing, swimming, working hard at his daily occupation,

Corners of mouth ulcerated, fever-blisters around mouth; exanthema on chin.

**Aggravation.**—Before a storm; cold, wet weather; at night, especially after midnight; anything cold. **Rest.**

**Amelioration.**—Warmth; warm, dry weather, wrapping up, warm or hot things; motion; change of position; moving the affected parts.

"The great characteristic of Rhus is that, with few exceptions, *the pains occur and are aggravated during repose and are ameliorated by motion.* This statement, however, requires some explanation. In addition to the symptoms of Rhus, which resemble paralysis, there are also groups of symptoms resembling muscular and articular rheumatism. These rheumatic symptoms come on with severity during repose and increase as long as the patient keeps quiet, until they compel him to move. Now, on first attempting to move, he finds himself very stiff, and the first movement is exceedingly painful. By continuing to move for a little while, however, the stiffness is relieved and the pains decidedly decrease, the patient feeling much better. But this improvement does not go on indefinitely. After moving continuously for a longer or shorter period, and finding comfort therein, the paralytic symptoms interpose their exhausting protest, and the patient is compelled, from a sensation of lassitude and powerlessness, to suspend his movements and to come to repose. At first this repose, after long-continued motion, is grateful, since it relieves, not the aching and severe pains, but only the sense of prostration. Before long the pains come on again during this repose and the patient is forced to move again as before."—DUNHAM.

The *pains* of Rhus are aggravated by rest, while the pains of Bryonia are relieved by rest. It is the languor and paralysis of Rhus that are relieved by rest, not the pains.

**Type.**—Every type. Quotidian; tertian, double tertian; quartan, double quartan. First two stages often irregular.

**Time.**—5, 6, 7, and 8 P.M. All periods, except forenoon. Morning fever without chill 6 to 10 A.M. Evening paroxysm predominant; that at 7 P.M. lasts all night (Nux v., Lyc., Puls.).

**Cause.**—Rheumatic exposure, especially getting wet when overheated; after a drenching from rain and neglecting the precaution of changing the wet clothes; too frequent cold bathing in ponds or streams; "going in swimming" too often in midsummer. Living in damp rooms; sleeping in damp beds; fevers occurring in damp, wet weather.

**Prodrome.**—Yawning; stretching and aching of the limbs; increase of saliva in the mouth; burning in the eyes and painful weariness of the limbs. "**A dry, teasing, fatiguing cough, coming on first sometimes hours before, and continuing during the chill** (**Samb.**). I have often cured intermittents with Rhus, guided by this symptom alone."—DUNHAM.

**Chill.**—Begins on only one side, the right by preference (Bry.). The arm and leg of this side first feel the cold. Shaking chill about 5 P.M., even in a warm room or by a hot stove, with thirst and salivation, relieved by covering up in bed (not relieved by covering, **Nux v.**); salivation and all symptoms disappeared during sleep or on rising. *Stretching and pain of the limbs, shivering over the whole body, with much thirst, cold hands, heat and redness of the face;* in the evening in bed shivering; in the morning perspiration over the whole body, with pressure in the temples. *Chilliness and heat in the evening; the face very hot, though the cheeks were cold to touch and pale; with very hot breath.* Shaking chill on going from the open air into a warm room, without thirst (reverse of **Puls.**). *Shivering heat* and *perspiration* over body at the same time (chill and heat alternating or simultaneously **Ant. t., Ars., Calc. c.**), without thirst. Shaking chill in open air, not relieved by covering. *Internal coldness of limbs* (like falling asleep) *but no trace of external coldness.* Extremely cold hands and feet. Chill in all the limbs for an hour at 6 P.M., with diarrhœa (without thirst), then violent heat and profuse perspiration lasting three hours, with thirst. **Severe chill at 7 P.M., as though dashed with ice-cold water (Ant. t.), or as if the blood were running cold through the vessels; cold when he moves; increased by eating and drinking;** *became hot by lying down and covering, pain between the shoulders and stretching of the limbs during fever at night; sweat in morning.* Chill at 8 P.M., without thirst, with diarrhœa and cutting pains in abdomen with the heat, for several hours, with thirst; followed by light sweat, sleep and morning diarrhœa. **Cough during chill;** dry, teasing, fatiguing (dry, racking, with pain and pleuritic stitches in chest, **Bry.**). **Great restlessness in chill** (in all stages, **Ars.**). The restlessness is because he finds that tossing about relieves, not from mental anguish, as in Arsenicum.

**Heat.**—*With thirst. General heat at 10* A.M., *with yawning, drowsy, tired feeling; as if dashed with hot water;* **excessive heat, as from hot water running through the blood-vessels,** *without thirst,* but with *throbbing, dull headache,* pressure and swelling at pit of stomach, and *diarrhœa with cutting pain in abdomen.* **No cough in heat, but urticaria breaks out over entire body with violent itching, increased by rubbing,** *with great heat and thirst, drinks little and often;* lips dry. (Urticaria as chill passes off, Apis—before and during chill, Hepar—during heat and sweat, Rhus—during heat only, Ign.) She was too hot internally and chilly externally. Head and hand hot, rest of body chilly, or *vice versa.* Heat on the left side and *coldness of right side of body.* Hot, flushed face and burning heat of skin, yet not warm to the touch. Heat, after the chill, with *sweat, which relieves,* or chill in some parts and heat in others, both at the same time. **Restless, constantly changing position (Ars.).** *Shuddering on moving or uncovering.*

"The uticaria is intolerable; appears in spots or weals over the whole body; even the palms of the hands and soles of the feet, driving the patient frantic."—PEARSON.

**Sweat.**—*Profuse sweat, odorless and not exhausting* (**Samb.**). *Morning-sweats, not debilitating.* **Urticaria, with violent itching, which passes off with the sweat.** Sweat, with violent trembling. Night-sweat; sometimes sour; musty; putrid (rare). Sweat over whole body, except face (reverse of **Sil.**), or *vice versa.* **Sleep during sweat** (**Pod.**). Sweat does not relieve all pains (like **Natr. m.**).

**Tongue.**—Coated white, often on one side only; takes imprint of teeth (**Mer., Pod.**); with *red, dry, triangular tip.* Bread tastes bitter, after eating; food, putrid after eating. Hunger, without appetite; **craving for cold milk**; *cold water;* beer; to relieve the dry mouth. Aversion to alcoholic liquors and meat (reverse of **Puls.**).

**Apyrexia.**—Not characteristic. Symptoms of the paroxysms, continue in a modified form, particularly of the skin. *Continual motion only relieves. Constant restlessness, cannot sit quiet, turns in bed frequently without finding an easy place* (because bed is so hard, **Arn.**). Hydroa on upper lip, not as pearly, but as characteristic as **Natr. m.**

In July, 1881, I cured three cases of ague in one family, where hydroa on upper lip was characteristic. **Natr. m.** had been given in each case without success, and one prescription of Rhus cured. Since verified by W. A. Allen and A. McNeil.

### Natrum mur.

**Time.**—4 to 9; 10 to 11 A.M.; 4 to 7 P.M. Fever without chill at 10 to 11 A.M.

**Cause.**—Exposure to emanations from salt or fresh water, streams, ponds; near recently turned-up (especially virgin) soil.

**Prodrome.**—*Dreads the chill.* Languor, headache, thirst, nausea and vomiting.

**Chill.**—With thirst; blue lips and nails; bursting headache; severe, shaking; chattering of teeth and tearing in bones; nausea and vomiting, and some-

### Rhus tox.

**Time.**—10 A.M.; 7 *P.M.* and evening, lasting all night.

**Cause.**—Rheumatic exposure, especially by cold bathing. Swimming.

**Prodrome.**—Burning in eyes; stretching and pain of limbs; dry, teasing, fatiguing cough.

**Chill.**—Mixed and irregular; severe chill, as if ice water were dashed over him, or blood running cold through the vessels. Coldness of *left tibia, arm*

times unconsciousness. *Begins in fingers and toes.*

**Heat.**—With thirst; increased headache, unconsciousness and excessive weakness. Long and severe. Nausea and vomiting.

**Sweat.**—With thirst; profuse, gradually relieving all pains. Chilly.

**Tongue.**—Mapped; herpes like ringworm on the tongue; yellow coating; salt taste. Aversion to bread. Longing for salt. Hydroa around the mouth, like strings of pearls.

and *left side of body.* Shaking chill on going from open air into a warm room. Dry, teasing, fatiguing cough.

**Heat.**—Excessive heat, as if dashed with hot water, or as if hot water were running through the vessels. Urticaria over entire body, itching violently. Restless, constantly changing position, without finding an easy place.

**Sweat.**—Over whole body, except face, or *vice versa.* Profuse, but not debilitating. Violent trembling during sweat.

**Tongue.**—Coated white, or on one side white; red, dry, triangular tip. Aversion to alcoholic liquors. Putrid taste after eating or drinking. Hydroa on upper lip.

## CLINICAL.

Mr. S., an artilleryman, æt. 24, small stature, full habit, brown hair was taken in November last with a quartan fever, Paroxysm came on in the evening, with predominating chill, much thirst during chill and heat; throbbing pain in forehead before and after heat; chronic miliary eruption on back of left hand. Rhus$^6$, two doses, cured him in eight days. No return.—Dr. Segin, *Hom. Clinique.*

Aug. 13th, T. L., æt. 64.—Saw patient about 10 A.M.; he had been shaking an hour, during which time was almost frantic, frequently changing position in bed, groaning and complaining of drawing, tearing, crampy pains in muscles of both limbs, which passed off down posterior portion of thighs, to calves of legs. *Fever* was intensely high; pulse accelerated, but weak; face and whole body red; slight thirst during both chill and fever, most during chill; fever followed by sweat and headache. He was suffering too intensely to answer my questions, except as to pains in his hips. We must relieve his suffering or he should die. The intense drawing, tearing, crampy pains in both hips, running down to calves were so characteristic that I gave him a single dose of Rhus tox.$^{200}$, dry on the tongue. In from ten to fifteen minutes easier, and in less than half an hour entire relief, followed by perspiration and sleep. August 15th, slight chilliness at same hour; slight pain in hips, little or no thirst or fever; Sac. lac. August 21st, symptoms reappeared, but much less severe. Single dose Rhus$^{1700}$, (Fincke), dry on the tongue. January 1st, no more medicine; no return.—A. P. Skeels, *H. M.*,—II, p. 493.

## SABADILLA.

**Characteristic.**—Suited to persons of light hair, fair complexion, with a weakened, relaxed muscular system.

Worm affections of children.

Nervous diseases: twitching, convulsive tremblings, catalepsy; from worms.

Nymphomania from ascarides.

Most symptoms, especially throat, go from right to left (Lyc., Pod.).

Headache: from too much thinking too close application or attention; from tænia.

Follows Bryonia well in pleurisy, and has cured after Aconite and Bryonia failed.

**Aggravation.**—Cold; sensitive to cold air; during rest; forenoon.

**Type.**—Quotidian; tertian; quartan. Periodicity well marked; paroxysm returns at same hour with great regularity (**Aran., Ced., Gels.**). Stages irregular, incomplete.

**Time.**—3, 5 P.M.; 9 and 10 P.M. Afternoon and evening.

**Chill.**—Without thirst, and often without subsequent heat. *Violent chilliness*, at 5 P.M., over the back as if *dashed with cold water* (**Ant. t., Rhus**); *relieved by warm stove* (**Ign.**—*not relieved by heat of stove*, **Ver. a.**). Chilliness at 9.30 P.M., has to go to bed, followed by shaking chill; after half an hour, alternately hot and cold for half an hour; afterwards profuse perspiration. Recurring fits of shuddering coming and going quickly (Nux m.). *Chill always runs from below upward* (reverse of **Ver. a.**). **Dry, spasmodic cough, with pain in ribs and tearing in all the limbs and bones** (dry, teasing cough *before* and *during chill*, Rhus—*during chill and heat*, racking cough with pleuritic stitches, **Bry.**). Chill beginning in hands and feet. *Thirst begins* as chill leaves. **Chill predominates.**

**Heat.**—With slight thirst *for warm drinks* (**Casc., Ced.**), *before heat begins* (between cold and hot stages), little after. Mostly on head and face; flushes of heat with redness of face, alternating with shivering; yawning; stretching; delirium. Sweat, often *during* or *with the heat* (**Pod.**). Redness and burning of face; hands and feet cold.

**Sweat.**—Profuse sweat about head and face, which were hot to touch, rest of body cold. Sweat after midnight, towards morning;

*sweat of soles of feet.* Sleep only during sweat (see Pod., Rhus—after chill, **Nux m.**). Sweat in axillæ.

**Tongue.**—Coated white in centre; tip bluish and sore, as if full of blisters; as if scalded.

**Apyrexia.**—Constantly chilly; loss of appetite; eructations sour, rancid; vomiting of bile and bitter mucus; oppressive bloatedness of the stomach; pain in chest; *debility.* Sour eructations (**Lyc.**).

The gastric symptoms predominate as in Nux and Pulsatilla.

## CLINICAL.

Case I.—Patient, a boy, æt. 6. Towards 4 p.m., complained of feeling cold and asked to go to bed; went to sleep soon and only awakened at end of four hours; then ordinarily had a little sweat and asked for a drink. One drop Sab.$^3$ promptly relieved.—Dr. Segin, *Homœop. Clinique.*

Case II.—A gardener at Mendon, æt. 55, large, robust, jaundiced hue, had fever for several weeks of a quartan type, paroxysm coming on *invariably at* 3 *P.M. Chill* lasted two hours, with some thirst; *heat* violent, of three hours duration, and sweating for four hours. No thirst in heat or sweat. *Apyrexia* clear. April 28th, Sab.$^{30}$, one dose; following day, attack light. May 1st, fever missed, but at *the same hour* a weak trembling sensation in the limbs. May 3d, one dose Sab.$^{30}$. No return.—Dr. Gueyraid, *Homœop. Clinique.*

## SAMBUCUS.

**Characteristic.**—Adapted to diseases of scrofulous children: air passages.

Persons formerly robust and fleshy suddenly become emaciated.

Bad effects of violent mental emotions; anxiety, grief, or excessive sexual indulgence.

Œdematous swellings in various parts of the body, especially in legs, instep, and feet.

Dry coryza of infants; nose dry and completely obstructed; breathing much impeded; snuffles.

Dyspnœa; child awakens suddenly, nearly suffocated, face livid, blue, sits up in bed, turns blue, gasps for breath, which it finally gets; spell passes off, but is again repeated; child inspires, but cannot expire.

Cough dry, suffocative, with crying, worse about midnight.

**Aggravation.**—During rest; midnight; after eating fruit.

**Amelioration.**—Sitting up in bed. Motion: most of the pains occur during rest and disappear during motion (Rhus).

Follows well after Opium in fright. Antidotes abuse of Arsenic.

**Type.**—Irregular.

**Time.**—3, 4, 5 and 6 P.M. Afternoon and evening.

**Prodrome.**—Cough, *deep and dry, for half an hour*, with nausea and thirst (dry, teasing, fatiguing cough, **Rhus**). *Sweat* (**Carb. v., Nux v.**).

**Chill.**—Without thirst. Coldness creeps over the whole body, especially hands and feet, which are cold to touch. Shaking chill creeping over whole body, though face was warm. *Hands and feet icy-cold;* the rest of body warm as usual. *Chill lasts half an hour. Spasmodic, deep, dry cough* from lower part of chest, without expectoration; *may occur during chill if absent in prodrome.* Rarely occurs both before and during chill (see **Rhus**).

**Heat.**—Without thirst: dread of uncovering. *Sensation of burning heat in the face, with warmth of body, and icy-coldness of the feet, without thirst. Dry heat on falling asleep.* Intolerable dry heat all over the body, with dread of uncovering: thinks he would take cold or have an attack of colic *if uncovered* (**Hepar**). **Dry heat while he sleeps.**

**Sweat.**—**Profuse sweat breaks out on the face, without thirst, while awake, from 7 P.M. to 1 A.M.**; stood in drops upon the face, and extends over the entire body during waking hours; on going to sleep again the dry heat returns (sweat when he sleeps, stops when he wakes, **Thuja**). *Profuse nondebilitating sweat, day and night,* with relief of all symptoms (**Natr. m.**).

**Apyrexia.**—*Profuse sweat continues during this stage;* may become weakening from its profuseness alone, which is out of all proportion to the chill and heat.

Sambucus is almost the only remedy which has *dry heat while asleep*, **profuse sweat while awake,** then *dry heat again when he sleeps. The profuse sweat* is *rarely debilitating*, and *never in proportion to its profuseness;* always without thirst. Cinch. has *profuse, debilitating* sweat with *great thirst;* the reverse of Sambucus. *Deep, dry, racking cough before the chill, for half an hour,* with nausea and thirst, *is char-*

*acteristic* (Rhus has dry, teasing cough, like Rumex crispus, before and during chill.).

## CLINICAL.

CASE I.—Irregular paroxysm occurring every other day. Quinine had no effect. *Cough deep and dry for half an hour*, with nausea and thirst. *Chill* for half an hour, without cough, nausea or thirst; slight fever with moist skin; profuse sweat at night not debilitating. Apyrexia complete. Prescribed for the profuse sweat at night, not debilitating, Sambucus, a drop dose of the tincture, which resulted in a perfect cure, no other attack occurring.—CARROLL DUNHAM, *N. A. J.*, —XXI, p. 108.

CASE II.—Mrs. H——. Chills and fever; type quotidian. Paroxysm commenced at 3 P.M., with hard, dry cough, from lower part of the chest, racking and shaking the whole body, and producing a pain over the whole head, which is relieved by pressure or having the head tightly bound up. No expectoration with the cough. Great thirst for large quantities of water very often. Longing for acids.

*Chill.*—Severe and shaking, continuing for *half an hour*. Lips and nails blue. Nausea and vomiting, aggravated by drinking, the substances vomited having a bitter, sour taste. Bitter, sour taste in the mouth during the paroxysm. Tongue coated white, chills running down the back. Back and limbs ache, particularly during the chill, and worse when they come in contact with the bed. Cough, headache and thirst continued.

*Heat.*—Great, with stupor and prostration. Thirst and cough continue, but no headache. Pains in the back and limbs. Great difficulty in speaking. With the heat a profuse perspiration.

Delirium.—Is distressed because she imagines some one in bed with her. This oppresses her respiration, as she has to breathe for two. Continual talking. Sense of suffocation, with a fluttering at the heart. Great distress in the region of the heart, whence the cough seems to proceed. Moaning and weeping during sleep.

*Sweat.*—At night a drenching sweat, smelling sour-fetid, staining yellow, not debilitating. Ineffectual desire to urinate, passing water once in twenty-four hours, a small quantity of turbid, loam-colored urine.

Attempts to cover the totality of the symptoms with any one remedy, resulted in the conviction that it was impossible. Eup. perf., Bryon., Ipec., Arsen., Calcar., and Sabad, were successively given without benefit. Dr. Dunham now suggested that the "hard, dry cough before the chill," "the half-hour chill," and the "profuse, non-debilitating sweat at night," reminded him of a case he had cured with Sambucus. The cough and sweat, however, seemed the characteristics in this case, and Sambucus $^{1000}$ was given. To my surprise and gratifi-

cation, I found the entire train of symptoms removed, till the seventh day, the cough returning, was removed by a repetition of the remedy.
—S. SWAN, M.D., *N. A. J.*,—XXI, p. 106.

## SARRACENIA.

**Type.**—Quotidian; tertian.

**Time.**—5 P.M.; afternoon and evening.

**Chill.**—General chills between shoulder-blades. Horripilations between shoulder-blades in afternoon or evening. Coldness of extremities, as from deficient circulation. Chills, heat and sweat at 5 P.M., of a tertian or quotidian type. Chills, with cold perspiration and a desire to lie down after meals.

**Heat.**—Beginning in the afternoon and *lasting all night* (**Lyc., Puls., Rhus**). Fever, with heat and redness of the face, burning in the stomach, great prostration, delirium and loss of consciousness. Burning heat of the skin, with *excoriation* and *fissures*, as if it had been *excessively stretched*. Heat and continual burning in the legs; heat in the whole right lumbar region. *General heat*, with dryness of the skin, excessive thirst, and *as if hot vapors rise up to the brain*. Heat in the feet, as if *he had been cut*.

**Sweat.**—Copious night-sweat. Great sweat on the limbs, especially in the evening and during rest.

**Tongue.**—Coated brownish-white. Bad taste in the mouth, with loss of appetite.

## SECALE.

**Characteristic.**—Best adapted to women of thin, scrawny, feeble, cachectic appearance, and irritable, nervous temperament.

Women of very lax muscular fibre; everything seems loose and open; no action, vessels flabby; passive hemorrhages, copious flow of thin, black; watery blood; the corpuscles are destroyed.

Hemorrhagic diathesis; the slightest wound causes bleeding for weeks (Phos.); discharge of sanious liquid blood, with a strong tendency to putrescence, tingling in the limbs and great debility, particularly when the weakness is not caused by previous loss of fluids.

Leucorrhœa; green, brown, offensive.

Boils; small, painful, with green contents; mature very slowly and heal in the same manner; very debilitating.

Unnatural appetite; even with exhausting diarrhœa he is hungry.

Diarrhœa; involuntary, profuse, watery, putrid, brown; discharged with great force; very exhausting; urine suppressed.

Eneuresis; of old people, pale, watery, bloody.

Burning; in all parts of the body, as if sparks of fire were falling on them.

Cholera collapse; face pale, sunken, distorted, particularly around the mouth.

Senile, dry gangrene; cannot bear heat.

**Aggravation.**—Heat; warmth; from covering up. All affected parts; during fever, diarrhœa, cholera, menses, pregnancy, abortion, parturition, hemorrhage, ulcers, gangrene, the burning pains (reverse of Arsenic.).

**Amelioration.**—In the cold air; getting cold; rubbing; uncovering.

**Type.**—No periodicity.

**Time.**—At all periods.

**Prodrome.**—Vomiting.

**Chill.**—*With thirst. Violent, shaking,* followed by violent heat, with anxiety, delirium and almost *unquenchable thirst. Shaking chill,* with creeping coldness in different parts of body, as from snow (**Petr.**). **Intense icy-coldness of the skin,** *particularly of face and extremities* (**Camph., Meny., Nux v., Verat.**). Cold limbs, cold skin, *with shivering; pale, sunken face,* with coldness of back and abdomen. Temperature of body diminished (**Camph., Verat.**). *Lips bluish* (**Nux.**).

**Heat.**—*With thirst* and hot skin. *Burning heat, interrupted by shaking chills, then internal burning heat,* with *great thirst.* During heat great pain in stomach, abdomen, limbs (cramps and pain in stomach and abdomen, with vomiting and purging, **Elat., Verat.**). *Severe, long-lasting, dry heat, with great restlessness and violent thirst* (**Ars., Natr. m., Rhus**).

**Sweat.**—*All over the body, except the face* (**Rhus**—reverse of, **Sil.**). General sweat, relieving all the symptoms (**Natr. m., Samb.**). *Profuse cold sweat on cold limbs. Cold, clammy sweat over whole body. Sweat from head to pit of stomach.*

**Pulse.**—Accelerated during heat; generally slow, contracted, at times intermittent; often unchanged even with the most violent attacks.

**Tongue.**—Sticky, yellow coating; tongue *deathly pale* (mucous membrane of mouth and tongue pale, **Ferr.**); or clean, with dry, red tip; or red tip and edges, centre coated. Desire for sour things; lemonade (**Eup. purp.**). Disgust for food, meat and fats.

**Apyrexia.—Aversion to heat or to being covered.** *May feel cold, but does not wish to be covered* (**Camph.**). **Face pale, drawn, collapsed, hippocratic.** Great tendency to typhoid.

## SEPIA.

**Characteristic.**—Adapted to persons of dark hair, rigid fibre, but mild and easy disposition (compare Pulsatilla).

Diseases of women; particularly those occurring during pregnancy, child-bed, and lactation; or diseases attended with sudden prostration and sinking faintness (Murex, Nux m.).

"The washerwoman's remedy;" complaints that are brought on by or are aggravated after laundry work.

Pains extend from other parts to the back; are attended with shuddering (with chilliness, Puls.).

Particularly sensitive to cold air, "chills so easily;" lack of vital heat, especially in chronic disease (in acute disease, Ledum).

Sensation of a ball in inner parts; during menses, pregnancy, lactation; with constipation, diarrhœa, hemorrhoids, leucorrhœa and uterine affections.

Coldness on the vertex (Verat.—heat of vertex, Cal., Graph., Sulf.).

Indifference; even to one's family; to occupation.

Indolent; does not want to do anything, either work or play, even an exertion to think.

Yellowness of the face; conjunctivæ; yellow-spots on the chest; a yellow saddle across the upper part of cheeks and nose.

Herpes circinnatus in isolated spots on upper part of body (in intersecting rings over whole body, Tell.).

Painful sensation of emptiness in the epigastrium, not relieved by eating (Murex, Phos.).

Constipation during pregnancy (Alum.); stool hard, knotty, in balls, insufficient, difficult; pain in rectum during and long after stool (Nitr. ac.); sense of weight or ball in anus, not relieved by stool.

Urine; deposits a reddish, clay-colored sediment, which adheres to the vessel as if it had been burnt on; fetid, so offensive must be removed from the room.

Eneuresis; the bed is wet almost as soon as the child goes to sleep; always during the first sleep.

Prolapse of uterus and vagina; pressure and bearing down as if everything would protrude from pelvis, must cross her limbs to prevent it; with oppression of breathing (see Lilium, Murex).

Should not be alternated with Pulsatilla.

Often indicated after Silicea, Sulfur.

**Aggravation.**—At rest; in afternoon or evening; cold air; sexual excesses.

**Amelioration.**—Warmth; hot applications; violent exercise.

**Type.**—Many types; quotidian most common. **Monthly** (**Nux v.**, **Puls.**—every six or twelve months, **Lach.**). Quotidian; tertian; quartan.

**Time.**—9 or 10 A.M.—4 to 6 P.M. Indefinite periods; time not marked.

**Cause.**—In women, uterine diseases, menstrual delays, suppression or irregularities are often present. Constitutional chronic disease usually found.

**Chill.**—*With thirst. Shaking chill for an hour in the evening*, with brown, acrid-smelling urine; *he must lie down.* **Chilliness from every motion,** *though in a warm room* (**Nux v.**). Chill commencing in *fingers* and *toes* (**Natr. m.**), in *chest* (**Apis**) and *between shoulder-blades in back* (**Caps.**). Violent headache *during chill,* **external warmth is unbearable** (**Puls.**). *Icy-coldness of the whole body,* she could not get warm even in a warm room. *At* 11 *A.M. a shaking chill, beginning with very cold feet, thence over whole body; she had to lie down,* became hot at 4 A.M., and slight sweat during night over whole body. Chill, with icy-cold hands and warm feet, or *vice versa.* **Very cold feet, with headache, evening and in the morning. Icy-cold and damp feet all day, like standing in cold water**

up to ankles (Lyc., Puls.—icy-coldness of right limb, as if standing in cold water, Sabi.). *Coldness, with* **deadness of the limbs and fingers.**

**Heat.**—With less thirst than in chill. *Attacks of flushes of heat,* **as if hot water were poured over one (Rhus), with redness of face,** *sweat of the whole body,* **with anxiety, without thirst or dryness of throat.** *Flushes of heat from the least exercise.* Violent rising of heat to the head, alternating with chilliness in lower limbs. **Heat ascends (Natr. m., Verat.).** Face hot from talking. Feet hot at night. **Vertigo,** *unable to collect one's senses.*

**Sweat.**—*Profuse in the morning* **after awaking** (see **Samb.**). *Sweat worse from least exertion, mental* or *physical, walking, writing, eating* (**Bry., Psor., Sulf.**); smelling like elder blossoms. Cold night sweat on *breast, back, thighs* and *male genitals*. Sour night-sweat. Sweat from above downwards to calves of legs, *every third night.*

**Pulse.**—Pulsations in all the blood-vessels (Natr. m.); violent beating after waking, from mental emotions; pulse full, quick, intermitting, with an occasional hard "thump" of the heart.

**Tongue.**—Coated white, with vesicles in old cases. Food tastes too salt (Carb. v., Cinch.). Aversion to meat (**Arn.**).

**Apyrexia.**—Canine hunger, or complete loss of appetite.

## CLINICAL.

A girl, æt. 16, tall, slender, fair, light hair and eyes, had ague for six months, commencing in fall of the year. First two months it was tertian, but under allopathic treatment it assumed present form. Every four weeks to the day she was taken in the morning with a severe chill, lasting two or three hours, followed by very high fever equally long as chill; and this succeeded by profuse sweating; the entire paroxysm consumed nearly all day. The attack was repeated a second and third time, with an intervening well day; after which ague disappeared until expiration of four weeks from commencement. The girl had never menstruated. This was all that could be learned from person applying for medicine; patient was not seen. Quinine had been given without effect. Sepia, for two weeks. No return of ague, but instead menses, with entire return of health.—HAMILTON RING, *A. J. H. M. M.,*—I, p. 261.

## SILICEA.

**Characteristic.**—Adapted to the nervous, irritable, sanguine temperament; persons of a scrofulous diathesis.

Constitutions which suffer from deficient nutrition, not because food is lacking in quality or quantity, but from imperfect assimilation (Calcarea); oversensitive.

Scrofulous, rachitic children with large heads; open sutures; much sweating about the head, which must be kept warm by external covering; large bellies; weak ankles, slow in learning to walk.

Persons of light complexion; fine, dry skin; pale face; weakly, with lax muscles.

Diseases: caused by suppressed foot-sweat; exposing the back to any slight draft of air; from vaccination (Thuja); chest complaints of stone cutters, with total loss of strength.

Want of vital heat even when taking active exercise (Ledum, Sepia).

Has a wonderful control over the suppurative process, whether it be the soft tissue, periosteum or bone; maturing abscesses when desired or reducing excessive suppuration (chiefly affecting soft tissues, Hepar).

Children are obstinate, headstrong, cry when kindly spoken to (see Iodium).

Inflammation and suppuration of the lymphatic glandular system in any part of the body.

Vertigo; as if one would fall forward, from looking up (Pulsatilla—looking down, Kalmia, Spigelia).

Chronic, sick headaches, since some severe disease of youth; rising from the nape of the neck to the vertex, as if coming from the spine and locating in one eye, especially the right, relieved by pressure and wrapping up warmly.

Constipation, before and during menses; difficult, hard, with great straining, as if rectum was paralyzed; stool that has already protruded recedes again.

Complementary to Thuja.

Graphites, Fluoric acid, Hepar follow well.

## SILICEA.

**Aggravation.**—Cold; motion; during menses; during new moon; uncovering, especially the head.

**Amelioration.**—Warmth, especially from wrapping up the head; all the symptoms, except gastric which are relieved by cold food (see Lyc.).

**Type.**—Periodicity not characteristic. Stages ill defined.

**Time.**—Midnight to 8 A.M.; 10 A.M. to 8 P.M. Evening chill from 5 to 6 P.M. **Chilly all day.** Fever without chill 12 to 1 P.M.

**Cause.**—If the fever can be traced to a suppressed foot-sweat, Silicea is the first remedy to be thought of.

**Chill.**—Without thirst, **on every movement (Arn., Nux. v.), very chilly all day;** *in the morning fell asleep from excessive weariness. Very chilly even in a warm room. Cramp-like chill in the evening in bed,* with shivering. *She did not dare to put her foot out of bed on account of consequent chilliness* (**Bar. c., Canth.**). **Shaking chill at 6 P.M.;** *was obliged to lie down and could not get warm in bed for a long time.* **Icy-cold shivering frequently creeps over the body,** *not relieved by heat of fire* (**Phos.**). **Affected parts feel cold. Coldness with ravenous hunger (Cina).** *Coldness of knees and arms;* finger-nails *white* (coldness of knees, **Apis., Carb. v., Phos.**). *Nose cold as ice.* **Icy-coldness of the feet and legs as far as the knees.**

**Heat.**—*With thirst,* and chilliness, at 11 A.M. **Violent heat in the head, and dark redness of the face** (face of a mahogany red, **Eup. perf.**). **Fever in evening, worse at night (Cina).** *Afternoon paroxysm, consisting of heat with intense thirst and very short breath.* **Great heat all night, with catching respiration.** *Heat returning periodically during the day,* followed by slight sweat.

**Sweat.**—**Profuse and general at night (Cinch.). Sweat only on the head or head and face** (reverse of **Rhus, Sec.**). *Sweats periodically;* 6 *A.M.*, 3 to 5 *P.M.*, 11 *P.M. Sweat only on the head, running down the face. Profuse night-sweat, offensive, sour, debilitating; worse after midnight; from least exertion* (**Sep., Sulf.**). **Offensive sweat of feet, they become sore while walking (Graph.).**

**Tongue.**—Clean or coated with brown mucus. Loss of taste and appetite; or taste of blood, of soap-suds; rotten eggs; oil. *Sensation* *as if a hair were lying on the forepart of the tongue.* Disgust for meat. Averse to warm food; desire only for cold things (see Lyc.).

**Apyrexia.**—The constitutional symptoms developed during this stage are numerous and always reliable.

## SPIGELIA.

**Characteristic.**—Adapted to anæmic, debilitated subjects, of rheumatic diathesis; scrofulous children afflicted with ascarides and lumbrici (Stannum).

Body painfully sensitive to touch; part touched feels chilly; touch sends shudder through the whole frame.

Rheumatic affections of heart.

Nervous headache; periodical, beginning (in A.M.) at cerebellum, spreading over head and locating in eye, orbit, and temple of left side; pain pulsating, violent.

Intolerably pressive pain in eyeballs; could not turn the eyes without turning the whole body.

Prosopalgia; periodical, left-sided, orbit, eye, malar bone, teeth; from morning till sunset; pain tearing, burning; cheek dark red.

Toothache from tobacco smoking.

Pains in chest are stitching, needle-like.

Dyspnœa, must lie on right side or with head high (Cac., Spong.).

Chest affections, with stitch pains synchronous with pulse, worse from motion.

**Aggravation.**—From motion; noise; touch; inspiration; turning the eyes.

**Amelioration.**—Lying on right side with the head high (see Spong.).

**Type.**—Quotidian; periodicity marked.

**Time.**—Morning; at same hour. Evening paroxysm is rare.

**Cause.**—Rheumatic exposure; or occurring in connection with periodic neuralgia of head, face or chest.

**Chill.**—*Every morning, at same hour;* alternates with heat or perspiration, especially on the back.

*Sudden creeping chills,* at one time only in the feet, at another only in the head and hands, at another on the back or chest and abdomen, at another over whole body, without thirst. Chill spreads from the chest (Apis., Carb. an., Sep.); least movement of the body causes chilliness.

**Heat.**—Especially in the back; in flushes at night; on the face and hands with chill in the back. Heat in back, hands, abdomen, gradually increasing until he becomes hot all over. Thirst for beer, not water (**Nux v.**).

**Sweat.**—Putrid-smelling night-sweat. Sweat of hands clammy; cold all over body; on slightest covering (**Cinch.**).

**Pulse.**—Irregular, generally strong but slow; trembling.

**Tongue.**—Coated yellow or white; cracked. Taste like putrid water. Ravenous hunger with nausea and thirst. Desire for alcoholic drinks.

## STAPHISAGRIA.

**Characteristic.**—For the bad effects of onanism, sexual excesses, loss of vital fluids, chagrin, mortification, unmerited insults.

Onanism: persistently dwelling on sexual subjects; constantly thinking of sexual pleasures.

Spermatorrhœa; features sunken; guilty, abashed look; emissions followed by backache, weak legs, prostration and relaxation or atrophy of sexual organs.

Apathetic, indifferent, low-spirited, weak memory from sexual abuses.

Mechanical injuries from sharp cutting instruments, post-surgical operations; colic from lithotomy or ovariotomy (see Bismuth, Hepar).

Styes, chalazæ, on eyelids, on upper lids, one after another, leaving hard nodosities in their wake.

Toothache; during menses; sound as well as decayed teeth; painful to touch of food or drink, but not from biting.

Teeth are black or show dark streaks through them; cannot be kept clean; crumble, decay on edges. Scorbutic cachexia.

Ostitis of phalanges, with sweating and suppuration.

Arthritic nodosities of joints, especially the fingers (Caul., Colch.).

**Type.**—Quotidian; tertian.

**Time.**—9 A.M.; same time every day. 3 P.M., evening.

**Prodrome.**—Ravenous hunger for days (see **Cina, Sil.**).

**Chill.**—Without thirst. **Chill predominates.** *Shaking chill of whole body,* with hot cheeks, cold hands, warm forehead, **without subsequent heat or thirst (Sep., Sulf.).** Shivering over whole body, *without thirst* or **subsequent heat.** Chill with goose-flesh about 3 P.M., which was relieved by exercise in open air. Chill ascends from the neck over the head and face, or transient shivering running down the back (transient chills run up the back, **Sulf.**). Chill worse in a warm room (**Apis**).

**Heat.**—With thirst; at night; could not sleep after 3 A.M., with shaking chill at 9 A.M. Great heat at night, especially of the hands and feet, must be uncovered (**Sulf.**—external heat is unbearable, **Puls.**). Heat without subsequent sweat. Burning heat at night (**Ars., Sepia**).

**Sweat.**—Profuse in afternoon, without thirst, but with heat over the whole body (**Nux v.**). Warm night-sweat on abdomen, feet, genitals. Night-sweat of bad odor, like rotten eggs; with desire to uncover. Sweats when sitting quietly (**Psor.**). *Cold sweat on forehead and feet.*

**Pulse.**—Very fast, but small and trembling.

**Tongue.**—White coating; food tastes bitter. Gums white, spongy, ulcerated, bleed when touched.

**Apyrexia.**—**Extreme hunger, even when stomach is filled with food;** putrid taste in mouth, gums bleed easily; constipation. Longing for fluid food, soup, bread and milk (longing for eggs, **Cal. c.**).

## STRAMONIUM.

**Characteristic.**—Adapted to diseases of young plethoric persons; especially children, in chorea, mania, fever.

Delirium; simulates Belladonna and Hyoscyamus, yet differs in degree. The delirium is more furious, the mania more acute, while the congestion though greater than Hyoscyamus is much less than Belladonna, never approaching a true inflammatory condition.

Convulsions with consciousness (without, **Bell., Cic., Hyos.**); renewed by sight of a light, a mirror, or water.

Desires light and company; worse in the dark and solitude; awakens with a shrinking look, as if afraid of the first object seen.

Painlessness with most complaints.

Disposed to talk continuously (Cic., Lach.).

Imagines all sorts of things; that she is double, lying crosswise, etc. (see Petr.).

Desire to escape, in delirium (Bell., Bry., Opium, Rhus). No pain with most complaints.

Twitching of single muscles or groups of muscles, especially of upper part of body.

**Aggravation.**—In the dark; when alone; looking at bright or glistening objects; touch; after sleep; attempting to swallow.

**Amelioration.**—From company; light; warmth.

**Type.**—Quotidian; double quotidian.

**Time.**—6 to 7 A.M. At all periods, day or night.

Fever without chill, *noon* and *midnight* (11 A.M. and 11 P.M., **Cac.**).

**Chill.**—Without thirst. Shaking chill through whole body, with single jerks, partly of whole body or only single limbs, elbows and knee-joints. Chilliness runs *down* along the back as from cold water (as if dashed with cold water, **Rhus, Sab.**). *General coldness of the whole body*, with red face (Arn.), hot head, and twitchings of the limbs. *Chills*, with **great sensitiveness to uncovering** (excessively sensitive to cold air, **Camph.**—chill through and through from the slightest uncovering in warm air, **Thuja**). *Skin icy-cold, and covered with cold sweat, hands and feet livid* (Verat.). *Face, hands* and *feet* **blue and cold (Camph., Verat.). Coldness of the limbs.** *Hands and feet extremely cold, bluish* and *almost immovable; coldness and paralysis of limbs* (**Nux v.**—numbness of limbs, **Ced.**).

**Heat.**—With thirst. Violent fever at noon, returning at midnight (11 A.M., returning at 11 P.M., **Cac.**). Heat of head and face, then coldness of whole body, then general heat, with anguish; sleeps during heat (**Apis, Ign.**—falls asleep during heat and sweats profusely, **Pod.**). Nausea and vomiting in evening followed by violent, anxious heat. Heat over whole body from the least motion (least motion relieves the heat, **Caps.**). Dry, glowing heat over whole body, with redness of head and face, and coldness and paleness of the rest of the body (**Bell., Opium**). Skin hot and burning, with sweat at same time (**Sep.**). During heat, pains became violent if he put out a finger from under the cover (chilly, if she puts a limb from under the cover, **Bar. c., Canth.**). **Covers up closely.** During chill, *heat in head and face;* during the hot stage, *cold feet and legs;* during sweat, *cannot bear to be uncovered. Vertigo; delirium; epileptiform convulsions* (**Hyos.**).

**Sweat.**— *With thirst* (Ars., Cinch.). Profuse sweat, with burning in the eyes and dim vision. During sweat, good appetite, diarrhœa, distention of abdomen, and colic. *Cold sweats over whole body.* Perspiration of forehead and face, *rest of body red, dry and hot.* **Oily sweat** (**Phos.**—as if mixed with oil, **Cinch.**).

**Tongue.**—Clean or whitish-coated, with red papillæ; or swollen, dry and difficult to protrude. Juicy fruit tastes dry; *food tastes like straw.*

During fever, in children, they cry out in sleep; start suddenly, twitch and jerk; eyes half open; pupils dilated; urine suppressed.

Stramonium, like Nux v., cannot bear to be uncovered in any stage; but not for the same reason. The Nux patient is cold and chilly, if uncovered in the slightest, even cold on moving in bed; while the Stramonium patient is cold, and with the coldness comes immediately violent pain.

## CLINICAL.

E. C., æt. 28, had sunstroke twice, afterwards was subject for some time to epileptic convulsions, which only occur at present during febrile stage of paroxysm. Has had quotidian ague four or five times in last three months, each time suppressed by Quinine. *Chill* usually began at 9 or 10 A.M., with pain in the head and limbs, great thirst, headache, nausea and vomiting. *Fever* comes on slowly, with congested face, eyes heavy and dry, and general muscular twitchings. During convulsion the eyes become bright and staring, body rigid, jaws locked, frothing at the mouth, with sensibility. Duration of paroxysm from five to fifteen minutes, after which he is unconscious of all that transpired. Sometimes three or four spasms in succession. When I saw him, June 2d, he had been having chills, followed by convulsions, for four consecutive days. Had terrible headache, high fever, and presenting symptoms heralding approaching convulsions. He received one drop Stram. tincture in water. In fifteen minutes heat and redness of face and head disappeared, and he was free from pain and conversing freely, as well as any member of the family. He was cured with a single dose.—Dr. Fahnstock, *Am. Obs.,*—1872, p. 364.

## SULFUR.

**Characteristic.**—Adapted to persons of a scrofulous diathesis, subject to venous congestions, especially of portal system.

## SULFUR.

Persons of nervous temperament, quick motioned, quick tempered, plethoric, skin excessively sensitive to atmospheric changes (Hep., Psor.).

Most suitable for lean, stoop-shouldered persons who walk and sit stooped. Standing is the worst position for Sulfur patients; cannot stand; walk stooping like old men.

Dirty, filthy people, prone to skin affections (Psor.).

Children cannot bear to be washed or bathed (in cold water, Ant. c.); emaciated, big-bellied; restless, hot, kick off the clothes at night (Hep.); have worms, but indicated remedy fails. When carefully selected remedies fail to produce a favorable effect, especially in acute disease, it frequently serves to rouse the reactive powers of the system (in chronic diseases, Psor.).

Scrofulous chronic diseases that result from suppressed eruptions.

Complaints that are continually relapsing; patient seems to get almost well, when disease returns again and again.

Sick headache, every week, or every two weeks, prostrating, weakening (see Sang.), with hot vertex and cold feet.

Constant heat on top of head; cold feet with burning soles; wants to find a cool place for them; puts them out of bed to cool them off; cramps in calves and soles.

Hot flushes during the day, with weak, faint spells.

Weak, empty, gone or faint feeling in the stomach about 11 A.M.; cannot wait for dinner.

Diarrhœa; after midnight; painless, driving out of bed early in the morning; as if the bowels were too weak to retain their contents.

The discharge both of urine and fæces is painful to parts over which they pass.

Drowsy in afternoon, after sunset; wakefulness the whole night (Nux v.).

Nightly suffocating fits; wants doors and windows open.

Complementary to Aloe.

**Aggravation.**—At rest; standing; after midnight; warmth of bed; washing, bathing; changeable weather.

**Amelioration.**—Heat; dry, warm weather; drawing up the limbs; lying on the right side.

**Type.**—Quotidian; double quotidian; tertian. In regular paroxysms. Yearly (**Ars., Carb. v., Lach., Natr. m., Thuja**).

**Time.**—Not characteristic; at all periods. Morning; afternoon; evening; night. Evening predominant; 8, 9, 10 A.M., 12 M.; 1, 2, 5, 6, 7, 8, 9, 11 and 12 P.M.

**Prodrome.**—Evening fever without chill. *Thirst* (**Caps., Eup., Puls.**—but *can only drink* in prodrome and apyrexia, **Cimex**).

**Chill.**—Without thirst. **Frequent internal chilliness.** *Chilliness, with headache in the evening* (**Sep.**), disappearing after lying down. Aching in forehead with restlessness, relieved when sweat comes on. *Chilliness and shivering over whole body,* **without subsequent heat or thirst** (**Bov.**). Chilliness and rigor, with blue nails, pale face, heavy, giddy head, not relieved by heat of stove, but by lying down. Chilly in open air, as if naked. Shivering on slightest movement in bed (**Nux v., Stram.**). Coldness transient, of the *nose, hands, feet, chest, arms, back, abdomen.* **Chilliness in the back,** *in the evening for an hour, without subsequent heat.* **Chilliness constantly creeps from the sacrum up the back, without subsequent heat or thirst,** sometimes relieved by warmth of stove. **Icy-coldness of the genitals.** Coldness through all the limbs. Hands and feet very cold, with livid, pale face. Shaking chill for half an hour in the P.M., with blue face and cold hands and feet; subsequent heat and perspiration (**Ars., Bell., Rhus**). Headache, vertigo, delirium. Chill begins in hands, fingers, feet and toes (**Bry., Carb. v., Natr. m., Sep.**).

**Heat.**—With thirst. *Frequent flushes of heat in the face, with shivering sensation over the body* (**Sep.**). **Burning heat of the palms of the hands and soles of the feet;** or *cold feet, with hot, burning soles; was obliged to put them out of bed to find a cool place.* Heat and redness of face, with burning in single parts, as on malar bones, around the eyes, ears, nose, mouth. **Orgasm of the blood, and violent burning of the hands.** Alternate heat (of body and face) with chilliness (**Ars., Calc. c.**). *Frequent flushes of heat, ending in moisture and faintness.*

**Sweat.**—*Copious morning-sweat, setting in after waking* (sweat while awake, dry heat when sleeping, **Samb.**). **At night profuse sweat all over the body and restless sleep** (sweat all night without relief, **Kali c.**). Profuse sweat on occiput. *Perspiration on slightest* *motion* or *manual labor* (**Bry.**—sweat on least exertion or every mental effort, **Sep.**). *Profuse sweat* when **walking**, *reading, riding, writing, talking. Profuse sour night-sweat*, of a sour, burnt odor (**Lyc.**), vomiting; morning diarrhœa; tenesmus.

**Tongue.**—Coated white or yellow, which wears off during the day, and becomes red and clean in evening. Bitter taste in mouth in morning; food tastes natural. Longing for sweets, beer, brandy. Aversion to meat. Milk disagrees, causes sour taste, sour eructations.

**Apyrexia.**—Great prostration after every paroxysm (**Ars.**), with thirst for beer. Burning heat on vertex. Early morning diarrhœa. Feels as if he was just convalescing from a severe illness.

Sulfur bears the same relation to chronic cases that Ipecacuanha does to acute, viz.: if the indications for the remedy be not clear and well defined, *Sulfur may clear up the case, or completely cure it alone.* Intermittent fever is a terrible searcher after weak organs; and Sulfur is frequently required in all forms of the disease—acute and early, or chronic and later—to combat some latent malady aroused during the course of the fever. If we would use Sulfur more and Quinine less, our success would be much more satisfactory, both to our patients and ourselves.

"The antiperiodic virtue of Sulfur does not apply simply to pyrexial intermittents, but it also comprehends intermittent neuralgias, which consist of attacks of pain on the right side of the face and head, which begins at the maxillaries and finally extends along the orbital nerves, and thence involves the whole side of the head, there being no dental caries. The pains begin toward evening, last three to four hours, then cease, reappear later, and again cease up to the hour of attack in the evening. Psoric subjects; after the suppression of an exanthem; after the abuse of Quinine."—A. CHARGE, M.D.

Sulfur worn next the skin, in the form of flowers of Sulfur, is an effective antidote to the malarial poison which is supposed to produce intermittent fever, typhus and diphtheria, as well as cholera.*

---

* "Just as the milk of Sulfur applied to the skin (worn in the stockings) is the best preventive of cholera, so Carb. v. is the best preventive of yellow fever."—C. HG.

"In Memphis, in 1873, charcoal came much into favor as a prophylactic; out of more than fifty persons who took it and were constantly exposed to the fever, not one was attacked; the usual dose was half a teaspoonful of the crude powder, two or three times a day."—DR. MORSE.

## CLINICAL.

An old school M.D. passed through a stage of bilious fever last September. Was treated by a brother allopathist, *secundum artem;* suffered so much as to alarm friends. He recovered seemingly; but after a month's respite, was seized with intermittent fever; had two paroxysms, tertian; suffered much—sent for me. Found the chief symptom to be gastrosis that nothing could allay, and *diarrhœa driving him out of bed early in the morning.* Sulf. $^{200}$, one powder cured him. In a day or two went to the Mississippi bottom duck shooting; camped out; violated prescribed regimen, declaring he would test the cure; but he not only remained well but gained in strength and health to date, December.—C. P. JENNINGS.

## THUJA OCCIDENTALIS.

**Characteristic.**—Adapted to hydrogenoid constitution of Grauvogl, which is related to sycosis as effect to cause.

Thuja bears the same relation to the sycosis of Hahnemann—figwarts, condylomata and wart-like excrescences upon mucous and cutaneous surfaces—that Sulfur does to psora or Mercury to syphilis.

Acts well in lymphatic temperament, not very fleshy, dark complexion, black hair, unhealthy skin.

Bad effects of vaccination (Silicea).

Vertigo; when closing the eyes.

Headache; as if a nail had been driven into parietal bone (Coffea, Ignatia); or as if a convex button were pressed on the part; from sexual excesses; from tea (Selenium).

Abdomen: as if an animal were crying; motion, as of something alive: protrudes here and there like the arm of a fœtus.

Distressing, burning pain in left ovarian region, when walking or riding, must sit or lie down (Crocus), worse at each menstrual nisus.

Diarrhœa: in early morning; expelled forcibly, with much flatus (Aloe); gurgling, as water from a bung-hole.

Sweat, only on uncovered parts.

Skin: looks dirty; brown or brownish-white spots here and there; warts, seedy, pediculated; eruptions, only on covered parts, burn after scratching.

The flesh feels as if beaten off the bones (as if scraped, Rhus).
Complementary to Silicea.
Follows well after Nitric acid.

**Aggravation.**—At night; from heat of bed; at 3 A.M. and 3 P.M.; from cold, and cold damp air; alcohol; narcotics.

**Amelioration.**—Warmth; in the open air.

**Type.**—Quotidian, same time every day. Yearly (Carb. v., Lach., Sulf.).

**Time.**—3 **A.M.**, **characteristic**; 10 *A.M.*, 3 *P.M.*, 5, 6, 7, 7.30 *P.M.* After midnight.

Fever without chill 10 to 11 A.M., or 10 to 11 P.M. (Cac.—12 M. and 12 P.M., Sulf.).

**Cause.**—The indication is more certain if the system be contaminated with sycotic or gonorrhœal poison.

**Prodrome.**—Chilly and weak some time before the paroxysm.

**Chill.**—With thirst. **Chill beginning in the thighs.** *Violent shaking chill, for a quarter of an hour, about 3 A.M.*, followed by thirst, then profuse perspiration all over except on the head. *Shaking chill, with much yawning; warm air seems cold* and the *hot sun does not warm him.* **Shivering through and through, from the slightest uncovering of the body in warm air** (shivering from the slightest contact with the open air, **Nux v.**—great aversion to cold air, **Camph.** —chill as soon as he gets out of bed, **Canth.**). Chilliness every evening from 6 to 7.30, with excessive heat of the body, dryness of the mouth, and thirst. Chill of *left side of the body*, which felt cold to the touch (**Carb. v., Caust., Lach.**). About 7 P.M., *shaking chill, beginning in thighs*, with *blueness of nails, chattering of teeth, rapid* and *difficult respiration*, for half an hour; then *thighs hot, like a glowing coal*, with *cold hands and feet;* gradually became warm, though had a shaking chill *every time he moved* (**Nux v.**); fell asleep after two hours, and awoke in a profuse perspiration, had to change his shirt eight times up to 3 A.M., with headache and mild delirium and some thirst. Morning headache, chill at 10 A.M., lasting till noon, followed by heat, nausea, *constant one-sided headache*, and repeated bilious vomiting and diarrhœa in the evening. Chill internal, with external heat and violent thirst—chill, then sweat (**Ant. t.**).

**Heat.**— *With thirst, neither preceded nor followed by chilliness. Sensation of burning heat in the face,* which causes neither *real heat, redness* nor *perspiration, with icy-cold hands.* Burning heat only in the face and cheeks, lasting the whole day (**Bell.**, **Calc. c.**). Dry heat of covered parts. Heat mornings, chill afternoons. *Deadness of fingers* (**Ced.**, **Sep.**).

**Sweat.**—Only on uncovered parts; or all over, except the head (reverse of **Sil.**). Sweat, *when he sleeps, stops when he awakens* (reverse of **Samb.**). *Chill, then sweat* (**Ant. t.**, **Ipec.**). *Profuse night-sweat, staining the clothes yellow,* as if saturated with oil (**Bell.**—as if mixed with oil, **Cinch.**). *Sour-smelling or fetid sweat almost every night* (**Arn.**, **Lyc.**, **Natr. m.**). *Scrotum, perinæum* and *inner surface of the thighs* dripping with sweat (**Hep.**, **Petr.**). Profuse night-sweat, so that he changes his shirt several times at night. *Congestion of blood to the head.*

**Pulse.**—Full and accelerated in the evening; slow and weak in the morning.

**Tongue.**—*Swollen, clean or red, the tip is painfully sore to the touch.* Vesicles or blisters on the margin. Bitter, sour taste; had to get up in the night and rinse out the mouth (**Nux v.**).

*Thuja* helped in some cases, where the fever consisted in mere chills, with external and internal coldness (with thirst in same), followed by general sweat, without any previous heat.—*Ann.*,—II, p. 398.

## CLINICAL.

Andrew Mc——, æt. 26, a resident of East Saginaw, Michigan. Eight years ago, had intermittent fever, which was "broke up" with massive doses of *Quinine*, only to return from time to time, especially every Spring and Autumn, only to be again suppressed in a similar manner with *Quinine.* When fever first appeared, paroxysm came every alternate day, at 10 to 11 A.M., attended with bone pains, violent headache, and at times nausea and vomiting.

February, 1882.—Has now had chills and fever every day for seven weeks. Chill from 5 to 7 P.M.; severe, shaking; must sit close to stove, although external heat does not relieve. Chill begins in *knees and thighs*, and gradually extends to hips, thence over body, lasting from one to two hours. Some thirst in chill, but drinking aggravates. Heat, with thirst; drinking refreshes; continues until 1 or 2 A.M.; very restless; severe headache. Sweats profusely on his legs, where chill began; less on his body; never on his head; when he sleeps, ceases when he awakes. Tongue clean; appetite and digestion good; and feels perfectly well as soon as paroxysm is over. The chill beginning in knees and thighs, the time of its appearance, the character of the sweating stage, and the entire freedom from ill-feeling during apyrexia, determined the selection of Thuja$^{30}$, four doses during intermission. Cured.—H. C. ALLEN, *Medical Advance*, XII.,—p. 296.

## VERATRUM ALBUM.

**Characteristic.**—Adapted to diseases with rapid sinking of the vital forces.

Cold sweat on forehead, with nearly all complaints.

Mania; with desire to cut and tear everything, especially clothes.

Cannot bear to be left alone; yet persistently refuses to talk.

Attacks of fainting, from least exertion (see Carb. v.).

Sensation of a lump of ice on vertex.

Face; pale, blue, collapsed; features sunken; red while in bed, becomes pale on getting up (see Aconite).

Constipation; stools large, hard; from inactivity of rectum; in children when Nux vomica, though indicated, fails to relieve.

Cholera; vomiting and purging; stool profuse, watery, gushing, prostrating, after fright.

Dysmenorrhœa, with vomiting and purging (Amm. c.).

Bad effects; of opium eating, tobacco chewing.

**Aggravation.**—After drinking; ice cream; before and during stool.

**Amelioration.**—Uncovering head; sitting or lying.

**Type.**—Quotidian; tertian; quartan. Congestive; pernicious; sinking. Periodicity strongly marked.

**Time.**—6 *A.M.* Characteristic—certain. Fevers of nursing children; coldness predominates.

**Prodrome.**—Sweat often marks the commencement of paroxysm (Nux v.).

**Cause.**—Choleraic. Intermittents occurring during cholera epidemics. Often the genus epidemicus.

**Chill.**—*With thirst.* Daily chill, with violent shaking, vertigo, delirium, nausea, paleness of the face, and spasms. *Severe, long-lasting, congestive chill, not relieved by external warmth* (**Aran., Camph.**). **Chill, with coldness and thirst,** for half an hour, *without subsequent heat,* with great weakness of thighs and limbs (every other day). **Internal chilliness running from the head to the toes of both feet, with thirst.** Shaking chill, with sweat, at first warm but soon passes off into general coldness. *Coldness of the whole body, increased by drinking* (**Ars., Caps., Eup., Nux**); *lessened* by getting out of bed (increased by even putting hands from under bedclothes, **Bar. c., Canth.**). Coldness at times; heat, with profuse sweat at others. *Chill and heat alternating on single parts*, now here, then there (**Puls.**). Great coldness over the back and through shoulders into arms. **Face cold, collapsed. Extremities cold.** Coldness in limbs, shoulders and arms, as if cold air were *streaming through the bones. Skin cold and clammy.* Vomiting and diarrhœa (nausea, vomiting and purging, **Elat.**). **Predominant external coldness.** Coldness of the feet, *as if cold water were running into them.*

**Heat.**—With thirst, mostly internal; with no desire to drink, or continued thirst for cold drinks, the beverages are never cold enough. Heat ascends from extremities to head (chill descends). Heat streaming up the back into the occiput (chills running in successive waves from sacrum to occiput, **Gels.**). Head hot, dull, confused; first *warm*, then **persistent cold sweat on the forehead.** *Redness and heat of the face; burning* and *redness in the cheeks*, with contracted pupils and cold feet (**Opium**—with dilated pupils, **Bell.**). Blood runs cold through the veins (**Rhus** — runs hot, **Ars.**).

**Sweat.**—*Without thirst*, which is *profuse, cold* and clammy (profuse sweat, *with thirst*, **Ars., Cinch.**). **Sweat always with deathly pale face**; *offensive, bitter-smelling, staining yellow. Easily prespires on every motion* (**Bry., Hep.**). **Cold sweat on the forehead; after every stool; after vomiting of mucus.** Sweat often begins before the chill and continues through paroxysm until next chill.

**Tongue.**—Coated white or yellowish-brown; **cold,** *red tip and edges; swollen.* Voracious appetite. *Craves cold fruits, ice water, juicy food, wants everything cold.* Aversion to warm things. Hunger and appetite between paroxysms of vomiting.

**Pulse.**—Small, weak, slow, and growing continually weaker during the apyrexia.

**Apyrexia.**—There is great general exhaustion and rapid sinking of strength; oppression of the chest; deep sighing; face pale and cold, *with sweat on forehead.* The heart's impulse very weak in the intermission, as well as during the paroxysm; fainting; there are cramps in the stomach, abdomen and limbs; great thirst if much vomiting and diarrhœa, and *vice versa;* extremities persistently cold. Skin bluish, cold, inelastic, with deficient reaction.

We may require to compare Elaterium with Veratrum which it resembles in the suddenness of its onset, the profuseness of its evacuations, and its great prostration. But the characteristic predominance of the cold stage will serve to distinguish between them.

Like Camphor, the cold stage is so well marked that it overshadows all the others; the hot stage is light and often wanting altogether. When the hot stage is present the temperature is rarely elevated, and is often actually diminished during heat. There is such a general lack of vital heat, and slow and weak reaction, that the patient scarcely recovers from one paroxysm ere another begins.

The above makes one of our best pictures of the " sinking," " congestive," or " pernicious " forms of intermittent fever. The patient thinks he will die; and the physician shares his fears. The allopath now resorts to stimulants for the present; and Quinine to prevent the return of future paroxysms. Shall we, on that threadbare plea of pseudo-homœopaths, that "there is not time for homœopathic remedies to act," follow his example? Those are not lacking "in faith," but *in knowledge*, who "desert their colors under fire." The homœopath who knows his Materia Medica will *cure such cases* without resorting to "rational" (?) uncertainty. If he do not know his Materia Medica, he is justified in resorting to anything to try to save his patient; but the treatment should go by its right name, and the failure to cure should be properly credited. Every homœopath is responsible *for not knowing* what he professes to practice.

"Among the great number of intermittent fevers there is a formidable pyrexia called *pernicious*, because it may carry off the patient in the second or third paroxysm; he dies probably from the excess of poisoning. This extremely violent pyrexia forms no exception to the rule; and, like all other pyrexiæ, finds its most prompt and certain remedy in the drug which is most homœopathic to it. But here a delicate question arises which should be solved at once: What shall we do in the presence of a pernicious fever in which we have reason to fear sudden death, in the second or third paroxysm? Find the homœopathic remedy. Without doubt, principles are inflexible, and I know no means more powerful to combat the radicalism of the false than to oppose to it the radicalism of the true.

"We have a law of cure which has always shown itself triumphant when rigorously applied. Why should we be unfaithful to it? I see no reason. The violence of the disease? But the more urgent the haste, the more highly ought we to value the shortest road. Now, the most prompt and certain means of curing any disease whatever, however pernicious we may suppose it, consists in opposing to it the homœopathic remedy. Then, instead of renouncing in this emergency the application of our law, it is best to conform to its requirements. The greater the danger, the greater this obligation."—A. CHARGE, M.D.

"When we have to do with an art whose end is the saving of human life, any neglect to make ourselves thoroughly masters of it, becomes a crime."—HAHNEMANN.

## CLINICAL.

CASE I.—Man, æt. 30. Has had several chills, every other day. Chill commences with coldness in abdomen, spreading thence all over body, frequent, thin, watery stools; coldness became general, but no shaking; breathing much oppressed and labored; stools become bloody, finally nothing but pure blood running from the bowels steadily (involuntarily); part of time blood thin and bright red, afterwards dark and thick. *Prostration is excesssive; speechlessness.* The chill had lasted eight hours and the patient seemed on the point of death. Veratr.$^{200}$ in water, a teaspoonful every half hour, was given. In about three-quarters of an hour he began to feel warm; in two hours he was in a quiet sleep. No return of chills. China$^{200}$ was given twice daily for remaining weakness.—J. G. GILCHRIST, *Med. Inv.*,— VII, p. 79.

CASE II.—"The only remedy with which I have ever succeeded in relieving severe congestion *during chill.* It has more coldness than heat (reverse of Arsenic), cold perspiration and great prostration, and is almost the only remedy that will modify a paroxysm after it has set in."—C. PEARSON, *U. S. M.* and *S. J.*,—April, 1866.

# MINOR REMEDIES.

**ÆTHUSA.**—Adapted to diseases of children, especially during dentition.

Great intolerance of milk in nursing children; it is thrown up almost as soon as swallowed, curdled or not curdled, by a sudden spasmodic vomiting, then weakness causes drowsiness for a time.

A drawn condition about nose and mouth—a well-marked *linea nasalis*—giving the face an expression of pain and anxiety.

Sensation: of a band around the head and chest (Cac., Sulf.); of head, chest, back, as if in a vise; as if head, face and hands were swollen.

Great weakness; children cannot stand; cannot hold up head (Calc. p., Sil.).

Convulsions and spasms, with clinched thumbs, red face, eyes turned *downwards*.

The febrile symptoms usually occur in the morning and are accompanied with great lassitude and tendency to delirium, which disappears during sweat.

**Chill.**—Violent, without thirst, through whole body, with general and external coldness. Coldness of abdomen, objective and subjective; of extremities; with red face; with horripilation; with rigors and stiffness of the limbs.

**Heat.**—General, with complete adipsia.

**Sweat.**—From least bodily exertion; on going to sleep; cannot bear to be uncovered during sweat (Acon., Nux v.); relieves delirium.

**ALSTONIA.**—This remedy has frequently proved efficacious in chronic cases in which the paroxysms have been repeatedly suppressed by Quinine. It will sometimes postpone the day of chill, and may change or convert an anticipating into a regular type. But sufficient data have not yet been accumulated to properly assign this remedy its place in the therapeutics of intermittent fever.

The paroxysm occurs in the forenoon—from 9 to 11 A.M. The thirst comes on during the prodrome and heat (during prodrome and sweat, Cinch.).

**Heat.**—With headache, backache, and thirst for large quantities of water, which is thrown up sometimes as soon as it reaches the stomach (Ars., Natr. m., Phos.).

The sweating stage is not marked. Our knowledge is empiric, chiefly clinical.

**AGARICUS.**—Best adapted to persons with light hair and complexion; muscles and skin lax. Old people with indolent circulation.

Burning, itching and redness of various parts, like chilblains; of ears, nose, face, hands feet.

Sensation: as if ice-touched, or ice-cold needles pierced the skin (hot, burning needles, Ars.).

Chorea; all degrees, from simple involuntary motions and jerks of single muscles to a dancing of the whole body.

Involuntary movements while awake; cease during sleep.

Spine: sensitive to touch; worse mornings; before thunder-storm; from every motion, every turn of body; burning, shooting pains deep in spine.

**Chill.**—General, through whole body; from above downwards (Verat.); in open air; on slightest movement, or from raising the bed-clothes; in back as if water were running down.

**Heat.**—Almost wanting; chiefly on upper part of body. Swollen veins.

**Sweat.**—*Profuse;* greasy, but not offensive (Cinch.); all night; during sleep; from slight exertion or bodily effort; on front of body, especially about the legs. The face, neck and chest were wet with cold perspiration. The sweat, though profuse, is not debilitating.

**ASAFŒTIDA.**—In phlegmatic, scrofulous persons, who are subject to venous, hemorrhoidal congestions (see Sulf.).

Syphilitic patients who suffer from bone diseases and abuse of mercury.

Scrofulous children are clumsy, bloated (Apis).

Pain like from splinters (Hep., Nitr. ac.); attended with numbness.

Globus hystericus; sensation in the œsophagus as if the peristaltic motions were reversed.

**Time.**—8 to 9 A.M.; 3 to 4 P.M.

**Chill.**—Chill, coldness, dryness of skin. Chills run over the body, especially back and loins, from time to time. Chill every day at 3 to 4 P.M., with cold feet, cold hands and bluish nails; salivation and eructations smelling of garlic.

**Heat.**—*Of the face, after eating,* with anxiety, sleeplessness, cold hands and feet, *and unbearable stitches in the head,* but without thirst.

**Sweat.**—Cold on forehead and limbs.

**BENZINUM.**—There is nothing marked about the cold or hot stages of the *Benzinum* fever; indeed, the heat is often wanting. But like *Petroleum* and all its products, Benzinum has both profuse and partial sweat. Sweat of single parts is very characteristic.

**Chill.**—From extremities of fingers and toes to chest, head and vertex.

**Sweat.**—At night, *copious, general, warm* and *very exhausting* (Cinch.); followed toward morning by perspiration only *on the breast,* in the *axillæ* and *on the side not lain upon* (reverse of Acon., Bry., Nitr. ac.).

**CALADIUM.**—Phlegmatic persons, with lax muscular fibre.

Asthma: after eating, with frequent eructations of very little gas, *as if the stomach were full of very dry food;* when rash on forearm disappears; in alternation with rash on chest; with great oppression, as if mucus would suffocate him.

Sudden corrosive itching on small spots, nose, cheeks, toes; must touch the parts, but cannot scratch them.

Complementary to Nitric acid.

**Chill.**—Without thirst; in the evening or after midnight; beginning in abdomen and extending to fingers and toes, which were icy-cold.

**Heat.**—With thirst; internal; as from oppressive heat; disappears during sleep; of hands, face, abdomen, with cold feet, before midnight; after midday sleep, then sweat.

**Sweat.**—Towards evening, with prostration, yawning, sleepiness. After heat, *sickly sweat, which attracts the flies very much* (Sumbul). Amelioration of all complaints as soon as the sweat breaks out (Natr. m.).

**CANCHALAGUA.**—Especially for vernal intermittents (Gels., Lach., Sulf.).

**Chill.**—*Severe,* especially down the spine (Verat.); violent, with chattering of the teeth; with extreme paleness of the face, hands and lips; all over body, especially in bed at night; with nausea, vomiting of mucus colored with bile.

**Heat.**—In whole body, better in open air.

**Sweat.**—Not profuse, but causes a shrivelling of the fingers and toes, like a washerwoman's (Ant. c., Merc., Verat.). Face, lips and hands cold.

**Apyrexia.**—Excellent appetite as soon as paroxysm is over. Constipation, stool hard, dry, knotty.

**CARBOLIC ACID.** — *Miasmatic fevers,* with enlargement of spleen. Intermittent and remittent fevers occurring in the autumn, of a low, intractable form, or with a marked tendency to typhoid; tongue coated dark brown; sordes on the teeth.

**Chill.**—Without thirst; in the open air. Chilly and sleepy, though sitting in a warm room with a hot fire; from the face downwards; with flushed face.

**Heat.**—Severe; alternating with chills of short duration.

**Sweat.**—At night; copious, was covered with perspiration.

**CASCARILLA.—Chill.**—*With thirst for warm drinks* (for warm drinks in prodrome, Eup. perf.); slight when walking in the open air, which immediately disappeared on standing still, but returned after walking again.

**Heat.**—*With thirst and desire for warm drinks* (Ced., Eup. purp.); anxious of the whole body, and a slight sweat followed by sleepiness.

**Sweat.**—Slight, on the back, when walking in the open air. Profuse at night, drenching the clothes, but not debilitating.

"Cannot drink anything but hot drinks during fever."—A. O. HARDENSTEIN.

The thirst and desire for warm drinks is as marked as under *Cedron,* and both remedies have proved very efficacious in the treatment of intermittents occurring in the lower Mississippi valley. The late Dr. Hardenstein, of Vicksburg, relied upon *Cascarilla* when he found this symptom present, and says it rarely failed to cure.

**COLCHICUM.**—The following instructive case should have appeared in its proper place in the clinical record of *Colchicum:* In the autumn of 1866, L. C., æt. 30, was attacked with ague of the.quotidian type. The case lasted some eighteen days, a chill every day, and every day alike. It began at 10 A.M. with violent thirst, intense headache, greatly aggravated by the slightest motion, so that the patient lay on his right side with his head almost down to his knees, and moved only when the distress was so intense he could not avoid it. Wanted to be covered, but no relief from the covering. Chill lasted about an hour, and was followed by intense heat lasting about two hours, with continuance of thirst and headache, when the sweat began, with immediate relief of all the symptoms. He received a single dose of *Bryonia*$^{200}$. The next day the chill returned and I got this additional symptom: *he could not bear the sight or smell of food.* This suggested *Colchicum,* but, careful not to spoil the case by too hasty prescriptions, I gave Sac. lac. I took time to study *Colchicum.* My attention being given almost wholly to the fever symptoms, I concluded *Colchicum* did not cover the case, and.gave *Natr. m.*$^{200}$, one dose. The chill returned the next day; but Hering says *Natrum* is a slow acting remedy, and I thought we must give it time. I waited four days with just the same chill every day. Soon it appeared that every day the chill began with a desire for cold water, immediately after swallowing which he begins to be cold in the stomach, the coldness at once becoming general. It is not necessary for me to mention the various remedies he received, as I floundered day after day trying to cure intermittent fever, with that symptom of the appetite prominent before me all the time. At length a friend called, and I asked him to go with me to see the case. He did so, and, making his examination, took copious notes of the symptoms, till he struck that symptom of the appetite, when he whispered to me " *Colchicum.*" " Yes," I said, "but that is the only symptom of it in the case." He finished his examination, and we gave Sac lac. The next morning my friend called at my office and said: "That case is *Colchicum* or *Cocculus;* I am not sure which." "Well," I said, "if you say *Colchicum,* here goes;" and putting a vial of Fincke's 21 M. in my pocket, I went at once to see my patient. I found him in a chill, as usual. I gave him Sac. lac. in solution, once in two hours, and left a powder of *Colchicum* 21 M. to be taken as soon as the paroxysm was over. He never had another chill.

*Moral.*—Treat the patient, not the disease.—Wm. A. Hawley, M.D. *Advance,*— XIII, p. 204.

**CORNUS FLOR.**—Has been used in fevers of a supposed miasmatic origin.

**Prodrome.**—The paroxysm is preceded for days by sleepiness; sluggish flow of ideas; headache of a heavy, dull character; nausea, vomiting, loss of appetite; bilious or watery diarrhœa.

**Chill.**—Severe, with cold, clammy skin, nausea, vomiting and violent pains in abdomen.

**Heat.**—With thirst; bursting, throbbing headache; pronounced cerebral fulness and at times stupor; skin hot but moist; pulse full, rapid, hard.

**Sweat.**—Often wanting. When present is aggravated or brought on by slight exercise and is attended by great debility.

**Apyrexia.**—With more or less gastric irritation and painful diarrhœa. Weak, languid, with loss of appetite. "When all the stages seem aborted and the patient says his chills amount to nothing."

**CROCUS.**—Adapted to the nervous, hysterical subject.

Spasmodic contraction of single sets of muscles (Hyos., Stram.).

Sensation of something living, jumping, in various parts, especially in stomach, abdomen, arms.

Hemorrhage; epistaxis, hæmoptysis, menorrhagia, the blood dark, almost black, tenacious, stringy.

**Aggravation.**—Motion (hemorrhage).

**Amelioration.**—Open air (symptoms almost entirely disappear).

**Chill.**—With thirst; in the afternoon, increasing toward evening; with shivering from the back down the legs.

**Heat.**—*With thirst;* internal flushes with pricking and crawling in the skin; principally of head and face, with paleness of cheeks. Violent heat over whole body, worse in the head, with intense redness of face and distention of blood-vessels (Cinch., Cham.), great thirst without much dryness of the mouth.

**Sweat.**—Scanty; only on the lower half of body; or only at night, then cold and debilitating.

**CUPRUM.**—Complaints which may be traced to a repercussed eruption or suppressed foot-sweat, as a possible cause.

**Chill.**—Over whole body, most severe on the extremities. Icy-coldness of the whole body, and severe cramps in extremities.

**Heat.**—Internal, debilitating, exhausting. Flushes of heat, with burning of the soles (Sulf.).

**Sweat.**—Cold at night; clammy.

**CYCLAMEN.**—Great lassitude, particularly of the knees (Cocc.). Enervation of the whole body, burdensome to move even a limb.

The derangements of the digestive tract and female sexual organs are often accompanied by semi-lateral headache (usually left side), attended with nausea, vomiting, vertigo, obscuration of sight or absolute blindness.

**Aggravation.**—At night, when at rest; while reposing; fat food.

**Chill.**—*Without thirst;* in the evening; *with great sensitiveness to cold air and uncovering* (Bar. c., Calc. c., Canth.). Alternate chill and heat.

**Heat.**—Without thirst; principally of the face; succeeds the chill. Sensation of heat through the whole body, particularly in the face and on the hands; the hands continue cold a long time. General heat after eating. Heat of various parts, with swelling of veins of hands.

**Sweat.**—At night, during sleep; not profuse, but offensive. Slight sweat over whole body on waking from sleep at night.

**Tongue.**—Coated white or yellowish-white. Taste flat, putrid, offensive, qualmish, with disgust for food, especially fat food (Ant. c., Ipec., Puls.).

The fever is partial in all its stages. The chill generally predominates, and like its cognate Pulsatilla, usually occurs in the evening, and is without thirst. *Thirstlessness characteristic.*

**EUCALYPTUS.**—For many years this has been a popular remedy in Australia, Italy, Algiers, some places in Spain and in Provence, France. The leaves possess a very penetrating odor, which is diffused to a great distance, and it appears to possess the power of antidoting marsh miasm and thus exercising a preventive action. The Abbé Féles Charmatant, missionary priest to the African missions, Algiers, writes: "I will give you some facts about our *Eucalyptus* plantations at Maison-Carrée, which is now become our Mother-House. This estate was, six years ago, an immense territory covered with brush, dwarf-palms, and rendered very unhealthy by the neighborhood of the stagnant waters of Harach. In 1869 and 1870, as fast as the brush was destroyed, we planted a considerable quantity of *Eucalyptus* in groups, or beside paths the whole length of our fields and gardens, and the result was most marvellous; for the intermittent fever, which often stopped our orphans in their agricultural labor, has gradually disappeared, so that to-day this domain, formerly the most subject to fevers, is now one of the most healthy suburbs of Angiers."

Fevers of a **relapsing**, obstinate and prolonged character; of a miasmatic origin, in which the spleen becomes affected early in the disease. It is at first swollen and sensitive, then becomes more resistant, harder, bunchy on its surface. Vertigo is pronounced in all its stages. There is a dull congestive headache; malaise; rheumatic pains of a jerking, tearing, stitching character, worse at night.

Our pathogenesis of this remedy has not been sufficient to give us any definite indications for its use. It is used as a substitute for Quinine, by the other school of practice.

**EUPHORBIUM.**—Usually a morning paroxysm.

**Chill.**—Of the whole body in the morning; while walking in the open air. Constant chilliness, with constant sweat. Shivering; over the whole body; over the back, with glowing cheeks and cold hands.

**Heat.**—Great, the whole day; all the clothes seemed burdensome, even his whole body was too heavy for him, as if he had carried a great load.

**Sweat.**—*In the morning*, from the feet over the whole body; some thirst. Morning-sweat; on the neck, thighs and legs; sometimes cold on the legs.

**HYDRASTIS.**—Nearly all complaints are attended with weakness and great physical prostration (Ars.).

Affections of mucous membranes; the secretions are increased and become tenacious, ropy (Kali b., Teucr.); erosions.

Cachectic persons, with marked disturbance of gastric and hepatic functions.

Faintness, sinking, goneness at the stomach, and violent palpitation of the heart.

**Chill.**—Morning or evening; especially in the back or thighs, with aching; around shoulders and chest; pulse slow.

**Heat.**—In flushes, over face, neck and hands. Great heat of the whole body, at 10 P.M., followed by great debility.

**Sweat.**—Profuse, offensive of the genital organs.

**KALI BROM.**—Acts more satisfactorily in children than in adults. Especially adapted to large persons inclined to obesity. Acne of the face in young fleshy people of gross habits.

*Painful flushings of the face*, at the climacteric.

**Type.**—Quotidian.

**Chill.**—Chilliness, and a general feeling of coldness, more pronounced about the extremities.

**Heat.**—Like the cold stage, this is not very strongly marked. Heat in the face, and fugitive flushings here and there.

**Sweat.**—Abundant and viscid, all over the body. This stage is unusually long lasting and exhausting.

**LACHNANTHES.**—Torticollis: neck stiff, head drawn to one side; pain in the nape as if dislocated, when turning the neck or bending the head backward.

Sensation: as if a piece of ice was lying on the back between the shoulders; of burning, in sacrum, in spine four inches above the small of back, of palms of hands and soles of feet.

**Chill.**—With thirst; body icy-cold, relieved by hot flatirons, but not by external covering (Caps.); head burns like fire (see Arn.).

**Heat.**—Dry, feet burn; restless tossing about with rumbling in abdomen. Burning heat, red face, worse on right side; after heat, circumscribed dark redness of face, also worse on right side (see Chel., Sang.). Flushes of heat alternating with chilliness. Evening fever without chill, worse from 6 to 12 P.M., with red cheeks and red face (worse on upper part of face). Fever with somnolency (Apis).

**Sweat.**—After 12 P.M.; after a restless sleep. Morning-sweat. Skin cold, damp, clammy and sticky. Sweat with vertigo.

**LAUROCERASUS.**—Painlessness with most complaints (Stram.).

Diseases attended with rapid sinking of the vital forces (Camph., Verat.).

Deficient reaction, want of energy of vital forces, especially in affections of the chest.

Long-lasting fainting spells.

Irresistible sleepiness; after dinner; in the evening.

**Chill.**—With thirst; in the afternoon or evening. Violent chill and coldness, with shivering, not relieved by external warmth; coldness and shaking chill, not relieved by heat of stove, alternating with burning heat. Deficient animal heat (Led.). Vertigo; stupor, and apoplectic symptoms (Opium).

**Heat.**—After the chill; from evening till midnight; descending the back (see Verat.).

**Sweat.**—During and after the heat; after eating; rarely profuse.

**MARUM.**—Very indolent both mentally and physically.

**Chill.**—Over whole body, with icy-cold hands, and frequent yawning and stretching; *always after eating* (Bell., Kali c., Nux v.—after eating and drinking, Asar.); from talking about unpleasant things.

**Heat.**—Frequent feeling of flushing heat in the face, without external redness. Increased heat and exaltation in evening, *with great loquacity* (Lach.). Great mental excitement and loquacity during fever heat.

**NATRUM SULPH.**—Should be thought of for the intermittents which are brought on, or are always made worse by the damp, moist atmosphere at the seashore (Arsenicum, Natrum mur.).

**Time.**—Afternoon or evening paroxysm.

**Chill.**—Internal, with yawning and stretching; with coldness the whole night; in the evening; as if fever would set in, with desire for a warm stove. Chilliness; generally in the evening, going off in bed; at night waking with shaking and chattering of the teeth, as from coldness. During chill forehead and hands are warm.

**Heat.**—Frequent flushes of heat, towards evening. Dry heat over whole body as if perspiration would break out, several afternoons.

**Sweat.**—Profuse, without thirst or subsequent weakness; on the scrotum while sitting, towards evening.

**PARIS QUAD.**—Headache aggravated by thinking. Contractive, pressive pain in forehead, as if scalp were constricted and the bones scraped sore; *eyes feel as if projecting, with a sensation as if a thread was tightly drawn through the eyeball and backward into the middle of the brain.*

Dull pain in nape of neck; feels stiff and swollen on turning it; weary, as from a great weight lying upon it; worse from exertion, better from rest and in open air.

**Chill.**—Mostly towards evening; in the chest, abdomen and lower limbs, with gooseflesh, yawning and icy-cold feet; with internal trembling. Coldness of the whole right half of the body, from the head to the feet, while the other half was of natural warmth (see Rhus). Small icy-cold spots here and there in the skin. The coldness produces a drawing, contracting sensation in skin and all parts of the body as if drawn together by the cold.

**Heat.**—Starts from nape of neck and descends the back; in the face; with sweat of upper part of body. The fingers are alternately hot and cold as if dead and of a dead color (Ced., Sep. Stann.).

**Sweat.**—In the morning, when waking, with biting-itching that compels scratching; profuse; on waking, about 3 A.M.

**PETROSELINUM.**—In the herbarium of Horstius, as early as 1630, this remedy is mentioned as having cured catarrhal, quotidian and tertian fevers. But like all similar cures, they were purely empirical and practically worthless. Vesical or urinary symptoms are usually present as valuable concomitants. There is frequent desire to urinate, recurring nearly every half hour, caused by a crawling, stitching, titillating in the fossa navicularis. *Drawing, burning, sticking in fossa navicularis,* **that after urinating changed to a cutting-biting** (see Canth.).

**Type.**—Quotidian by preference; tertian. Periodicity strongly marked; the stages are regular both in their evolution and succession (Quinine). Adapted to acute, non-miasmatic fevers, which appear to depend upon defective assimilation or perverted innervation.

**Apyrexia.**—There are twitching, jerking pains in the epigastrium, flatulent eructations, colic, nausea and vomiting; stools white, clay-colored (Pod.).

**PHELLANDRIUM.**—Adapted to persons of a feeble, irritable, lymphatic constitution, with weak and deficient reaction.

**Time.**—From 4 to 10 P.M.—4, 6, 7, 8, 9, 10 P.M.

**Chill.**—Coldness and chilliness, with frequent shaking, about 8 P.M., continuing even after lying down; internal, could scarcely get warm in bed until midnight, though the skin was not cold to the touch. Shivering; as if dashed with cold water (Rhus, Saba.); not relieved by warmth of stove. Chilliness and shivering over whole body, with gooseflesh on the arms and cutting pains in epigastric region.

**Heat.**—Of the head and face, with burning and redness of the face.

**Sweat.**—Slight; intermingled with heat; often wanting altogether.

There may be present as concomitants catarrhal and pulmonary affections, loss of appetite, emaciation, sleeplessness, diarrhœa and night-sweats.

"Jn. Frank reports (*Path. Med. Trans.*, Paris, 1835) that he cured, without a failure, the intermittent fevers which prevailed during the spring and summer of 1801 with *Phellandrium*. But, he adds, immediately after that, in the following years, the same means employed in the same disease failed. What more evident proof of the necessity of absolutely and always individualizing in pathology and therapeutics? The law of cure is immutable; there is no caprice about it; caprice is the appanage of physicians! *Phellandrium* cured the fever of 1801; with the testimony of Jn. Frank no one has a right to doubt it; and if it failed in the following epidemics it was because the medical constitution was no longer the same; and, not knowing how to individualize, Jn. Frank has left us a memento, but a sterile one. If, however, he had left us the minutely exact portraiture of the fever of 1801, he would have left us the characteristics of *Phellandrium*, and the success which he obtained, instead of being lost to us, might have been repeated."—A. CHARGE, M.D.

**ROBINIA.**—Gastric symptoms are usually prominent. There is excessive acidity of stomach; the child smells sour (Rheum). Eructations and vomiting of intensively sour fluid, setting the teeth on edge (Lyc., Sulph. ac.). Sick headache, with irritability, despondency and acid eructations and acid vomiting (with sweet saliva, sweet vomiting, Iris).

**Chill.**—Especially in afternoon and evening; feels frozen, as if the blood did not circulate (Lyc.). Hands cold.

**Heat.**—With intense thirst; frothy saliva; pasty, nauseous taste; cerebral congestion; soporous sleep, violent cramps of extremities and great prostration. Heat and sensation of drowsiness over the whole body; face pale, with circumscribed redness of cheeks, headache, nausea, colic and thirst (see Lachn.).

**Sweat.**—Copious, oily, fetid, especially on the scalp and face.

**SABINA.**—Great lassitude, weariness, heaviness, with despondency.

**Chill.**—Chilliness all day; one chill after another, on lying down in the evening. Shivering, with obscuration of sight, followed by sleepiness. Shuddering, with gooseflesh. Cold feeling in right limb, as if it were standing in cold water (see Sep.).

**Heat.**—Burning, of the whole body, with great restlessness. Flushes of heat in face, rest of body chilly; with icy-cold hands and feet.

**Sweat.**—Night-sweats. Sweats easily; on the feet.

**SARSAPARILLA.**—Dark hair and complexion. Scrofulous and sycotic affections.

Especially adapted to tettery eruptions, worse in spring and summer; and to affections of urinary tract.

Urine: passes gravel or small calculi; blood with last of urine; sand in urine or on diaper, child screams before or while passing it (Bor., Lyc.); passes in a thin, feeble stream; dribbles while sitting, standing passes freely. *Severe pain at conclusion of urination.*

**Aggravation.**—During chilliness.

**Amelioration.**—Soon as he becomes warm (during heat); in open air, if he does not move about.

**Time.**—Mostly in forenoon (Eup. perf., Natr. m., Nux v.).

**Chill.**—Predominates (day and night): chilliness and frequent shuddering, running from feet upward; of whole body, especially of the feet; not relieved by heat of stove.

**Heat.**—In the evening, with ebullitions of blood and palpitation of heart. Feels better in the evening when heat comes on.

**Sweat.**—Only on the forehead; in the evening; during fever heat.

**STANNUM.**—Pain begins lightly, increases gradually to its highest part, then gradually declines.

Excessive prostration of mind and body, must sit or lie down. Great weakness in the chest; great loss of strength in arms and legs; the arms have no strength in them; the legs cannot support the body; when about to sit down falls upon the chair in the attempt.

**Chill.**—Over whole body at 10 A.M.; with coldness in the hands, deadness of the fingers, and numbness of their tips (Paris, Sep.); in the evening over the back; slight, but with chattering of the teeth, as from convulsion of masseter muscles; only in left arm, or only in left leg; knees and feet very cold (Carb. v.).

**Heat.**—From 4 to 5 P.M., with sweat; of single parts, back, chest, abdomen, limbs. Anxious heat as if sweat would break out. Burning heat in limbs.

**Sweat.**—Profuse after 4 A.M. every morning. Morning-sweat, mostly on the neck, nape of the neck, and forehead; smells mouldy, musty; debilitating from least movement.

**TARAXACUM.**—**Mapped tongue,** *which is covered with a white film, with a sensation of rawness in it; afterwards this film comes off in pieces, leaving dark red, tender, and very sensitive spots* (see Lach., Natr. m.).

**Time.**—8 P.M.; at night, with gastric ailments.

**Chill.**—Great chilliness after eating, and especially after drinking (Bell., Caps., Kali c., Lob., Marum). Long-lasting chill; when he falls asleep, sweat breaks out, mostly on the head. Nose, hands and tips of fingers are icy-cold.

**Heat.**—Sensation of heat, and heat in face, with redness (Lach.).

**Sweat.**—With thirst; *copious;* at night; with pain in spleen; all over body on falling asleep in the evening (Cinch.); *debilitating night-sweats,* causing biting of the skin.

The abundant, debilitating, nocturnal perspiration is the guiding symptom of *Taraxacum*. It occurs invariably at night, and differs from *Cinchona* in that the latter, although abundant and debilitating, comes on night or day when covering up. The condition of the tongue will further serve to distinguish between them.

**VALERIANA.**—For nervous, irritable, hysterical subjects, in whom the intellectual faculties predominate and who suffer from hysterical neuralgia of the limbs.

Headache, with violent pressure in the forehead, followed in a few minutes by sticking in the forehead, over the orbits; soon the sticking changes again to pressure, and so on in constant alternation; the sticking is like a darting, tearing, jerking, as if it would pierce from within outward.

**Chill.**—Short; *with thirst;* begins in neck and runs downward (heat begins in neck and runs down the back, Paris); with fainting during chill (in heat, Acon.).

**Heat.**—Long-lasting, severe, *with thirst* and dull headache; with restlessness and neuralgia of the limbs; indigestion; often with sweat on the face. In evening; spells of fugitive heat; after eating; with thirst. Hot stage predominates.

**Sweat.**—Profuse, especially at night, but not debilitating; from exertion, with *violent thirst;* often attended with or followed by heat. Better after sweat.

# REPERTORY.

## TYPE.

**Anticipating:** Ant. t. **Ars.** Bell. **Bry.** Chin. s. Cinch. Eup. perf. *Gamb.* Ign. **Natr. m. Nux v.**
——, every day, two hours: Cham.
——, —— other day: Natr. m. Nux v.
——, —— —— ——, one hour: **Ars.**
——, —— —— ——, several hours: Ant. t.
——, one to three hours, each attack: Chin. s.
——, two to three hours, each attack: Cinch.
——, rarely: Bell. Ign. Mer.
——, or postponing: **Bry.** Gamb. **Ign.**
——, converted into a regular: Alston.
**Apoplectic:** Laur. Nux v. Op.
**Autumnal:** *Æsc.* Bap. **Bry.** Carb. ac. *Cinch.* **Colch. Natr. m.** Verat.
**Changing:** *Elat.* Eup. perf. **Ign.** Meny. **Puls.**
——, frequently: *Elat.* Ign. *Puls.*
——, no two attacks alike: *Puls.*
——, after abuse of quinine: Arn. Ars. *Elat.* **Eup. perf.** Ign. *Ipec.*
**Congestive:** Apis. **Arn.** Bell. Cac. *Camph.* Elat. Hyos. **Nux v. Op. Verat.**
**Day,** every, at precisely same hour: Anac. *Ang.* **Aran.** Cac. **Ced. Gels.** *Sabad.* Stan. (see Psor.) *Spig.*
——, at different times of: Eup. purp.
——, every other: Ant. c. **Aran. Ced.** *Chin. s.* Cinch. *Natr. m.*
——, —— ——, in evening: **Lyc.**
——, —— seven: *Amm. m.* Canth. *Cinch. Lyc.* Meny. Plant.
——, —— fourteen: *Amm. m.* **Ars.** Calc. Chin. s. *Cinch.* **Lach.** Plant. Puls.
——, —— twenty-one: *Chin. s.* Mag. c.
**Endemic:** Ars. **Ced.** Chin. s. Cinch. Eup. perf. Gels. *Nux v.*
**Epidemic:** Ant. t. Arn. *Ars.* Bap. Bry. *Chin. s.* Colch. Elat. *Eup. perf.* **Ipec. Natr. m.** Phel. Rhus. Verat.

**Epileptic:** Cup. Hyos. *Lach.* **Op.**
**Intermittents,** acute: *Ars.* Bap. *Bry.* **Chin. s.** Cinch. *Gels.* Ign. **Natr. m.** *Nux v.*
——, chronic: Alum. Apis. Calc. Carb. v. Graph. Hep. Kali c. Lach. Lyc. Natr. m. Nux v. Phos. Psor. Sep. Sil. Sulf.
——, of children: **Ars. Cham.** Cina. Crotal. *Gels.* **Lach.** *Op.*
——, of old people: Alum. Bar. **Op.**
**Malarial:** Alston. **Arn.** Canch. Carb. ac. **Chin. s.** *Cinch.* Corn. f. Eucalyp. Eup. perf.
**Menses,** after the: **Nux v.** Sep.
**Monthly:** Nux. m. **Nux v.** Puls. Sep.
**Paroxysm,** irregular: **Ars.** Eup. perf. Ign. *Ipec.* Meny. **Nux v.** Puls. Samb.
——, ——, stage irregular: **Ars.** *Ipec.* **Nux v.**
——, ——, —— ——, *long chill, little heat, no thirst:* **Puls.**
——, ——, —— ——, short chill, long heat, no thirst: **Ipec.**
——, ——, one stage wanting: *Apis,* Aran. **Ars.** Bov. Camph. Dros. Meny. Mez. Verat.
——, regular: Chin. s. Cina. Cinch.
——, ——, stages irregular: *Opium.*
——, ——, first two stages irregular: *Rhus.*
——, ——, stages regular: **Chin. s.**
——, ——, stages regular, apt to run into each other: Ars. Nux v. Puls. Pod.
——, increasing in severity: Ars. *Bry.* Eup. perf. *Natr. m.* Nux v. **Puls.**
**Periodicity,** marked: Æsc. Ang. **Aran.** Cac. Caps. **Ced.** *Cina.* **Gels.** Pod. Spig.
**Periodicity,** not marked: Acon. Amb. Amm. m. Bell. Camph. Canth. Carb. an. Carb. v. Caust. Chel. Cic. Col. Mag. c. Psor.
**Postponing:** Alston. Cina. Cinch. **Gamb.** Ign. *Ipec.*
**Pernicious:** *Apis, Arn.* **Camph.** Cur. *Nux v.* Op. **Verat.**
**Quartan:** Acon. Anac. Ant. c. *Arn.* **Ars.** Bell. Bry. Carb. v. Cinch. Cina. Clem. Coff. *Elat.* **Hyos.** Ign. **Iod.** Ipec. Lach. Lyc. **Meny.** *Natr. m.* Nux m. *Nux v.* Plant. Pod. **Puls.** Rhus. **Sabad. Verat.**
——, double: *Ars.* Cinch. **Dul.** Eup. perf. *Eup. purp.* Gamb. Lyc. Nux m. Puls. Rhus.
**Quotidian:** Acon. Æsc. Anac. Ant. c. Ant. t. Apis, *Aran. Ars.* Bap. Bary. c. Bell. Bry. *Cac.* Calc. *Cap.* Carb. v. *Ced.* Cham. Cic. *Cina.*

Cinch. Con. **Cur.** Dros. Elaps. Elat. Gamb. *Gels.* Graph. Hep. Ign. Ipec. Kali b. Kali c. Lach. Lob. Lyc. Mag. c. *Natr. m.* Nitr. ac. **Nux v.** Petros. Phos. Plant. *Pod.* Polyp. *Puls.* **Rhus.** Sabad. Sarr. Spig. Stan. Staph. Stram. Sulf. Verat

———, double: Ant. c. Apis. Bap. *Bell. Cinch.* Dul. **Elat.** *Graph.* Led. *Stram. Sulf.*

**Relapsing:** Ars. Eucalyp.

———, after abuse of Quinine: **Ars.**

**Remittent:** **Ars.** Bap. Ant. t. Carb. ac. Chin. s. Pod.

———, of children: Ant. c. Gels.

———, resembling: Bap. Ced. Pod.

———, prone to become: Ant. t. Eup. purp. Phos. ac. Phos.

———, intermittent becomes: Eup. purp. *Gamb. Pod.*

———, becomes intermittent: Gels. Phos.

———, ——— intermittent or typhoid: Ant. t. Phos. ac.

———, prone to become typhoid: *Ant. t.* **Ars. Bap.** Carb. ac. Mez. Phos. **Rhus.** *Sec.*

———, ——— ——— ——— ——— and typhus, after abuse of Quinine: **Ars.**

**Septimani:** *Amm. m.*

**Sinking.** (See Pernicious.)

**Spasmodic,** with epidemic pertussis: Dros. Kali c. Hyos.

**Spring:** *Ars. Canch.* Carb. v. *Gels.* **Lach.** Sep. Sulf.

———, and Autumn: Lach. Sep.

———, early: **Ant. t.** *Lach.* Sulf.

**Summer:** Caps. Casc. Ced. Natr. m. Nux v. Polyp.

———, excessive heat of: **Bap.**

**Tertian:** Æsc. Alum. Anac. Ant. c. *Apis,* **Aran.** Arn. **Ars.** Bar. c. **Bell. Bry.** Calc. **Canth.** Caps. Carb. an. Carb. v. **Ced.** Cham. Chin. s. Cic. Cina. **Cinch.** Dros. Dul. Elat. Eup. perf. Fer. Gamb. Gels. Hyos. Ign. Iod. **Ipec.** Lach. **Lyc. Mez. Natr. m.** Nux m. **Nux v.** Plant. Petros. *Pod. Polyp.* **Puls.** Rhus. *Sabad.* Sarr. Sulf. Verat.

———, double: Æsc. Ars. Cinch. Dul. Elat. Eup. purp. Gamb. Lyc. Nux v. Rhus.

**Weekly.** (See Days, every seven.)

**Winter:** Ant. t. Natr. m. Polyp. Psor. (cough).

**Yearly:** *Ars. Carb. v.* **Lach.** *Natr. m.* Psor. *Sulf.* Thuja.

———, half: Lach. *Sep.*

## TIME.

**Autumn:** Æsc. *Ars.* Bap. Carb. ac. **Colch.** *Nux v.* **Sep.**
——, hot days and cool nights, in: Acon. Colch. Mer.
——, and Spring: Lach. **Sep.**
**Bed,** in: *Alum.* Amm. m. Ars. Bov. Bry. Calc. Carb. an. Chin. s. Dros. Fer. *Hep.* Laur. *Mer.* Nux v. **Phos.** Sil. Sulf.
——, ——, in morning: Chin. s. Graph. Nux v.
——, ——, at night: Canch.
**Day,** all: *Alum.* **Sil.**
——, during, fever at night: Alum.
——, ——, at any time: **Ars.** Camph. Kali c. *Plant.* Sars.
—— and night: Sars.
**Evening:** Acon. Æsc. **Alum.** Agar. Amm. c. *Amm. m.* Aran. **Arn.** Ars. Bell. *Bov.* Bry. *Calad. Calc.* Carb. ac. Carb. v. Ced. Cham. Chel. Chin. s. **Cina.** Cocc. Cycl. Dul. Fer. *Gamb.* Graph. **Hep.** Hyd. *Ign.* Kali b. *Kali c. Lach.* Lachn. *Lyc.* Mag. c. *Mag. m.* Mer. Mez. *Nitr. ac.* Nux v. *Petr.* **Phos.** Phos. ac. Plat. Psor. **Puls. Rhus.** Sabad. Samb. Sarr. **Sep.** Sil. Stan. Staph. Stront. **Sulf.** Tab.
——, at sunset: *Ign.* Puls. Thuja.
——, in bed: Alum. Amm. c. Bov. Carb. an. Chin. s. Fer. *Dros.* Hep. Nux v. **Phos.** Sil. *Sulf.*
——, ——, going off in bed: *Natr. s.*
——, with the pains: *Cycl.* Ign. **Puls.**
**Forenoon:** Alston. Amb. Ang. *Arn.* Calc. Con. Eup. perf. Euph. Led. **Natr. m. Nux v.** Sil. Stan. Stront.
**Midnight:** Ars. Canth. Caust. **Sulf.**
——, after midnight: Ars. Op. Thuja.
**Morning:** Ang. Apis. Arn. **Bry.** Calc. Con. Cycl. Dros. **Eup. perf.** Euphor. Fer. Gels. Graph. *Hep.* Hydr. Kali c. Led. *Lyc.* Mer. **Natr. m. Nux v.** Phos. **Pod. Sep.** Sil. *Spig. Sulf.* Thuja. Verat.
——, early in: Arn. *Chin. s,* Graph. Lyc. *Natr. m.* **Nux v. Verat.**
——, to noon: *Eup. perf.* **Natr. m.**
**Night,** at: *Alum.* Amb. Arg. **Apis.** Bell. Bov. Carb. v. Caust. Fer. Gamb. Hep. Iris. *Kali iod.* Mag. s. **Mer.** Mur. ac. Natr. s. Nitr. ac. Nux v. Op. Phos. *Sars.* Sil. Staph. *Sulf.* Thuja.
——, in bed: Canch.
——, never at: Cinch.
**Noon,** at: *Ant. c. Elat.* Elaps. *Eup. perf. Lach. Lob.* Mer. Nux v. Sil. *Sulf.*

**Noon, after:** Alum. Anac. Ant. c. Arg. *Arn.* **Ars.** Bap. Bar. *Bor.* Bry. Chel. Chin. s. Cic. Cina. Cocc. Croc. Dig. Eup. perf. Gels. Graph. Kali b. Lach. **Lyc.** Mercurialis. *Natr. m.* Nitr. ac. *Nux v.* Op. Petr. Phos. ac. Phos. **Puls.** *Ran. b.* Rob. Sabad. Samb. Sarr. Sil. Staph. Sulf. Thuja.

**Paroxysm returning at:**

—— 1 A.M.: **Ars.** Canth. Puls. Sil.

—— 2 A.M.: **Ars.** Canth. Hep. Lach. Puls. Sil.

—— 3 A.M.: Amm. m. Canth. Ced. Led. Natr. m. Sil. **Thuja.**

—— 4 A.M.: *Alum.* Amm. m. Arn. **Ced.** Con. Natr. m. Sil.

—— 5 A.M.: *Bov. Cinch.* Con. Dros. *Natr. m. Polyp.* Sep. Sil.

—— 6 A.M.: *Arn. Bov.* Dros. Graph. *Hep.* Natr. m. *Nux v.* Sil. Stram. **Verat.**

—— 7. A.M.: *Bov.* Dros. **Eup. perf.** Fer. Graph. Hep. Natr. m. Nux m. *Nux v.* **Pod.** Sil. Stram.

—— 7 to 9 A.M.: **Eup. perf.** Natr. m. *Pod.*

—— 7 to 9 A.M, one day, 12 M. next day: **Eup. perf.**

—— 8 A.M.: *Bov.* Cocc. Dros. **Eup. perf.** Lyc. Mez. Natr. m. Pod. Puls. Sulf.

—— 8 to 9 A.M.: Asaf. *Eup perf.*

—— 9 A.M.: Alston. Ant. t. **Eup. perf.** Ipec. Kali c. Lyc. Mag. c. Mez. *Natr. m.* Phos. ac. Sep. Staph. Sulf.

—— 9 to 11 A.M.: *Alston,* **Natr. m.** Polyp. *Stan.*

—— 10 A.M.: Alston. Ars. Bap. Cac. Carb. v. Chin. s. Colch. Eup. perf. Led. **Natr. m.** Petr. Phos. ac. *Polyp.* Rhus. Sep. Sil. **Stan.** Sulf. Thuja.

—— 10.30 A.M.: Cac. Caps. *Lob. Natr. m.*

—— 10 to 11 A.M.: Ars. **Natr. m.** Nux v.

—— 10 to 2 P.M.: Mer. Sulf.

—— —— 3 P.M.: Sil. Sulf.

—— 11 A.M.: *Bap.* **Cac.** Carb. v. Cham. *Chin. s.* Hyos. *Ipec.* Lob. **Natr. m. Nux v.** Op. *Polyp.* Puls. *Sep.* Sil. Sulf.

—— 11 A.M., one day, 4 P.M. next: Calc.

—— 11 A.M. to 12 M.: Kali c. Kobalt.

—— 11 A.M. to 4 P.M.: Gels.

—— 11 A.M. and 4 P.M.: **Cac.**

—— 12 M.: *Ant. c.* Elat. Elaps. Eup. perf. Fer. *Kali. c. Lach.* Lob. Mer. Nux v. *Sil. Sulf.*

—— 12 M. to 2 P.M.: *Ars. Lach.*
—— 1 P.M.: **Ars.** Cac. Canth. *Cina.* Elat. Eup. perf. *Lach.* Mer. Nux m. Phos. Polyp. **Puls.** Sil. Sulf.
—— —— to 2 P.M.: **Ars.** Eup. perf. Natr. m.
—— 2 P.M.: **Ars.** *Calc.* Canth. Cic. Cur. *Eup. perf.* Gels. Plant. Sil. Sulf.
—— 2.30 P.M.: Led.
—— 3 P.M.: **Ang. Ant. t. Apis.** Ars. Asaf. *Canth.* **Ced. Chin. s.** Cic. Coff. Con. Cur. Fer. Lyc. Petr. Polyp. Sabad. Samb. Sil. **Staph.** *Thuja.*
—— —— to 4 P.M.: Apis. Asaf. Polyp.
—— —— to 6 P.M.: Ars. Eup. perf.
—— 4 P.M.: Æsc. Anac. **Apis.** Asaf. Bov. Canth. Caust. **Ced.** Cham. Con. Gamb. Gels. Graph. Hell. *Hep.* Ipec. Kali iod. **Lyc.** Mag. m. Natr. m. Nux v. Petr. Phel. Phos. ac. Polyp. **Puls.** Samb. Sep. Sil.
—— —— to 7 P.M.: Natr. m.
—— —— to 8 P.M.: Bov. Graph. Hell. *Hep.* Kali iod. **Lyc.** Mag. m. *Sabad.*
—— 4 to 10 P.M.: Phel.
—— 5 P.M.: Alum. Amm. m. Apis. Ars. Bov. Canth. Caps. Carb. an. *Ced.* Cinch. Con. Eup. perf. Gamb. Gels. Graph. Hell. Hep. **Kali. c.** Kali. iod. Mag. c. Natr. m. Nux m. Nux v. *Rhus.* Sabad. Samb. Sarr. Sep. Sil. Sulf. **Thuja.**
—— 5 to 6 P.M.: Caps. Kali. c. Phos. Sulf. Thuja.
—— —— to 8 P.M: Alum. Carb. an. Gamb. Natr. m.
—— 6 P.M.: Amm. m. *Ant. t.* Ars. Bell. Bov. Canth. Caps. Carb. an. *Ced.* Gamb. Graph. Hell **Hep. Kali c.** Kali iod. Lyc. Mag. m. Natr. m. Nux m. Nux v. Petr. Phel. Phos. ac. Phos. *Rhus.* Samb. Sep. *Sil.* Sulf. Thuja.
—— —— to 8 P.M.: Kali iod. Sulf.
—— 7 P. M.: Alum. Amm. m. *Bov.* Calc. Canth. Carb. an. *Ced.* Gamb. Graph. Hell. **Hep.** Kali iod. **Lyc.** Mag. c. Natr. m. Nux v. Petr. Phel. Phos. ac. Phos. **Rhus.** Sil. *Sulf.* Thuja.
—— 7.30 P.M.: Thuja.
—— 8 P.M.: Alum. Ars. Bary. c. *Bov.* Canth. Carb. an. Coff. Elaps. Gamb. Graph. Hell. Hep. Kali iod. Mag. c. Mag. m. Nux v. Phel. Phos. ac. *Rhus.* Sil. *Sulf.* Tarax.
—— 9 P.M.: Ars. *Bov.* Canth. Carb. an. Gamb. Gels. Hydr. Mag. c. Mercurialis. Nux m. Nux v. Phel. Phos. ac. Polyp. Sabad. Sulf.

—— 10 p.m.: Ars. *Bov.* Canth. Carb. an. *Chin. s.* Elaps. Hydr. *Kali iod.* Mag. c. *Petr.* Phel. Phos. ac. Sabad.
—— 11 p.m.: Ars. **Cac.** Canth. Carb. an. Sulf.
—— 12 p.m.: *Ars.* Canth. Caust. Sulf.

**Fever, without chill, returning at:**
—— 12, midnight: Stram. Sulf.
—— 12 to 3 a.m.: **Ars.** Kali c.
—— —— 2 a.m.: Ars.
—— 1 to 2 a.m.: Ars.
—— 2 to 4 a.m.: Kali c.
—— 3 a.m.: **Ang.** Thuja.
—— 4 a.m.: Arn.
—— 6 to 10 a.m.: Rhus.
—— 7 a.m.: Pod.
—— 9 a.m.: Kali c.
—— 9 to 12 m.: Cham.
—— 10 a.m.: **Natr. m.** *Rhus.* Thuja.
—— 10 to 11 a.m.: **Natr. m.** *Thuja.*
—— 11 a.m.: *Bap.* Cac. Calc. **Natr. m.** Thuja.
—— 12 m.: *Stram. Sulf.*
—— 12 to 1 p.m.: Sil.
—— 1 to 2 p.m.: **Ars.**
—— 2 p.m.: **Puls.**
—— 2 to 3 p.m.: Cur.
—— 3 p.m.: Coff. Cur. Fer. Lyc. Nicc.
—— 3 to 4 p.m.: **Apis.** Clem. Lyc.
—— 4 p.m.: **Anac.** *Apis.* Ars. Graph. Hep. Ipec. Kali b.
—— 4 p.m., lasting all night: Ars. Hep. Puls.
—— 5 p.m.: Con. Kali b. Kali c. Petr. Sab.
—— 5 and 5.30 p.m., pricking in the tongue: Ced.
—— 5 to 6 p.m., very ill-humored: Con.
—— 6 p.m.: Calc. Carb. v. Caust. Kali c. **Nux v.** Petr.
—— 6 to 12 p.m.: Lachn.
—— 6 p.m., lasting all night: *Nux v.* Lyc. Rhus.
—— 6 to 7 p.m.: Calc. Nux v.
—— 6 to 8 p.m.: Caust. Ant. t.
—— 7 p.m.: Æsc. Bov. Lyc. *Calc.* **Nux v.** *Rhus.*
—— 7 to 8 p.m.: Amb.

—— 7 to 12 P.M.: Æsc.
—— 8 P.M.: Coff. Fer. Hep. Sulf.
—— 10 P.M.: *Ars.* Hydr. Lach. Petr. Sab.
—— 11 P.M.: **Cac.**

## CAUSE.
### Attack brought on by:

**Acids,** abuse of, or after taking: Lach.
**Alcohol,** abuse of: Led. *Nux v.*
**Anger:** *Bry.* **Nux v.**
**Anxiety:** Ars. *Gels.*
**Arsenic,** abuse of: *Ipec.*
**Choleraic,** occurring during cholera epidemics: Elat. Verat.
**Coffee,** abuse of: Cham. Nux v.
**Diet,** indiscretions in: Ant. c. Cycl. *Ipec.* Puls.
——, —— ——, may produce relapse: Ant. c. *Ipec.*
——, —— ——, eating pork; rich, fat food: **Puls.**
——, —— ——, —— late suppers; irregular, unseasonable: *Nux v.*
**Eating,** after: Bell. Carb. an. Kali c. Marum. Tarax.
——, ——, and drinking: Asar. Tarax.
**Exertion,** physical: Ars. Eup. perf. Mer. Sil. Sulf.
——, too much mental, too little physical: Nux v.
**Exposure:** *Acon.* Ang. Ant. c. *Aran.* Arn. Ars. Bar. Bry. Cac. *Calc.* Canth. Carb. v. *Ced. Chin. s.* Cinch. Dros. Dul. Eucalyp. Eup. perf. Hep. Kali c. Led. Lach. Natr. m. Rhus. Sep. Spig. Zinc.
——, to cold, or cold and debility: Led.
——, cold bathing, too frequent: Ant. c. *Rhus.*
——, —— vegetables or fruit, handling: Calc. Val. Zinc.
——, draught, to a: *Acon.* Bar. Canth. Hep.
——, ——, —— when heated: **Acon.**
——, margins of streams or ponds, from living on: **Natr. m.**
——, malarial influence, to: *Arn.* Carb. ac. Ced. *Chin. s.* Cinch. Cur. *Eucalyp.* Eup. perf. *Natr. m.* Natr. s.
——, marshy regions, in: Ced. Chin. s. Eucalyp.
——, swamps, in: *Ang.* Ced. *Chin. s. Natr. m.*
——, ——, ——, tropical countries, in: *Ang.* **Ced. Natr. m.**
——, sleeping in damp rooms or beds, from: *Aran.* Carb. v. *Rhus.*

**Exposure**, soil, freshly turned up, to: **Natr. m.**
——, water, standing in: Aran. *Calc.* Led. Rhus.
——, water, working in: *Calc.* Rhus.
——, working in clay: **Calc.**
——, wet, from getting: Acon. Aran. *Bry.* Dul. **Rhus.** *Sep.*
——, ——, —— ——, when overheated: *Acon.* **Rhus.**
——, working in the rain, from: *Aran.* **Rhus.**
——, rains, during: Aran. Ced. Cur. Fer. Dul. Zinc.
——, seashore, residing at; **Natr. m.**
——, ——, exposure at: Natr. m. Natr. s.
——, ——, visits to: *Ars.* Natr. s.
——, sun, to: *Cac.*
——, sun, heat of: *Cac.* Lach.
**Fright**: Acon. Gels. Op.
**Gonorrhœa**: Thuja.
**Grief**: *Gels. Ign.*
**Ground.** (See Soil, freshly turned).
**Hours**, irregular, late: **Nux v.**
**Joy**, excessive: Coff.
**Malarial.** (See Exposure.)
**Opium**, abuse of: Cham.
**Overheated**, from becoming: *Ant. c.* **Carb. v.**
**Paludal**: **Arn.** Carb. ac. Casc. Ced. Chin. s. Cinch. **Eucalyp.** Eup. perf. *Natr. m.*
**Perspiration**, suppressed from: Acon. Cup. *Sil.*
——, ——, from a draught: **Acon.**
——, ——, of feet: *Cup.* **Sil.**
**Quinine**, abuse of: Alston. Arn. Ars. Carb. v. Ipec. Natr. m.
**Rheumatic**: Acon. *Aran. Bry.* Led. **Rhus.** *Spig.*
**Room**, when in a: Ars.
——, warmth of: *Apis.* Ars. *Ipec.*
**Sycosis**: *Thuja.* Sars.
**Tobacco**, abuse of: Bell. Nux v.
**Touched**, from being: Spig.
**Weather**, cold, damp, rainy: Aran. Dul. Rhus.
——, damp, suddenly becoming cold: **Dul.**
——, dry, whether hot or cold: *Bry.*
——, dry and cold: Acon. Hep.

**Weather**, hot days and cool nights: **Acon.**
——, —— —— and cool damp nights in Autumn: Colch. *Mer.*
——, warm during: *Ant. c. Ars. Bell.* Bry. *Calc.* **Caps.** Carb. v. **Ced.** *Cina. Ipec.* **Lach.** Natr. m. Puls. **Sulf.** *Thuja.*
**Whooping-cough**, during epidemic: Dros. Kali c.
**Worms**, or intestinal irritation: Cina. Spig. Sil.

## PRODROME.
### Conditions, occurring during:

**Anguish**: Cinch.
**Anticipation**, of any unusual ordeal, may hasten chill: Gels.
**Anxiety**: Ars. Cinch.
**Back**, aching in: Carb. v. *Eup. perf.* Ipec. **Pod.** Rhus.
——, pain in, above right ilium: Eup. perf.
——, —— severe in lumbar region: *Æsc.* **Pod.**
**Bilious**, symptoms strongly marked: **Pod.**
**Bones**, pains in: Cinch. *Eup. perf.* Eup. purp. Natr. m.
——, —— ——, of extremities: Eup. purp.
——, —— ——, —— ——, as if broken: **Eup. perf.**
**Bowels**, pain in: Ars. Elat. Eup. perf.
——, —— ——, cutting like knives: Ars.
**Chest**, pain in: Ars. Plant.
——, —— ——, cutting: Ars.
——, —— ——, erratic: Plant.
**Chilliness**: Elat. Thuja.
——, and weakness some time before: *Thuja.*
—— and crawling, after drinking: Ars.
**Colic**: Cinch. Eup. perf.
—— pain in upper abdomen: Eup. perf.
**Cough**: Apis. **Rhus.** Rum. Samb.
——, dry, teasing, for hours: **Rhus.**
——, ——, hacking, in spells: *Eup. purp.*
——, deep, dry, for half an hour, with nausea and thirst: Samb.
**Covered**, desire to be: **Eup. perf.** Nux v.
**Debility**: *Ars.* Cinch. Corn. fl.
**Dreads** the attack: **Natr. m.**
**Diarrhœa**: *Ars.* Cina. *Puls.* Verat.
——, mental emotions, from: *Gels.*

**Diarrhœa**, mucous, at night: **Puls.**
———, in early morning: **Fer. Sulf.**
———, previous night without thirst, if morning chill: **Puls.**
**Drink**, can *now:* Cimex.
———, cannot, enough: *Eup. perf.*
———, desire to, some time before: *Caps.* Cinch. *Eup. perf.* Natr. m.
**Drinking**, causes nausea and hastens chill: *Eup. perf.* Nux v.
———, chilliness and crawling, immediately after: Ars.
———, creepings over the back, after: Ars.
———, vomiting, after: Ars. **Eup. perf.** *Natr. m.*
———, refreshes: *Arn.*
**Excitement**, mental: **Ced.**
**Emotion**, sudden mental, may hasten chill: Gels.
**Emptiness**, in head: Ars.
**Eyes**, blue margins around: **Cina.** Phos.
———, burning in: Rhus.
**Eyeballs**, painful soreness of: *Eup. perf.*
**Face**, heat of: Stram.
———, florid, animated: Ced.
———, pale: Ars. Cina. Fer.
———, ———, with blue margins around eyes: Cina.
**Feet**, cold: Carb. v.
**Fever**: Ced. Lyc. *Nux v.* Sulf.
———, evening, without chill: *Sulf.*
**Fright**, may hasten chill: Gels.
**Gaping.** (See Yawning.)
——— and quivering: Elat.
**Gastric** disturbances: *Ant. c.* Cycl. *Ipec.* Puls.
——— ——— may bring on a relapse: **Ipec.** *Ant. c.*
——— ———, eating pork, fat, rich food, from: **Puls.**
**Grief**, may hasten chill: **Gels.** Ign.
**Head**, heat of: Ced. **Stram.**
———, heaviness of: *Calc.*
———, ——— ———, and body: Calc.
———, pressive pain in: Ced.
———, throbbing in temples: Carb. v.
———, ——— and dulness in: Plant.
**Headache**: *Æsc.* Ars. **Bry.** Carb. v. Cinch. Ced. Corn. fl. Elat. Ipec. *Natr. m.* Plant. Rhus. *Thuja.*

**Headache,** bursting: Æsc. *Bry.*
——, stitching, jerking, throbbing, from before backwards, as if head would burst: **Bry.**
**Heat:** Ced. Lyc. *Nux v.* Sulf.
——, in evening: *Sulf.*
——, general: Ced.
——, flushes of: Lyc. Sulf.
**Heart,** palpitation of, with anxiety: Cinch.
**Hunger:** Cina. Cinch. Eup. perf. **Staph.**
——, canine: Cinch.
**Illness,** a general feeling of: Cinch.
**Joints,** drawing pain in: Calc.
——, aching in large: Polyp.
——, —— —— knees, ankles, elbows, wrists: Pod.
**Languor:** Ars. *Bap.* Natr. m. Polyp.
——, wants to lie down: *Bap.*
**Limbs,** drawing in: Ars. Bry. *Nux v.*
——, —— pain in thighs and legs: **Nux v.**
——, —— up and stretching out: Ars. **Nux v.**
——, —— pain as if in periosteum: *Arn.*
——, heaviness of lower: Cimex.
——, pain in: Carb. v. Elat. *Eup. perf.* Natr. m. *Nux v. Rhus.*
——, ——, tearing, in: *Carb. v.*
——, ——, ——, in hands, feet and kidneys: *Natr. m.*
——, paralytic weakness of: Nux v.
——, soreness of: Elat.
**Malaise:** Ars. Bap.
**Melancholy:** **Ant. c.** Ced. Puls.
——, spirits depressed, senses dull: Ced.
**News,** bad, may hasten chill: *Gels.*
**Nausea:** Arn. Cina. *Cinch. Eup. perf.* **Ipec.** Lyc. Natr. m. Puls. Samb.
——, and thirst, night before: **Eup. perf.**
——, —— vomiting: Lyc. Natr. m.
——, —— retching: Ipec.
**Periosteum.** (See Limbs.)
**Retching,** violent: Ipec.
**Sadness,** great: **Ant. c.**

**Saliva,** flow of: Ipec. Rhus.
**Shuddering:** *Ars.* **Ign.** Lach.
——, after thirst: Lach.
——, —— drinking: **Caps.**
**Sleep,** restless: Arn. *Cinch.*
——, ——, night before the paroxysm: **Cinch.**
**Sleepiness:** Ars. Corn. fl. Puls.
——, and drowsiness all day: Puls.
——, night before: **Ars.**
——, preceded for days by: Corn. fl.
**Sleeplessness:** Amm. m.
**Sneezing,** when exposed to cold air: Cinch.
**Sore,** bruised feeling: Arn. Bap.
——, —— —— of limbs: Elat.
——, —— —— of parts lain on: Bap.
**Stretching:** Æsc. Ant. t. Arn. *Ars.* Bry. *Eup. perf.* Ign. Ipec. *Natr. m.* Rhus.
——, of limbs: Ars. *Nux v.* Plant. Rhus.
——, and drawing in limbs: Bry.
——, —— aching in limbs: Rhus.
**Sweating:** Corn. fl. Nux v. Samb. *Verat.*
——, after exercise: Bry. Corn. fl. Psor.
**Taste,** bitter in mouth, for hours before: Hep.
**Thirst:** Alston. Amm. m. Ang. **Arn.** Ars. Bor. *Bry.* Cimex. Cina. Cinch. Eup. perf. Lach. Lob. *Puls.* Samb. *Sulf.*
——, and bone pains some time before: **Eup. perf.** *Natr. m.*
——, but hurts to swallow: Gels.
——, some time before: **Caps.** Cinch. Natr. m.
——, for large quantities of cold water: **Arn.** Eup. perf. *Bry.*
——, —— warm drinks: Eup. perf.
——, then shuddering: Lach.
**Trembles,** as after severe illness: Bap.
**Toothache:** Carb. v.
**Urine,** incontinence of, sets in before: Gels.
**Urticaria,** itching, stinging: *Hep.*
**Vertigo:** Ars. Bry. Natr. m.
**Vomiting:** Apis. Cina. *Eup. perf.* Fer. Lyc. Natr. m. Puls. Sec.
——, of bile: Cina. **Eup. perf.**

**Vomiting,** of ingesta: Cina. *Eup. perf.* **Fer.**
——, —— mucus: Puls.
——, —— water: *Natr. m.*
——, sudden: *Apis.*
——, sour: Lyc. Rob.
**Weakness:** *Ars.* Bap. Natr. m. Thuja.
——, weariness and inclination to lie down: Ars. *Bap.* Rhus.
**Woeful** mood: **Ant. c.**
**Yawning:** Æsc. Ant. t. Arn. Ars. Elat. *Eup. perf.* Cinch. Ign. Ipec. Natr. m. Nux v. Rhus.
——, mouth remains open for a time, when: Ant. t.

## COMMENCEMENT OF CHILL.
### Chill begins in:

**Abdomen:** **Apis.** Cur. *Ign.* Verat.
——, and extends to fingers and toes: Calad.
**Ankles,** between knees and: Cinch. Lach. Puls.
**Arms:** **Bell.** Dig. Hell. *Ign.* Mez. Plat.
——, both, in: *Bell.* Hell. Mez.
——, ——, at once, in, thence over the body: **Bell.**
——, upper arms and spreads to chest and back: **Ign.**
——, —— —— and thighs: Psor.
**Arm,** right: *Mercurialis.*
——, ——, and right side of chest: **Mercurialis.**
——, left: *Nux m.*
——, ——, and lower limbs: **Nux m.**
——, ——, and hand: Carb. v.
——, on which he lies: Carb. v.
**Back,** beginning in: Arg. m. Bap. Bov. Cac. Canth. **Caps.** Ced. Dul. Eup. perf. Eup. purp. *Gamb.* Gels. Kali iod. **Lach.** Led. *Lyc.* Natr. m. **Polyp.** Sarr. *Sep.* Spong.
——, —— ——, or running up the: **Canth.**
——, —— ——, passing up and down thence over body: Eup. purp.
——, —— —— dorsal region: *Eup. perf.* Gels. **Lach.** Natr. m.
——, —— —— interscapular region: **Caps.** Led. **Polyp.** Sarr. *Sep.*
——, —— —— lumbar region: **Eup. purp. Lach. Natr. m.**
——, spreads from the: *Eup. perf.*

**Body**, left side: Carb. v. Caust.
——, right side: Bry. Natr. m. Rhus.
**Chest**: *Apis.* Ars. *Carb. an.* Cic. Cina. Mercurialis. Nux v. *Sep.* Spig.
——, and extends down the legs and into the arms: Cic.
——, front of, in: **Apis.**
——, right side of, in: **Mercurialis.**
**Face**: Bar. Berb. **Caust.** Kreos. Petr.
**Feet**: Apis. Arn. Bar. *Chel.* Cimex. Gels. Hyos. Kali b. Mag. c. **Natr. m.** Nux m. *Nux v.* Sabad. Sarr. *Sep.* Sulf.
——, and legs: Kali b.
——, soles of: Dig.
**Fingers**: *Bry.* Coff. Dig. **Natr. m.** Nux v. *Sep.* Sulf.
——, tips of: **Bry.** Natr. m.
——, —— ——, and toes: **Bry.** Dig. Meny. Natr. m. **Sep.** Stan. Sulf.
**Foot**, right: Chel. Lyc. Sab.
**Hands**: **Chel.** Dig. Eup. perf. **Gels.** *Nux v.* Rhus. Sabad. Sulf.
——, palms of: Dig.
——, —— ——, and soles of feet: *Dig.*
—— and feet: Apis. Bry. Carb. v. Chel. Dig. Gels. **Natr. m.** Nux m. Op. Sabad. Sulf.
**Hand**, left: **Carb. v.** Nux m.
——, right: **Mercurialis.**
**Head**: *Bar.* Natr. m. Stan.
**Knees**: Apis. Thuja.
—— and thighs: Thuja.
**Legs**: Ced. *Cinch.* Kali b. *Nux m.* Thuja.
——, below the knees: Cinch.
——, lower: Nux m.
**Lips**: **Bry.**
**Mouth**, around the: Bry.
**Neck**: Staph. Valer.
——, nape of, running down the back: Valer.
**Scalp**, in: Mosch.
**Scrobiculus cordis**: Bell. *Calc.*
——, with spasms, or fixed, cold, agonizing weight: **Calc.**
**Thighs**: Ced. Therid. **Thuja.**
**Toes**: *Bry.* Coff. **Natr. m.** *Sep.* Sulf.
——, ends of: *Bry.* Natr. m.

## Chill; part affected, location of.

**Abdomen:** Æth. *Apis.* Ars. Calc. Cham. Chel. Colch. Cur. *Ign.* Meny. *Mer. Mercurialis.* **Mez. Op.** *Par.* Phos. ac. *Puls. Sec.* c. Sulf. Verat.

——, and chest: *Apis.* Spig.

——, to fingers and toes: Calad.

**Arms:** Bell. *Camph. Caust.* Cham. Cic. Dig. *Hell.* Ign. Kali b. **Mez.** Op. *Puls.* Sec. c. *Sil.* Sulf. Verat.

——, upper, and spreads to back and chest: **Ign.**

**Arm, left:** Carb. v. *Nux m.* Rhus. Stan.

——, right: **Mercurialis.**

**Ascends:** Acon. Amm. m. *Ars.* Benz. Caust. Cina. Coff. Eup. perf. *Gels.* **Hyos.** Kali b. *Sabad.* Sulf.

——, feet to chest, from: *Acon.* Benz.

——, extremities of fingers and toes to chest, head and vertex, from: *Benz.* Coff.

——, feet to neck and vertex, from: Benz. Coff.

——, upper part of body to head, from: Cina.

**Back, in, or on the:** Æsc. Agar. Alum. Ang. Apis. Ars. Asaf. Bell. Bov. **Cac.** *Camph. Canch. Canth.* Caps. Carb. an. Ced. Cham. Chel. Cocc. Coff. Con. Croc. Dul. **Eup. perf. Eup. purp.** *Gels.* Hydr. Hyos. Ign. Ipec. Kali b. Kali iod. **Lach.** Led. **Lob.** Lyc. Mag. c. Meny. *Nux v.* **Natr. m.** Op. Phos. **Polyp.** *Puls.* Sabad. Sarr. Sep. Stan. Staph. *Stram.* **Sulf.** Valer. Verat.

——, creeping up and down the: *Æsc.*

——, and abdomen: Cham.

——, water, were running down, as if: *Agar.*

——, running down the back and through the limbs: Colch.

——, running down the: *Agar.* Apis. Bell. Canch. **Canth.** Carb. an. *Caust.* Chel. Coff. Croc. *Eup. perf.* **Eup. purp.** Ipec. Lob. Phos. Staph. **Stram.** Valer.

——, —— —— ——, and terminating in pit of stomach: **Bell.**

——, —— —— ——, with heat in stomach: *Lob.*

—— and sides, over: **Meny.**

——, runs up the: *Æsc.* Amm. m. Ars. Eup. perf. *Eup. purp.* **Gels.** Hyos. Ipec. Kali b. Kali iod. **Lach.** Mag. c. Puls. *Sabad.* Sulf.

——, —— —— and down the: **Eup. purp.**

——, —— —— —— from sacrum to occiput in rapid successive waves: **Gels.** Lach. *Sulf.*

Back, constantly creeps from sacrum up the: **Sulf.**
——, interscapular region, in the: **Caps.** Eup. perf. Led. **Polyp.** Sarr. *Sep.* Sulf.
——, —— ——, like a piece of ice: Lachn.
——, lumbar region, in the: Asaf. **Eup. purp. Lach.** Led.
**Body,** all over the: Alum. Anac. Ant. t. Arn. Ars. **Camph.** Canch. Canth. Carb. an. **Carb. v.** Ced. Chel. **Chin. s.** Cic. Cim. **Cinch.** Cocc. Con. Cup. Cur. Dig. Dul. Eup. perf. Eup. purp. Euphor. Fer. Gamb. Gels. Graph. Hep. Hyos. **Ign.** Kali iod. *Lach.* Lachn. Marum. *Lyc. Meny.* Mer. *Mercurialis.* **Mez. Nux m. Nux v.** Op. Petr. Phel. Phos. ac. *Puls.* **Rhus.** Sec. c. *Sep.* Spig. **Staph.** *Stram.* **Verat.**

——, —— —— —— and head, with heat and redness of face: **Arn.** Cham.
——, —— —— —— alternating with heat of face: *Cham.*
——, —— —— —— with burning heat of face, which comes out of the eyes like fire: **Cham.**
——, —— —— except face, neck and genitals: *Amb.*
——, anterior parts of: Cham.
——, posterior parts of, only: Cham. *Ign.*
——, —— —— —— with heat of anterior: **Cham.**
——, upper parts over, of: **Meny.**
——, one side, of: Arn. Bar. **Bry. Carb. v. Caust.** Chel. Dig. Elat. Fer. *Lach.* **Lyc.** Natr. c. Natr. m. Nux v. Par. *Phos.* Puls. Rhus. *Sep.* **Sil.** Thuja. **Verat.**
——, left side of: **Carb. v. Caust.** Elat. Fer. *Lach.* **Lyc.** Rhus. Thuja.
——, right side of: Arn. **Bry.** Natr. m. Nux v. **Par.** *Rhus.* **Thuja.**
——, —— —— ——, from the head to the feet, the other half natural warmth: **Par.**
——, —— —— ——, with heat of left: **Rhus.**
——, on side on which he lies: *Arn.*
——, on icy-cold spots, here and there: *Par.*
**Cheeks:** Colch.
**Chest: Apis.** Carb. an. Cham. Cic. Cina. *Ign. Mercurialis.* Par. Sep. **Sulf.**
——, and abdomen: **Apis.** Par. *Sulf.* Spig.
——, —— extends to legs and arms: *Cic.*

**Chest**, right side of: **Mercurialis.**
**Descends:** Agar. Bar. Canch. Carb. ac. Caust. Cic. *Phos.* Valer. **Verat.**
——, from head to toes of both feet: **Verat.**
**Epigastrium:** *Arn.* Bar. **Bell. Calc.**
**Extremities:** Colch.
——, to face and head: *Acon. Benz.* **Gels.**
—— of fingers and toes, to chest, head and vertex: *Benz.*
**Face** of: **Bar. Berb. Caust. Cham. Ign.** *Petr.*
——, left side of, after midnight: *Dros.*
**Feet** of: Alum. Chel. Hyos. Ign. **Meny. Mez.** Nux v. Op. *Sep.* **Sil.**
——, soles of: **Dig.** *Meny.*
——, as if in cold water: Mag. c. Mer. **Meny.** Sep.
**Genitals**, icy-coldness of: **Sulf.**
**Fingers**, on the: Bry. *Meny.* Natr. m. **Phos.** ac.
——, tips of, on the: Bry. **Phos. ac.**
**Hands: Cac. Camph.** *Canth.* **Carb. v.** *Chel.* Colch. Dros. Fer. Hep. Hyos. Ipec. Led. *Lyc.* **Meny.** Mer. **Mez.** *Natr. m. Nux v.* **Op.** Polyp. **Phos. Sec. Verat.**
—— and feet cold, with warmth of rest of body: **Meny.**
**Head**, occiput in: *Dul.*
—— to extremities: **Verat.**
**Hips:** Mez.
**Hip**, right: Bry. *Mercurialis.* Rhus.
——, left: Carb. v. Caust. Thuja.
**Knees: Apis. Carb. v. Ign. Phos. Sil.** Stan.
——, icy-coldness of right: *Chel.*
**Legs:** *Caust.* Cic. Cocc. Coff. Colch. Ign. **Meny.** *Nux v.* Op. Par. Puls. **Rhus.** *Sec. c. Sil.* **Stram.** *Sulf.*
——, running up to back: Caust.
**Leg**, left: Carb. v. Caust. Stan. Thuja.
——, right, icy-coldness of: *Chel. Sab.* **Sep.**
—— —— as if standing in cold water: *Sab.* **Sep.**
**Loins: Asaf. Camph.** *Puls.* Thuja.
**Neck**, running down from: Par. Valer.
**Nose:** Colch.
**Parts**, single of: **Amb. Ars. Bell. Bry. Caust.** *Cham.* **Hep. Ign.** Led. **Lyc. Mez.** Nux v. Par. **Puls.** Rhus. Sep. *Sil. Spig. Thuja.* **Verat.**

Sacrum: Æsc. Asaf. Eup. purp. Puls. Sulf.
Shoulders: *Kali b.* Lach. *Polyp.* Verat.
Stomach, pit of: Arn. *Bell. Calc.*
———, ——— ——— most severely felt in: Arn.
———, chilly shivering in: *Colch.*

## CHILL AGGRAVATED.

Air, in a draft of: Caps. Carb. an. Dulc. **Nux v.**
———, in open: Anac. Agar. Ant. t. Ars. *Bar.* Canth. Cham. Chel. Cinch. Cycl. Dulc. Hep. Kali 'chl. *Mer.* Mosch. Nitr. ac. *Nux m.* Nux v. Petr. Plat. Polyp. *Puls.* Ran. b. Rhus. Seneg. Sep. Sulf. Zinc.
Awakes, as often as he: *Amm. m.*
Bed, by getting out of: Bar. *Canth.* Nux. v. *Sil.*
Dampness, by exposure to: Aran. *Calc.* Dul. *Rhus.*
Days, cold during: Acon. *Aran.* Cham. Ign.
———, rainy, during: *Aran. Cur.* Dul. Rhus.
Drinking, by: Alum. *Ars.* Asar. Cann. **Caps.** *Cinch.* Cocc. *Elaps. Eup. perf. Lob.* Lyc. Mez. **Nux v.** *Rhus.* Sil. Tarax. **Verat.**
Drinks, warm after: *Alum.* Cham.
Eating, after: Bell. Carb. an. Cocc. Euph. *Graph.* Kali c. Mar. *Rhus.* Tarax.
——— and drinking, after: Asar. Tarax.
———, during: Euph. Lyc. *Rhus.*
Evening, in the: Carb. v. Cycl. Kali c. *Puls.*
Exercising, when: *Ars.* Bar. Mer. Nux v. Sil. Sulf.
Motion, by: Acon. Agar. Alum. Ant. t. Apis. Arn. Bry. Camph. Canth. Ced. Cinch. Coff. *Cur.* Eup. perf. *Hep. Kali c. Nitr. ac.* Nux v. Rhus. Sep. Sil. Spig. Sulf. Thuja.
Rest, during: Dros. Rhus.
Rising, from stooping: Mer.
Room, in a: Apis. Bry. Ipec.
Smoking, by; Cocc. *Ign.*
Stove, near a warm: Alum. Apis. Cinch. Ipec. Nux v. Sepia.
Touched, when: Acon. Spig.
Uncovered: *Acon.* Agar. *Amm. m.* Arn. Bell. Carb. an. Cham. Clem. *Cycl.* Mercurialis. *Nitr. ac.* Nux m. Nux v. Stram. *Thuja.*
Undressing, when: Cham.

**Walking**, in the open air: Alum. Amm. c. *Ars.* Caust. Chel. Cinch. Kali chl. Mer. Nitr. ac. **Nux v.** Petr. Puls. Rhus. Tab.
**Warmth**, in: Alum. Anac. Ant. c. **Apis.** Ars. Bell. Bry. Bor. Canth. Caust. Cic. Cina. Cinch. Cocc. Dulc. Grat. Guaj. Iod. **Ipec.** Kreos. Laur. Mag. m. Meny. Mer. Mez. Natr. m. Nux m. Phos. Puls. Rhus. Ruta. Sep. Sil. Staph. Spong.
**Water**, by bathing with cold: Ant. c. Aran. Rhus.
**Weather**, in damp: Cur. Dul. **Rhus.**
**Wind**, in cold: *Acon.* Cur. Hep.

## CHILL AMELIORATED.

**Air**, in open: *Graph. Ipec.* Phosph. Puls. Sulf. ac.
**Bed**, covering up in, by: *Kali iod.* **Pod.** Rhus.
——, —— —— warmly in, by: **Pod.**
——, getting out of, by: Lyc. *Verat.*
——, warmth of, by: Kali iod.
**Covering**, by: Mercurialis. *Pod.* Rhus.
**Dinner**, before: Berb.
**Drinking**, after: **Caust.** *Graph. Ipec.*
**Eating**, after: Amb. *Cur.* Natr. c. Phos.
**Exercise** in open air, by: **Caps.** Mag. c. *Puls. Staph.* Sulf. ac.
**Flat-irons**, by hot: **Caps.** *Lachn.*
**Held**, by being: *Gels.* Lach.
——, firmly, by being: **Lach.**
**Lying down**, after: Kali c. Mercurialis. Rhus. Sulf.
**Motion**, on: Apis. Arn. Asar. Bell. **Caps.** Cycl. Mer. Mez. Nitr. ac. Nux v. Pod. Rhus. Sil. Spig.
**Pressed down upon**, by being: *Lach.*
**Rising**, on: Rhus.
**Sitting**, by: Ign. Nux v.
**Sleep**, after: Bry. Calc.
——, during: Rhus.
**Sunshine**, by exposure to: Anac. Con.
**Walking**, in the open air: **Caps.**
**Warmth**, external: **Ars.** Bar. Camph. Caps. Carb. an. Cic. *Cinch.* Con. Ign. *Kali c. Lach. Meny. Mez.* Nux m. Nux v. *Sabad.* Sulf.
**Wrapping up**, by, followed by severe fever and sweat: **Sil.**

## SYMPTOMS DURING THE CHILL.

### Chill absent:

Anac. Apis. Ars. Calc. Caust. Cham. Cina. Coff. Eup. perf. Fer. *Gels.* Hep. Ipec. Kali b. Kali c. Lachn. Lyc. Natr. m. Nux v. Petr. Rhus. Stram. Sulf. *Thuja.*

### Chill predominates:

Alum. Amm. m. **Ant. c. Aran. Arn.** *Bov.* **Camph. Canth.** Caps. Carb. v. *Ced.* **Chin. s.** Cim. Cina. **Cinch.** *Cocc.* Dig. *Dros.* Elaps. Hep. Laur. Led. *Lyc.* **Meny.** Mercurialis. **Mez. Nux v.** Petros. Petr. *Polyp. Rob.* Rhus. **Sabad.** Sec. c. Sep. **Staph.** Thuja. **Verat.**

—— afternoon, in the: Apis. Arn. **Ars. Lyc. Puls.** *Rhus.* Thuja.
—— noon at: *Ant. c.* Elat. **Sulf.**
—— morning, in the: *Bry.* **Eup. perf. Natr. m. Nux v.** *Pod. Sep.* Verat.
—— evening, in the: Alum. Arn. *Cina.* Cycl. Hep. *Phos.* **Puls.** Rhus. *Sulf.*
—— night at: Apis. *Merc.* Phos.

### Chill in General.

Acon. Æth. *Agar. Alum.* Alston. Amb. Amm. c. Amm. m. *Anac.* Ang. **Ant. c.** *Ant. t.* Apis. **Aran.** Arg. **Arn.** *Ars.* Asaf. Asar. Bap. Bar. Bell. Benz. Berb. Bov. Bry. Cac. Calad. Calc. **Camph.** Canch. **Canth.** *Caps.* Carb. an. *Carb. v.* Caust. *Ced. Cham.* Chel. **Chin. s.** Cic. *Cim. Cina.* **Cinch.** Coca. Coff. Colch. Col. Con. Corn. fl. Croc. Cupr. Cur. Cycl. Daph. *Dig.* Dros. Dulc. Elat. *Elaps. Eup. perf. Eup. purp.* Euphor. Evon. Fer. Gamb. *Gels.* Graph. Guaj. Hell. *Hep.* Hyos. *Ign.* Iod. *Ipec.* Kali b. *Kali c. Kali iod. Kreos. Lach.* Lachn. Laur. *Led.* Lob. *Lyc.* Mar. *Meny.* Mag. c. Mag. m. Mag. s. Mercurialis. Mer. **Mez.** Mur. ac. Natr. c. *Natr. m. Nitr. ac. Nux m.* **Nux v. Op.** Par. *Petr.* Phos. ac. Phos. Plant. *Pod.* Polyp. Psor. *Puls.* **Rob.** Rhus. Ruta. **Sabad.** Sab. Samb. Sarr. Sars. **Sec. c.** *Sep. Sil.* Spig. Stan. *Staph. Stram. Sulf.* **Tarax.** Therid. **Thuja.** Valer. **Verat.**

## Chill, Symptoms during.

**Abdomen,** bloated: Cina. *Kali c.*
——, cold: Æth. Apis. *Ars.* Cham. Chel. *Cinch.* **Meny.** Phos. ac. Puls. Sec. c.
——, coldness in, from pressure with the hand: **Meny.**
——, pain in: Aran. Ars. Bov. Bry. Calad. Calc. Cinch. Coff. Eup. perf. Ign. Lach. Meph. Mercurialis. Mer. Nitr. ac. Nux v. Phos. Pod. Puls. Rhus. Rumex. Sep.
**Air,** sensation of, being too hot: *Puls. Sep.*
—— of room seems too hot: *Apis.* **Puls. Sep.**
——, sensitiveness to cold: *Bar.* **Camph.** *Canth.* Caps. Carb. an. Caust. Coff. Cycl. *Dig.* Elaps. **Hep.** Kali c. Mer. *Mez.* Nux v. *Petr.* **Sil. Stram. Thuja.**
——, open, sensitive to: Ars. *Bap.* Camph. *Caps.* **Hep.** Mer. Mez. *Nux v.* Polyp. Sulf. Thuja.
——, warm, feels cold: **Thuja.**
**Anxiety:** Acon. Ars. Camph. Caps. Nux v. Puls. Verat.
**Appetite good:** *Chin. s.*
**Arms,** cold: Bell. Dig. Hell. Mez.
——, paralytic weakness of: Phos. ac.
——, distention of the veins of: **Chel.** *Meny.* (See Veins, Distended.)
**Back,** small of the, lameness of: Cocc.
——, pain in: Apis. Ars. Bell. Calc. *Caps.* Carb. v. Caust. **Chin. s.** Elat. *Eup. perf.* Hyos. Ign. Lach. Mosch. Natr. m. **Nux v.** Pod. Polyp. *Puls.* Zinc.
**Blood,** feeling as though it did not circulate: **Lyc.** Rob.
——, feeling as though cold: *Lyc.* **Rhus.**
**Bones,** pains in: Aran. Arn. Ars. Eup. perf. *Eup. purp.* Natr. m. Nux v. Polyp. Sabad.
—— aching in: **Arn.**
**Bowels,** aching in: Æth.
**Breath,** cold: **Carb. v.** *Verat.*
——, desire to take a long: Cimex.
——, hot: Anac. Camph. Cham. **Rhus.**
**Bruised,** feeling as if: **Arn. Bap.**
**Cheek,** heat of one: *Acon.* Arn.
——, redness of one: Acon. Arn. *Cham.* Ipec.
——, heat and redness of one: **Arn.**

**Cheek**, redness of one, other pale and cold: *Acon*. Cham. Ipec.
**Cheeks**, cold: Chel. *Cina. Petr. Rhus*. Sec. c.
———, dark red: *Alum*.
———, hot: *Acon*. Bry. Calc. Cham. *Cina. Cinch. Led*. Puls. Staph.
———, red: Alum. *Ars. Cinch*. Mercurialis.
**Chest**, oppression of: **Apis. Bry**. Cimex. Ipec. Lach. Mercurialis. *Mez. Natr. m. Puls*.
———, pains in: Ars. Bell. Lach. *Sabad. Rhus*. Seneg.
———, soreness of: Lach.
———, stitches in: **Bry**. Eup. perf. Kali c. Lach. *Rhus. Rumex.* Sabad.
**Colic**: Cocc. *Led*.
**Coma**: Bell. *Hep. Natr. m.*
**Convulsions**: *Lach*. Mer. Nux v.
**Coryza**: Calad. Elat.
**Cough**: Apis. **Bry**. Calc. Cina. Kreos. Phos. *Psor*. **Rhus**. Rumex. Sabad. *Samb* Sulf.
———, causes drinking: **Psor**.
**Covered**, cannot bear to be: **Camph**.
———, desire to be: Arn. Camph. *Eup. perf.* Natr. m. **Nux v**. Phos. Stram.
**Covering**, not relieved by: Cac. **Nux v**. *Phos*. Rhus.
**Cramps**: *Sil*.
**Cutis anserina**: Æsc. Ang. Bar. Carb. an. *Mercurialis*.
**Delirium**: *Arn*. Bell. **Natr. m**. Nux v. Sulf. Verat.
**Diarrhœa**: Ars. Elat. Phos. Rhus. Verat.
**Diseased parts**, coldness of: Caust.
**Drinking**, cough, dry, uninterrupted, with tickling in the larynx, after: Cimex.
———, headache, which almost deprives him of power to think, after: Cimex.
**Dyspnœa**: Apis. Arn. Cina. *Natr. m.* Nux v. Puls.
**Earache**: Graph. Gamb.
**Ears**, cold: Cic. Natr. m.
———, hot: Acon. **Ign**. Ran. b.
———, red: *Bell*. Ign.
———, ringing in: Ced. **Chin. s**.
**Elbows**, pain in: Ang. **Pod**.
**Epistaxis**: Kreos.

**Exhaustion:** Amb. Aran. Ipec. Mercurialis.
**Extremities,** cold and blue: *Camph.* Stram. Nux v. **Verat.**
——, cramps in: Ced. Cup.
——, icy, cold: **Camph.** *Canth.* Carb. v. *Ced.* Colch. Con. Hep. Ipec. Lyc. **Meny.** *Natr. m.* Nux m. **Nux v.** Phos. Samb. *Stram.* **Verat.**
**Eyes,** fixed: Acon.
——, pain in: Seneg.
——, sensitiveness of, to light: Nux v.
——, smarting of: Ced.
**Face,** bloated and red: *Amm. m. Bell.*
—— and hands bloated: *Lyc.*
——, blueness of: Natr. m. **Nux v.** Petr. **Stram.**
——, cold: *Camhp.* Chel. *Cina. Dros. Hep.* Ign. **Nux v.** *Petr. Puls.* Rhus. *Sec. c. Stram.* **Verat.**
——, ——, collapsed: *Camph. Verat.*
——, hot: Acon. Agar. Alum. Amb. Anac. *Apis.* **Arn.** Bell. Berb. Bry. Calc. Ced. Cham. Cinch. Col. Dig. *Dros.* Euph. *Fer.* Gels. Hell. *Hyos.* Jatr. Kreos. Lach. Led. Lyc. Mer. Mercurialis. Mez. Mur. ac. Natr. c. Nux v. Oleand. Puls. Ran. b. *Rhus.* Sab. Samb. Seneg. Staph. *Stram.* Sulf.
——, —— and red: Arn.
——, heat and redness of the, rest of body cold: **Arn.** Dig.
——, hot alone, rest of body cold: *Arn.*
——, pale: Ant. t. Bell. *Camph.* Canth. Cinch. Chin. s. *Cina. Dros.* Hep. Ign. *Nux m.* Nux v. *Puls. Sec. c.* Sulf. **Verat.**
——, ——, when lying down, red when sitting up: **Bell.**
——, pain (sticking) in left side of: Dros.
——, right half of, hot and dry: **Dros.**
——, red: *Acon.* **Amm. m.** Arn. Ars. **Bell.** Bry. Cham. Cinch. Dig. Fer. *Hyos.* **Ign.** Kreos. Led. Lyc. Mercurialis. Mer. Nux v. Puls. *Rhus.* Stram. Sulf.
——, ——, and pale alternately: Rhus.
——, ——, while sitting up: **Bell.**
**Fainting:** *Valer.*
**Feet,** burning and cold alternately: Graph.
——, cold: Acon. Alum. Ang. Ant. c. *Apis.* Asaf. *Bar. Bell.* Berb. Bov. Brom. Camph. *Canth.* Carb. an. *Carb. v. Caust.* Ced. Chel. Cim. *Cinch.* Coff. Cup. Dig. Dros. Eu, purp. *Fer.* Gels. Graph. *Hep.*

*Hyos.* Iod. Ipec. Kali b. Kali iod. Kreos. Lach. *Lyc.* Mag. c. **Meny.** Mer. *Mez.* Natr. m. *Nitr ac.* Nux m. *Op.* Par. Petr. **Phos** Plant. *Polyp. Psor.* Puls. Rhus. Sabad. *Samb.* Sarr. *Sec. c.* **Sep. Sil.** Stan. *Stram.* Sulf. *Thuja.* **Verat.**

**Feet,** cold, sweat on rest of body: Ant. c.
——— ——— with oppressed breathing: *Apis.*
———, cramps in: **Cup.** Elat. *Nux v.*
———, dead feeling of: Cim. Ced. **Puls.** Stram.
———, dropsical swelling of: Eup. perf. Kali iod.
———, heat of: Calad. Kali ch.
———, ——— ———, soles of: **Mer.**
———, icy-coldness of: *Ant. c.* **Meny.** *Phos.* Sep. **Verat.**
———, ——— ——— ——— soles of: *Nitr. ac.*
———, ——— ——— ——— ———, as if put in cold water: Mer.
———, ——— ——— ——— ———, and hands: Canth.
———, livid: Stram.
———, numbness of: Fer. Lyc. Nux m. Puls. Sep. Stan.
———, one cold, other hot: *Puls.*
———, pain in: Cup.
———, wet, feeling as though: Ipec. *Sep.*
———, water, feeling as though in cold: Gels. Merc. **Sep.**

**Fingers,** blueness of: Natr. m. Nux v. Petr.
———, cold and hot alternately: Par.
———, cold: Ang. *Apis. Cac.* Ced. Dig. Meny. *Natr. m.* Nux v. Par. Phos. ac. Plant. *Sep.* Sulf. Tarax. Verat.
———, stiffness of: Fer.

**Food,** aversion to: Kali c.
———, tastelessness of: Ars.

**Forehead,** cold sweat on: Cina. Cinch.
———, hot: *Acon.* Calc. Cinch. *Led.* Natr. s.
———, pain in: Eup. purp. **Natr. m.**
———, sweat on: Bry. Cina. Cinch. Dig.

**Frozen,** feeling as though: *Rob.*

**Gaping:** Alum. Cim. *Elat.* Lyc. *Nux v.*
———, with a sound resembling the neighing of a horse: **Elat.**

**Goose-flesh:** *Ang.* Bar. Bell. Bry. Camph. Canth. Carb. an. Croc. Crot. Hell. Laur. **Lyc. Natr. m. Nux v.** Par. Phos. Plant. Sabad. Staph. Thuja.

**Hair**, bristling of: **Bar.** Dulc. Grat. **Meny.**
**Hands**, blueness of: Gels. Natr. m. **Nux v.** *Stram.*
——, clenched: Cimex.
——, cold: Acon. Agar. Ang. Apis. *Arn. Cac.* **Camph. Canth. Carb. v.** Ced. *Chel.* Cinch. Coff. Con. Dig. *Dros.* Eup. purp. Euph. Fer. Gels. Hep. Hyos. Iod. *Ipec.* Kali b. Led. Lyc. **Meny.** Mer. Mez. Natr. c. *Natr. m. Nitr. ac.* Nux m. *Nux v.* Oleand. Op. Phel. Petr. Phos. ac. **Phos.** Polyp. Puls. Rhus. Samb. Sabad. Sarr. **Sec. c.** Sep. Stan. Staph. Stram. Sulf. *Tarax. Thuja.* **Verat.**
——, heat of: *Apis.* Ced. Cina. Ipec. Kali c. Mez. Nitr. ac. Natr. s. Sabad. Sep.
——, livid: Ced. Stram. Verat.
——, numbness of: Cim. Fer. Lyc. Nux m. **Puls. Sep.**
——, paleness of: Ced. Cinch.
——, one cold, other warm: Cinch.
——, —— and red, the other hot: *Puls.*
——, palms of, moist: Nicc. **Sticta.**
——, stiffness of: Kali c.
——, sweat cold, on: Cina.
——, veins of, disappearance of: Euph.
——, ——, distended: *Chel. Meny. Phos.*
——, wet, feeling as though: Ipec.
**Head hot**: Acon. Alum. **Arn.** Asar. **Bell.** Berb. Bry. Ced. Cina. Cinch. Eup. perf. Gels. Lachn. Natr. s. Nux v. Op. Rhod. *Stram.* Verat.
——, alone, hot: **Arn. Op.**
——, heat in the, rest of body cold: **Arn.**
——, painful, externally: Hell.
——, stitches in: Asaf.
——, sweat profuse about the: **Op.**
——, vertex constricted, feeling as though: Kali b.
**Headache**: Acon. Anac. Ant. t. *Aran.* **Bell.** Berb. Bov. Bry. Caps. Carb. v. Chin. s. Cim. Cina. Cinch. Cor. r. Dros. Elat. Eup. perf. *Eup. purp.* Fer. Graph. Ind. Ign. Kreos. Mez. **Natr. m.** Nux v. Petr. *Puls.* Sang. **Sep.** *Sulf.*
——, air, ceases entirely in open: *Aran.*
——, forehead: Eup. purp. **Natr. m.**
——, one-sided: Ign.

**Heart,** palpitation of: Gels. Phos.
——, icy-coldness about: Arn. Camph. Kali c. **Natr. m.** Oleand. Petr.
——, spasms and pains in region of: *Calc.*
**Held,** desire to be: Gels. **Lach.**
——, firmly, desire to be: **Lach.**
**Hoarseness:** Hep.
**Horripilation:** Æth. **Bar.** *Meny.* Psor. Sarr.
**Hunger: Cina.** Nux v. Phos. **Sil.** Staph.
**Hysteria:** *Eup. purp.*
**Hot drinks,** craving for: Ars. *Cas. Ced.* Eup. perf.
**Ice,** lying on, feeling as though: **Lyc.**
**Intestines,** coldness in, after drinking water: *Chel.*
**Irritability:** Anac. Caps. *Cina.* Gels. Hyos. Ign. Kali b. Kreos Nitr. ac. Plant.
**Jerkings:** Stram.
**Joints,** pains in: Cim. Hell. *Pod.* Polyp.
——, —— ——, large: Polyp.
**Kidneys,** pain in: Mill.
**Knees,** cold: **Apis. Carb. v.** *Ign.* **Phos.** *Sil.*
——, pain in: Ang. *Cim.* Pod.
**Lachrymation:** Elat.
**Lassitude:** Amb. Aran. Carb. v. Caust. Mercurialis. Natr. m.
**Leg,** coldness of left: Carb. v. Caust. Thuja.
——, —— —— right: *Bry.* Elaps. Sab. Sep.
**Legs,** coldness of, excessive: **Meny.** Sec. c. Stram.
——, cramps in: Cup. Elat. *Nux v.*
——, heaviness of: Therid.
——, lameness of: Ign.
——, numbness of: *Eup. purp. Nux v.*
——, pains aching, in bones of: Eup. perf. Eup. purp. Polyp.
——, position of, must change: Cim.
——, stretch out, inability to: Cim.
——, soreness of: Bell.
——, tired feeling of: Gels. Rhus.
——, weakness of: Seneg.
**Lie down,** desire to: Bry. Ced. Dros. Fer. *Lach.* Mer. Nux v. Puls. Sep. Sil. Therid.

**Lie down,** desire to be near the fire, and: **Lach.**
**Light,** dread of: Bell.
**Limbs,** coldness of: Acon. Æth. Amb. Ant. t. Arn. Ars. *Bell.* Berb. Calad. Calc. Camph. Canth. Carb. an. Carb. v. Caust. Cham. Chel. Cic. Cinch. Col. Con. Dig. Graph. Hell. Hyos. Ipec. Kali c. Laur. Led. Lyc. **Meny.** Mer. *Mez.* Natr. m. Nitr. ac. *Nux v. Op.* Phos. Plant. *Puls. Rhus.* **Sec. c.** Sep. **Stram.** Sulf. Thuja. Verat. Verb.
——, contraction of: Caps. **Cim.**
——, pain in: Acon. Ars. Bell. Bry. Dulc. Elat. *Eup. perf.* Eup. purp. Graph. Hell. Lach. Led. Lyc. Mercurialis. *Mez.* Natr. m. *Nux v. Op. Puls. Rhus. Sabad.* Sep. Sulf.
——, paralysis of: Stram.
——, —— —— upper: Phos. ac.
——, stretching and bending of: Alum.
——, trembling of: Bell. *Chin. s.* Con. *Sabad.*
——, twitchings in: *Nux v.* Stram.
**Lips,** blue: *Chin. s. Eup. purp.* Ipec. **Natr. m.** *Nux v. Sec. c.*
**Liver,** pain in the region of: Ars. Bry. *Cinch. Nux.* **Pod.** Verat.
**Loins,** pains in: Ars. Kreos. Lach. Nux v. Verat.
**Loquacity: Pod.** Marum.
**Moaning:** *Eup. perf.*
**Mouth,** dryness of: *Mez. Petr.* Thuja.
——, —— ——, posteriorly, saliva anteriorly: **Mez.**
——, foam at: Cina. (?) Therid.
**Mucus,** vomiting of: *Puls.*
**Muscles,** pain in: **Arn.** Bap.
**Nails,** blue: Apis. Arn. Ars. *Asaf. Carb. v. Cinch.* Cocc. Con. *Dros. Eup. purp.* Ipec. Mez. **Natr. m.** Nux v. *Petr.* Phos. ac. Sulph. *Thuja.*
——, finger, white: Sil.
**Nausea:** Arg. n. *Ars.* Bell. Bry. Chel. Cina. Cinch. Eup. purp. Ign. Ipec. Kali b. Kali c. Kobalt. Lach. *Lyc.* Lob. Mer. *Natr. m.* Petr. Puls. Rhus. Rumex. *Sabad.* Sang. Sep. Verat.
——, drinking, after: *Ars.* Arn. *Eup. perf.*
——, relieved by a swallow of water: *Lob.*
**Nervousness:** Cocc. Eup. purp.
**Noise,** dread of: *Bell.* **Caps.** *Hyos.*

**Nose,** cold: Apis. Ant. c. Ced. Chel. Colch. Iod. Meny. *Polyp.* Sil. Sulf. *Tarax.*
——, ——, tip of: **Ced.**
——, red: Bell.
——, sweat on, cold: Cina.
**Numbness:** Cinch. Fer. Lyc. Puls. *Sep.*
**Pain,** in parts rested upon: *Bapt.*
——, paroxysms of: Ars. Cinch. Eup. perf. Puls. Rhus.
**Paralysis,** sense of, in legs: Ars. Ign. Stram.
**Photophobia:** Hep.
**Ptyalism:** Caps.
**Pulse,** full: Ant. t. Chin. s.
——, hard: Cinch.
——, intermittent: Acon. Dig.
——, irregular: Ant. c. Cinch.
——, quick: Cinch.
——, slow: Meny.
——, thread-like: Acon. Apis. Chel.
——, weak: Ced. Gels.
**Pupils,** contracted: Acon. Gels.
——, dilated: Acon. *Bell.* Ipec.
**Recollect,** inability to: Ars. Caps. Stram.
**Respiration,** difficult: **Apis.** Ars. Gels. Kali c. Mez. Natr. m. Puls. Seneg. Thuja. Zinc.
**Restlessness: Ars.** Bell. Eup. purp. Plant. Rhus.
**Sacrum,** pain in: Ars. Gamb. Hyos. **Nux v.** Verat.
**Saliva,** spitting of: Alum. Caps. Rhus.
**Scapula,** pain under: Elat.
**Sensation,** loss of: Lach.
**Sight,** obscuration of: Bell. Cic. Hydr. ac. Sabad.
**Skin,** blue: Cinch. Mer. Natr. m. Nux m. *Nux v*
——, ——, and mottled: Crotalis. **Nux v.**
——, cold, damp, clammy: Lach. **Verat.**
——, coldness icy, of: **Sec. c.** *Stram.* Verat.
——, contracted, sensation of: Par.
——, dry: Ars. Asaf. Iod.
——, itching of: *Hep. Petr.*
——, painful: Camph. *Nux v.*

**Skin,** sore to touch: Camph. Cinch.
—, stinging: *Hep.* Samb.
—, warm to the touch: Ars. Elaps. Gamb.
**Sleep:** Amb. Ant. c. Ant. t. **Apis.** Cim. Gels. *Kali iod.* Lyc. Mer. Mez. *Natr. m.* **Nux m.** Nux v. **Op.** Pod. Psor. Sil.
—, deep, snoring: Laur. **Op.**
**Sleepiness:** Æth. Amb. Cim. Hell. Kali b. *Kali iod.* Mez. *Natr. m.* Nux m. Nux v. **Op.** Phos. Tarax.
**Sneezing:** Psor.
**Soreness,** feeling of: Arn. Bap. Camph.
**Spasms:** *Calc.* Camph. Verat.
—, clonic: Camph.
**Spine,** painful to pressure: **Chin. s.**
—, coldness of the: Canth. **Meny.**
**Spleen,** pain in the region of: Bry. **Chin. s.** *Eup. perf.* **Pod.**
—, stitches in: Bry.
—, swelling of: Caps. Cean. (?) Petr.
**Staggering:** Caps.
**Staring:** Cic.
**Stiffness,** and rigidity of the body: Op.
**Stretching:** Alum. Ars. Bry. Caps. Cim. Coff. Elat. *Eup. perf.* Ipec. Kreos. Laur. Marum. Mur. ac. Nitr. ac. Nux v. Petr. Polyp. *Rhus.*
**Stomach,** heat in: Lob.
—, pain in: Ars. Eup. perf. Lyc. Mercurialis. Sil. Sulf.
—, weight in, sensation of: *Bell.*
**Sun,** desire for the heat of: *Con.*
**Taste,** bitter: Alum. Ars. Eup. purp. **Hep.**
—, insipid: Aur.
**Teeth,** incisors—coldness of, sensation of: Gamb.
**Tendons,** short, feeling as though too: Cimex.
**Tenesmus:** Canth. Caps. Col. Mer.
**Thighs,** heat of: **Thuja.**
—, weakness of: Verat.
**Thirst:** Acon. *Alum.* Amm. m. **Apis.** Aran. **Arn.** *Ars.* Bell. *Bry.* Calad. *Calc.* Camph. **Caps.** *Carb. v. Chin. s.* Cinch. Croc. Cur. Dulc. Elat. Elaps. **Eup. perf.** *Eup. purp. Fer.* Gamb. Graph. **Ign.** Kali c. Kali iod. Lach. Lachn. Laur. *Led.* Lob. Mag. s. Mer. Mez. Mur. ac. Natr. c. *Natr. m.* Natr. s. Nitr. ac. Nux v. Plant. Psor. Puls. *Rhus.* Sec. c. *Sep.* Thuja. **Verat.**

**Thirst,** much: *Alum. Apis. Arn.* **Bry. Caps. Eup. perf.** Gamb. Graph. **Ign.** Led. Mez. **Natr. m.** Puls. Rhus.
——, quantity of water, large, which relieves: **Bry. Natr. m.**
——, —— —— small, frequent drinking: *Ars.* Cinch. *Eup. perf.*
——, without: Agar. *Ang.* Amm. m. Anac. *Ant. c. Ant. t. Aran.* Ars. Asar. Bar. *Bell.* Bov. *Cac.* Calad. *Camph. Canth. Carb. an.* Caust. Ced. *Cham.* Chel. *Cim. Cina. Cinch. Cocc.* Coff. Col. Cur. Cycl. *Dros.* Dulc. Elaps. Euph. *Gels.* Graph. Guaj. Hell. Hep. Hyos. *Ipec.* Kali b. Lach. Lyc. Meny. Mer. Mur. ac. Nitr. ac. Natr. m. Natr. c. Natr. s. Nux m. Nux v. Oleand. Petr. Phos. ac. Phos. Pod. *Puls.* Rhus. Sabad. Samb. Sil. Spig. *Staph.* Stram. Sulf. Therid.
**Throat,** rattling in: Camph.
**Throbbing,** through the body: Zinc.
**Toes,** coldness of: **Fer. Meny.**
——, pain in: Ang.
**Toothache: Carb. v.** Kali c. Graph. Rhus.
**Torpor,** of affected side: Puls.
——, —— —— parts: Caust.
**Trembling:** *Agn.* Anac. Ant. t. Ars. *Cina.* Cocc. Croc. Con. *Eup. perf.* Fer. Gels. Mer. iod. *Par. Petr.* Plat. Sabad. *Zinc.*
**Trismus:** Lach.
**Unconsciousness:** *Bell.* Camph. *Hep.* **Natr. m.** Nux v. Op. Puls.
**Uncovering,** pains from: **Stram.**
**Uneasiness:** Calc. Caps. Hyos. Sil.
**Urethra,** pains in: *Canth.* **Petros.** Sars.
**Urinating,** frequent: Canth. Hyper. Mer. *Petros.*
**Urine,** acid: Sep.
——, brown: Sep.
——, dark: Verat.
**Urticaria:** Apis. **Hep.**
——, over whole body when chills were suppressed: Elat.
**Veins,** distended: Ars. Bry. Calad. Caps. Caust. Cim. Cina. Elat. Eup. perf. Gamb. Kobalt. Laur. Lyc. Marum. **Meny.** Mer. Mez. Murex. Natr. m. Natr. s. Oleand. Par. Phos. Polyp. Sil. Thuja.
**Vertebræ,** pain in dorsal: **Chin. s.**
——, coldness in, sensation of: *Canth.*
**Vertigo:** Alum. Calc. Caps. Cinch. *Eucalyp.* Kali b. Laur. Natr. m. Nux v. Phos. Puls. Rhus. Sulf.

**Vomiting**, in all stages: **Eucalyp.** Verat.
**Vomiting**: Alum. Arn. *Ars.* Asaf. **Eup. perf.** Fer. Gamb. Ign. *Ipec.* Lach. Lyc. Natr. m. Nux v. Puls. Rhus. *Verat.*
——, of bile: Ars. Cina. Cinch. **Eup. perf.** Ign. Ipec.
——, drinking, after: *Arn.* **Ars. Eup. perf.** Nux v.
——, of ingesta: **Fer.** Ign. Eup. perf.
——, of mucus: Caps. Ign. **Puls.**
——, sour: **Lyc.** *Rob.*
**Warmth**, desire for, but does not relieve: Alum. Aran. Camph. *Cic.* Cina. Cocc. *Con.* Hep. **Lach.** Lyc. Meny. Nux v. Phos. Pod. Sil. Verat.
—— —— ——, especially heat of sun: **Con.**
——, —— —— without, or dread of open air: **Mez.**
——, external, unbearable: *Apis.* **Ipec. Puls. Sep.**
**Weakness**: Amb. Aran. Ars. Calc. Carb. v. Caust. Dros. Ipec. Lach. Laur. Mercurialis. *Natr. m.* Op. Phosph. Psor.
**Wrists**, tearing in: Phos. ac. **Pod.**
**Yawning**: Ars. *Bry.* Calad. Caps. Caust. Cim. *Cina.* **Elat. Eup. perf.** *Gamb.* Kobalt. Laur. Lyc. Marum. *Meny.* Mer. Mez. *Mur. ac.* Murex. **Natr. m.** Natr. s. *Oleand.* Par. Phos. *Polyp.* Sil. Thuja.

## CHILL, FOLLOWED BY:

**Anxiety**, internal, with short breath: Kali c.
**Bloating**, of hands and face: Lyc.
**Breathing**, oppressed: Cimex.
**Chest**, spasmodic pain in: Kali c.
**Cough**, dry, uninterrupted, from tickling in larynx: Cimex.
**Eyes**, redness of: Ced.
**Eyelids**, itching of: Ced.
**Face**, heat of: Dros.
**Feet**, coldness of: Petr.
**Fingers**, drawings in: Lyc.
**Hands**, icy-coldness of: Ced.
**Head**, heaviness of: Dros.
**Heart**, icy-coldness about the: **Natr. m.**
**Headache**, frontal: Ant. t. Ced. **Natr. m.**
——, throbbing, occipital: Dros.

**Heat**, with sweat and thirst: Ant. c. Ant. t. *Caps.*
—— and perspiration: Polyp.
**Itching**, violent, of the skin: **Petr.**
**Lips**, dryness of: Kali b.
**Mouth**, dryness of: Kali b.
**Nausea**: Acon. **Eup. perf.** Kali c.
**Nose**, coldness of the tip of, rest of face burning hot: Ced.
**Pains**: Kali c.
**Prostration**: Ars. *Natr. m.*
**Retching**, after drinking: Ant. t.
**Restlessness**: Apis. Camph.
**Shivering**: Lyc. Sep.
——, after drinking and while eating: Caps. Lyc.
——, —— every drink: Caps.
**Shuddering**: Caps.
**Skin**, itching of: **Petr.**
**Sleep**: **Apis.** Ars. Camph. Lyc. Mez. Nux m. Nux v. Sab.
**Sweat**: **Caps. Caust.** Dig. Kali c. *Lyc.* Rhus. *Thuja.*
**Thirst**: **Ars. Bar.** *Cim.* **Cinch. Dros.** Hep. Kali b. Mag. s. Puls. Sabad. Thuja.
——, yet cannot drink, makes headache unbearable: Cimex.
**Urticaria**: **Apis.**
**Vomiting**: Ant. t. **Eup. perf.** Kali c. *Lyc.* **Natr. m.**
—— and spasmodic pain in chest: Kali c.
——, of bile: **Eup. perf.** Kali c. **Natr. m.**
——, sour: Lyc.
——, after every draught: **Eup. perf.**
**Weakness**: Ars. Lyc.
**Weariness**: Cim. Lyc.
——, of the feet: Lyc.
**Wrists**, drawing in: Lyc.

### HEAT AGGRAVATED.

**Air**, in open: Cur. **Nux v.**
**Bed**, in: *Mer.*
**Carriage**, when riding in a: Graph. **Psor.**
**Drinking**, by: Calc. Cocc.

**Eating, after:** Amm. c. Brom. **Caust.** Cocc. Fluor. ac. Sep.
**Evening, towards:** Fer.
**Exercising, when:** Ant. c. Ant. t. **Camph. Cinch.** Cur. Nux v. Stram. **Sep.**
**Midnight, after:** *Dros.*
**Motion, by:** Alum. Ant. t. *Camph.* **Cinch.** Cur. Nux v. *Sep.* Stram.
**Night, at:** *Cina.* Cur. **Sil.**
**Sitting, while:** Phos. Sep.
**Sleep, in:** Dulc. Petr. Samb. Viol. tr.
———, after: Cina. Lach.
**Smoking, by:** Cic. Coff.
**Stooping, when:** Mer.
**Vexation, after:** Petr. Sep.
**Walking, when:** *Camph.* **Cinch.**
**Warmth, by:** **Apis.** Bry. **Ign.** Puls.
———, of room, by: Amm. m. **Apis.** Ipec. Natr. m.
**Weather, by damp:** Cur.

## HEAT AMELIORATED.

**Air, in open:** Canch. Natr. m.
**Carriage, by riding in a:** Nitr. ac.
**Eating, after:** Anac. Cinch. Cur. Fer.
**Heat, by artificial:** Ars. **Ign.**
**Motion, by:** **Caps.** Fer.
**Sitting, when:** **Bry.** Nux v.
**Speaking, when:** Fer.
**Uncovering, by:** Acon. Ars. Bov. Ign. Puls.
**Walking, when:** *Caps.*

## HEAT, ABSENT.

Amm. m. Agar. Aran. Benz. Bov. Camph. Caps. Caust. Cim. Cocc. Hep. Lyc. Mag. c. Mez. Phos. ac. Rhus. Sabad. Staph. Sulph. Thuja. Verat.

## HEAT, IN GENERAL.

Acon. *Æsc.* Æth. Alston. Alum. Amb. Amm. m. Anac. Ang. Ant. c. **Ant. t.** *Apis.* Aran. **Arn. Ars.** Asaf. *Bap.* Bar. **Bell.** *Bry.* **Cac.**

Calad. Calc. Canch. Canth. Carb. an. Carb. v. *Casc.* Ced. Cham.
*Chel.* **Chin. s.** Cic. Cina. **Cinch.** Coff. Con. Corn. f. Croc. Cup.
*Cur.* Cycl. Dig. Dros. Dul. Elat. *Elaps.* Eucalyp. **Eup. perf.** Eup.
purp. Euphor. *Fer.* Gamb. **Gels.** *Graph. Hell.* Hep. Hyos. *Ign.* Iod.
**Ipec.** Kali b. Kali c. **Kali iod.** *Lach.* Lachn. Laur. Led. Lob.
**Lyc.** Mar. Mag. c. Mag. s. Meny. *Mercurialis. Mer.* **Mez.** Mosch.
Mur. ac. *Natr. m.* Natr. s. *Nitr. ac.* Nux m. **Nux v.** *Op.* Par. Petr.
*Phos.* Plant. Pod. Polyp. Psor. **Puls. Rhus.** Rob. Sabad. Sab.
*Samb.* Sarr. **Sec. c.** *Sep. Sil.* Stan. Spig. Staph. Stram. Sulph. Tarax.
Thuja. Valer. Verat.

## HEAT, SYMPTOMS DURING.

**Abdomen,** coldness in: Zinc.
——, distended: Ars.
——, rumbling in: Lachn.
——, heat in: Apis. *Cac.* Calad. Canth. *Cic.* Cinch. Fer. Lach. Selen. Spig. Stan.
——, pain in: Ars. Caps. Carb. v. Cina. Elat. Ign. Nux v. *Rhus.*
——, pulsations in: **Kali c.**
——, weak: Anac.
**Adipsia,** complete: Æth.
**Air,** cold, sensitiveness to: *Bar.* Camph. *Cocc.*
——, as if there was none in the room (breathing difficult): Plant.
——, of room intolerable: **Apis.**
——, —— —— seems hot and close: Plant.
——, warm, sensitiveness to: *Cocc.*
**Anxiety,** with: Asaf. Casc.
**Appetite,** loss of: Cinch. Lach.
**Apples,** desire for: Ant. t.
**Arms,** cold: Kali b.
——, veins of, distended: *Chin. s.* Cinch.  (See Blood-vessels, Veins.)
**Back,** heat in, lumbar region: Sarr. Spig. Stan.
—— and loins, burning in: Kalm.
——, pain in: Alston. Arn. Ars. Caps. Carb. v. Chin. s. *Eup. perf.* Hyos. Ign. Kali c. Lach. Laur. Lyc. Natr. m. **Nux v.** Puls. Rhus.
**Beer,** desire for: *Nux v.* Spig.
**Bladder,** pain in: Cac.

**Blood,** feeling as though hot: *Ars. Bell.* **Rhus.**
**Blood-vessels,** distention of: *Bell.* Camph. *Chin. s.* **Cinch.** Croc. Puls.
**Body** red: Canth.
——, was too heavy, clothes seemed burdensome: Euphor.
——, upper part chiefly, heat of: Agar.
**Bones,** pain in: Ars. *Eup. perf. Eup. purp.* Ign. Mag. c. Natr. m. Puls.
**Breathing,** anxious and rapid: *Acon.* Puls.
——, deep: *Lach.*
——, oppressed: **Apis.** Ars. Bov. Cac. Carb. v. *Cim.* Elaps. *Ipec.* **Kali c.**
——, short: Cac. Cina. Con. *Sil.*
**Bruised,** feeling as though: *Arn.* Bap.
**Cheek,** heat and redness of one: Coff. *Ign. Ipec.* Puls.
——, red spot on the left: Lyc.
——, —— —— —— —— right: Lachn.
——, redness of one, the other pale: Acon. Bar. **Cham.** *Ipec. Puls.*
**Cheeks,** burning and dark red: Chel. Eup. perf. Mercurialis. Lachn.
——, red and hot: Carb. an. Chel. *Cina. Cocc.* Coff. Dig. **Eup. perf.** Fer. Kali c. Lach. Lyc. *Meny.* Mer. Nux v. Rhus. Rob. *Verat.*
——, red and hot subjectively, although objectively they are not warm: **Cinch.**
**Chest,** burning in: Amm. m. *Apis.* Cham. Puls. Seneg. Stan. Sulf.
——, oppression of: Acon. **Apis.** Ars. Berb. Bov. Carb. v. Ipec. Kali c *Lach.* Mer. Plant. Puls.
——, pain in: Ars. Caps. Carb. v. Cina. Cinch. Kali c. Nux v.
——, stitches in: Acon. **Bry.** *Kali c.* Nux v.
**Colic:** Caps. Carb. v. Elat. Rhus. Rob.
**Coma:** Arn. Cac. Ign. Laur. Op.
**Consciousness,** he almost loses: Phos. ac.
**Constipation:** Chin. s. Lyc. Natr. m. Nux v.
**Convulsions:** Cur. *Hyos.* **Nux v.** Op. **Stram.**
——, epileptiform: Hyos. *Stram.*
**Cough:** Acon. *Bry.* Dros. Cinch. Eup. perf. **Ipec.** Lob. Sulf.
——, with pleuritic stitches: *Acon.* **Bry.**
——, short, hacking, from tickling in throat-pit: Lob.
——, exciting, nausea and vomiting: **Ipec.**

**Cramps:** Cur. Cup. Rob.
**Deafness:** Lachn.
**Debilitating:** Cup.
**Debility:** Lob.
**Delirium:** Ant. t. **Arn.** Ars. Bell. Carb. v. **Chin. s.** Cina. Cinch. Coff. Gels. Hep. Ign. Lach. Lachn. **Natr. m.** Nitr. ac. Nux v. Op. Pod. *Psor.* Sabad. Sang. Sarr. Sec. c. Spong. **Stram.** *Verat.*
**Diarrhœa:** Cina. Con. Elat. Puls. *Rhus.* Thuja.
——, constant, on the days free from fever: **Iod.**
**Drinking,** repugnance to: Nux v.
**Drinks,** cold, feeling as though they were too: *Bell.*
——, ——, nausea after: Lyc.
—— little at a time: **Ars.** *Cinch.* Lyc.
——, warm, desire for: Ced. **Casc. Eup. purp.**
**Dyspnœa:** Acon. Anac. Apis. *Arn.* Ars. Bov. Cac. Camph. Carb. v. Cim. Crot. Elaps. Ign. Ipec. *Kali c.* Lob. Lyc. Phos. Puls. Sep.
**Ear,** heat and burning of one: **Ign.**
**Ears,** coldness of: Ipec.
——, heat of: *Caps.* Cinch. Dig. Elaps. Lach. Lyc. *Meny.*
——, humming in: Nux v.
——, pain in: Calad.
——, redness of: *Camph.* Caps. Cist. Elaps. **Ign.**
——, roaring in: *Nux v.*
**Eating,** after: Cycl. Valer.
**Epigastrium,** fulness in: Aran. *Ars.*
**Epilepsy:** **Hyos.** Stram.
**Excitability,** nervous: *Acon.* Con.
——, mental: Marum.
**Exhausting:** Cup.
**Extremities,** pains in: Elat. **Eup. perf.** Eup. purp. *Rob.*
——, twitchings in: Gels. Ign. Rob.
**Eyelids,** cannot open: **Gels.**
——, heat of: Chel.
——, swelling of upper: Apis. **Kali c.**
**Eyes,** pupils contracted: Laur. Op. Verat.
——, —— dilated: *Bell.* Hell. Stram.
——, rubbing of: Cina.
——, weakness of: Carb. v. **Natr. m.** Sep.

**Face,** burning, but not red: Plat.
———, ——— and redness of the: Phel.
———, ———, as if sweat would break out: Bap.
———, coldness of: Ang. *Ipec.* Puls. Rheum.
———, heat, flushes of, over the: Æsc. Bap. Cac. Carb. v. Cup. Hydr. Kali iod. Marum.
———, ———, ——— ——— in, rest of body chilly: Sab.
——— and hands, heat on, with chill in the back: Spig.
———, heat in, sensation of: Sep. Tarax. *Thuja.*
———, ——— ———, after eating: Asaf. Caust. Cham.
———, hot: Anac. Bell. Cac. Calad. Camph. Caps. Carb. v. Caust. Cham. Chel. Cic. *Cina.* Cinch. Cocc. Coff. Cycl. Dig. *Eup. perf.* Gels. Ipec. Kali b. Kali c. Lach. Laur. Lyc. *Mag. c.* Meny. Mercurialis. Mer. Nitr. ac. Par. Phos. ac. Phos. Plant. *Polyp.* Rhus. Sabad. Sab. *Samb. Sarr.* Sep. Sulf. Tarax. *Verat.*
———, paleness of: Ars. Bry. Caps. Cina. Croc. *Ipec.* Lyc. Rhus. Rob. Sep.
———, ——— ———, when rising up: *Acon.*
———, red: Acon. Alum. Amm. m. Asaf. **Bell.** Bry. *Cac.* Calc. Camph. Caps. *Carb. v.* Ced. Chel. *Chin. s.* Cic. **Cinch.** Cocc. Coff. Con. Croc. Cycl. Dulc. Elaps. Euph. **Fer.** Hep. *Ign.* Kali iod. Kreos. *Lachn.* Lyc. Mag. c. Mag. s. Meny. Mer. Natr. m. Nux m. Nux v. Op. *Petr. Polyp.* Puls. Rhus. Sabad. Sarr. **Sep. Sil.** Spig. Spong. *Stram. Sulf.* Tarax. Verat.
———, red and pale alternately: Acon. Bell. Bov. Caps. Croc. Ipec. Nux v. Op. Phos. Puls.
———, ———, when lying: *Acon.*
———, ——— and burning, one side of: Ign.
———, ———, right side of: Lachn.
———, redness of, dark: **Lachn.** Rob. **Sil.**
———, ——— ———, mahogany: **Eup. perf.**
———, sweat on: Dig. Dulc. Lob. Valer.
———, ——— ———, cold: Dig.
———, swollen: Amm. m. Ars. Bell. Cac. Chel. Cina. Lyc. Puls.
———, ——— and bloated, sensation of: Fer.
———, yellow: Ars. Cina. Eup. perf. Natr. m.
**Fainting:** **Acon.** Anac. **Arn.** Bell. Calc. Cur. Eup. perf. Mer. **Natr. m.** Nux v. Op. Phos.

**Fainting,** when rising up: **Acon.**
**Falling,** sensation of: **Gels.**
**Fanned,** desire to be: **Carb. v.**
**Fear:** *Acon.*
——, of falling: Gels.
**Feet,** coldness of: Anac. Ant. c. *Arn.* Asaf. Bell. Calc. Calad. Caps. Croc. Fer. Graph. Hydr. ac. Ign. Ipec. Kali c. Lach. Meny. Nux v. Petr. Phos. ac. Puls. Sabad. Sab. *Samb.* **Stram. Sulf.**
——, hot: *Led.* Mercurialis. Nux v. Plant. Polyp. Sarr. Staph.
——, pain in, from cold on uncovering: Nux v. Stram.
——, soles of, burning: Æsc. Canth. Cup. *Fer.* Graph. *Lach.* **Sulf.**
——, —— ——, ——, and palms of hands, must be uncovered: Æsc. Fer. **Lach.**
——, sweat on: Staph.
**Fingers,** heat of: Lyc.
——, alternately hot and cold: **Par.**
——, pain in: Elat.
**Food,** aversion to: Cinch.
——, cold, desire for: Phos. Verat.
**Forehead,** coldness of: Cina. Cinch. Puls.
——, hot: Chel. *Stram.*
——, sweat on: Ant. t. Ipec. Mag. s. Sars. Staph. **Verat.**
**Gagging: Cim.**
**Hands,** cold: *Arn.* Asaf. Canth. Caps. Cycl. Ipec. Nitr. ac. Puls. Sab. Thuja.
——, heat of: Agar. Bell. Calad. Chel. Cur. Cycl. Dig. Graph. Hydr. Kali b. Lach. *Led. Mag. c.* Mercurialis. *Nitr. ac.* Nux m. *Nux v.* Petr. Phos. Plant. **Puls.** Sab. Stan. Staph. **Sulf.**
——, —— —— one, the other cold: Cinch. Cocc. *Dig.* Puls.
——, —— —— ——, and coldness of the other, in alternation: Cocc.
—— heavy: Aran.
——, pain in, from cold when uncovered: Nux v. Stram.
——, palms of, hot: Æsc. Anac. Canth. **Fer.** *Lach.* Lyc. Mer. *Polyp.* **Sulf.**
——, perspiration on, cold: Nitr. ac.
——, sweat of: Bar. Hep. Nitr. ac. Plant.
——, veins of, distended: *Bell. Cinch. Hyos.* **Led.** Meny.
**Hard,** feeling as though the bed were: **Arn.** Bap. Mur. ac.

**Head,** coldness of: Bell.
——, hot: *Bell.* Cac. *Calc.* Camph. Carb. an. Caust. Chel. Cur. Dig. Eup. perf. Fer. Gels. Ipec. Kali iod. Lyc. *Mag. c.* Mercurialis. *Petr.* Phel. Phos. ac. Plant. Rob. Rhus. Sab. Sars. Sil. Staph. Stram. Verat.
——, pain in, lancinating: Cac.
——, sweat on: Mag. c.
**Headache:** Acon. Æsc. Agar. Alston. *Ang.* **Arn.** *Ars.* **Bell.** Berb. Bor. Bry. Cac. Calc. Caps. Carb. v. Chin. s. Cina. **Cinch.** Col. Corn. f. Crot. Dros. Dulc. Elat. **Eup. perf.** Graph. *Hep. Ign.* Kali b. Kali c. Lach. Lob. **Natr. m.** Nux v. Op. Plant. *Pod.* Puls. Rob. *Rhus.* Ruta. Sabad. Sep. **Sil.** Sulf. Valer.
——, one-sided: Spig. *Thuja.*
——, stitches in the temples: **Nux v.** Puls.
——, —— unbearable in the: Asaf.
——, as if it would burst: Æsc. Bell. Corn. f.
**Heart,** palpitation of: Acon. *Bar.* Calc. Mer. Sars. Sep. Sulf.
——, beats violently: Æsc.
**Hips,** burning in: Cur.
——, pain in: *Rhus.*
**Hoarseness:** Hep.
**Hunger:** **Cina. Cinch.** Cur. Eup. purp. **Phos.**
——, canine, or aversion to food: **Cinch.**
**Ice cream,** desire for: **Phos.** Verat.
**Irritability:** *Anac.* **Cham.** Bry. Plant.
—— in nursing children: **Anac.** Cham. Sil.
**Knees,** hot: Ign.
——, weak: Anac.
**Lachrymation:** Eup. perf.
**Leg,** pain in one: Gels.
**Legs,** coldness of: Carb. an. Meph. Sep. **Stram.**
——, heat in: Camph. Cur. **Led.** Sarr. Stan.
——, burning in, prevents sleep: Bap.
——, numbness of: Ced.
——, veins of, distended: **Chin. s.**
**Lie down,** feeling as though he must: Natr. m.
——, still, wants to: *Bry.* Gels.
**Light,** sensitiveness to: Bell. Stram.
**Limbs,** cold: Carb. an. Sep. **Stram.**

**Limbs,** hot, but feel cold: Bap.
———, heaviness of: Aran. Calc.
———, pain in: Ars. Bry. Calc. Caps. Carb. v. Cinch. Eucalyp. *Eup. perf.* Eup. purp. Lach. Lyc. Puls. Rhus. Sec. c. Sep. Sulf. Valer.
———, twitching of the: Op.
**Lips,** burning of: Cinch.
———, dryness of: Rhus.
———, fever blisters on: *Hep. Ign.* **Natr. m. Nux v.** Rhus.
———, ——— ———, upper, on: **Rhus.**
———, licks them, but does not drink: **Puls.**
**Liver,** pain in the region of: Ars. Cinch. Elat. *Nux v.*
**Loins,** pain in: Crot. Kali c.
**Loquacity:** *Carb. v.* **Lach. Marum. Pod.** Teucr.
**Lungs,** engorged, feel as if: Æsc.
**Milk,** desire for: Mer.
**Moaning:** Acon. Cham. *Eup. perf.* Lach. **Puls.**
——— during sleep: Eup. perf.
**Mouth,** burning in: *Æsc. Petr.*
———, dryness of: Ars. Chin. s. Cinch. *Nux m.*
———, fever blisters around: *Hep. Ign.* **Natr. m. Nux v.** Rhus.
———, frequent spitting of mucus from the: Æsc.
———, open: Op.
———, paleness around: *Cina.*
**Muscles,** twitching of: Gels. Ign. Iod. Op.
**Nausea:** Anac. Ant. t. Aran. Ars. Bor. Bry. *Carb. v.* Cham. Cim. Cocc. Dros. *Elat.* Eup. perf. Eup. purp. *Ipec.* Lyc. *Natr. m.* Nitr. ac. *Nux v.* Op. Phos. Rob. Sabad. Sep. Thuja. Verat.
**Neck,** pain in: Graph.
**Noise,** sensitiveness to: *Bell.* **Caps.** Gels.
**Nose,** cold: Ign.
———, hot, end of: **Caps.** Chel.
———, paleness around: **Cina.**
———, picking of the: *Cina.*
**Numbness:** Ced. Par. *Sep.* Thuja.
**Occiput,** heat in: Camph.
**Œsophagus,** pressure in: *Cim.*
**Pain,** in parts rested upon: *Bap.*
**Painfulness,** of body when touched: Puls. Spig. **Stram.**

**Painfulness,** of body when uncovered: Mer. **Nux v.** *Stram.*
**Pains,** on uncovering, violent: Nux v. *Stram.*
**Palate,** heat of: Dulc.
**Paralysis:** Cur.
**Photophobia:** Hep.
**Position,** desire to change: Arn. Bap. *Rhus.*
——, —— —— ——, because bed is hard: **Arn.**
——, —— —— ——, to relieve the pain, Rhus.
——, —— —— move, to a cool part of bed: Bap.
**Pulse,** full: Acon. Camph. Ced. Chin. s. Corn. f. Nitr. ac.
——, hard: Corn. f.
——, irregular: *Cinch.* Nitr. ac.
——, quick: *Acon.* Camph. *Cinch.* Corn. f. Dig. Iod. Rhus.
——, slow: Fer.
——, weak: Ant. t. Iod.
**Pupils,** dilated: *Bell.* Cina. Ipec.
**Recollect,** inability to: Ars. Natr. m. Phos. ac. Sep.
**Respiration,** rapid: Lob. Plant.
——, snoring: Con. **Op.** *Laur. Lob.*
**Restlessness:** *Acon.* Amm. c. *Arn.* **Ars.** Bap. Bar. Bell. Caps. Cham. Cina. Cinch. *Gels.* Ipec. Lachn. Mag. m. Plant. *Puls.* Rhus. Sab. *Sec. c.* Valer.
**Saliva,** profuse discharge of watery: Æsc. *Dros.*
——, frothy: Rob.
**Scapula,** pain under the right: Chel. *Nux v.* Pod.
——, —— —— —— left: Sang.
**Scrobiculus cordis,** pain in: Eup. perf.
**Shiverings,** from uncovering: Apis. Arn. Bar. **Nux v.** Stram.
**Shoulders,** pain between: *Rhus.*
**Sighing:** Ign. Puls.
**Sight,** obscuration of: Natr. m. Puls.
**Skin,** damp: Op. Verat.
——, dry: Acon. Æsc. Apis. Ars. Bar. Hyos. Ign. Iod. Ipec. Polyp. Sec. c.
——, excoriation of: Sarr.
——, fissures of: Sarr.
——, hot: Æsc. Apis. Ars. Bar. Bell. Corn. f. *Hyos.* Polyp.
——, itching of: Amm. m. Apis. *Ign.* Rhus.

**Skin,** itching of, worse from rubbing: *Rhus.*
——, pricking in: Croc. *Gels.* Nitr. ac. Polyp.
——, red: Ars.
——, stinging of: Amm. m. Cinch.
**Sleep: Ant. t.** Apis. Caps. Ced. *Cinch.* **Eup. perf.** *Gels.* Ign. **Lach.** Lachn. Laur. Lyc. **Mez. Natr. m.** *Nux m.* **Op. Pod. Rob.** Rhus. **Samb.** Stram.
——, disappears during: Calad.
——, at climax of heat: **Pod.**
——, deep snoring: Con. *Laur.* **Op. Rob.**
——, soporous: **Op. Rob.**
——, dreams during: Elaps.
——, inability to, after 3 A.M.: Ang.
——, startings in: *Cham. Cina.* Con. Gels. Lyc.
——, —— when beginning to: Ign. Puls.
**Sleepiness:** Apis. Asaf. Ced. Cinch. *Gels.* Hep. Ign. Lyc. Natr. c. Nux m. Op. Phos. Puls. Rhus. Stram. Verat.
**Sleeplessness:** Acon. Ang. Arn. Ars. Asaf. Bar. Coff. Con. Graph. Hyos. Natr. c. Puls. Staph.
**Smothering,** sensation of: **Apis.** Carb. v. Cimex.
**Sneezing:** *Chin. s..*
**Somnolency:** Ant. t. Arn. Ars. Cac. Dulc. Gels. Ign. Lachn. *Natr. m.* Nux m. Op. Phos. ac. Sep.
**Speech,** incoherency of: Cur.
**Spine,** painful to pressure: **Chin. s.**
**Spleen,** pain in the region of: Ars. Carb. v. Eucalyp. *Nux v.* Pod. Rob.
**Stomach,** heat in the pit of: Lach. Sarr.
——, pain in: Ars. Carb. v. Cina. Kali c. Rhus. Sec. c. Sep.
**Stool,** frequent: Lach.
——, urgency to: Caps.
**Stretching:** Æsc. Calc. Chin. s. Cin. Rhus. Sab.
**Swallow,** constant inclination to: Æsc.
**Swallowing,** difficulty in: Cic. Cim.
**Sweat:** Alum. Amm. m. Ant. c. Camph. Caps. Colch. Con. Mag. c. Stan. Staph.
——, profuse: **Colch.** Psor.
**Teeth,** chattering of: Ced.
**Temperature,** sensitiveness to change of: *Bar.* Calc. Hep. Psor.

**Thirst:** *Acon.* Alston. Amm. c. Amm. m. Ang. Apis. *Arn.* **Ars.** Bar. *Bell.* Bov. *Bry.* Cac. Calad. Calc. Canth. Caps. *Ced. Cham.* Chin. s. *Cina. Cinch. Coff.* Con. Corn. f. Croc. Cur. Elat. Elaps. Eup. perf. *Eup. purp. Hep.* Hyos. Ipec. Kali b. Lach. Lyc. *Mag. c.* Mer. **Natr. m.** *Nux v.* Phos. Plant. *Pod. Psor.* **Puls.** *Rob. Rhus.* Sab. Sarr. *Sec. c.* Sep. *Sil.* Staph. Stram. Sulf. *Thuja.* Valer. Verat.

——, large quantities of water, desire for: *Acon. Alston.* Bar. Bell. Bry. **Natr. m.**

——, —— —— —— ——, —— ——, which relieve: **Natr. m.**

——, water, desire for, but unable to drink: **Cimex.**

——, much: Acon. Alston. *Arn. Ars.* Bell. *Bry.* Casc. Cham. Chin. s. Cinch. Elat. *Hep.* Hyos. **Natr. m.**

——, slight: Cac. Sabad.

——, uncovering, aggravated by: Bar.

——, vomiting after drinking, with: Alston. *Ars.* Phos.

——, wanting: Æth. *Alum. Ant. t. Apis.* Asaf. Bar. Bov. *Calc. Camph. Caps.* Carb. an. *Carb. v. Caust. Cim. Cinch.* Cocc. Cycl. Dig. *Dros.* Fer. Gels. Hell. *Ign.* Ipec. Kali c. *Led.* Meny. Mur. ac. Nux m. Op. Phos. ac. Puls. Rhus. Sabad. *Samb.* **Sep.** Spig.

**Throat,** pain in: Phos. Phos. ac. Sep.

——, burning dryness and constriction of: Æsc.

——, sore when swallowing: Berb. Phos. ac.

**Toothache:** Carb. v.

**Trachea,** dryness of: *Petr.*

**Trembling:** Ars. Calc. Cist. Eup. perf. Kali iod. Mag. c. Sep.

**Unconsciousness:** Laur. **Natr. m.**

**Uncovered,** desire to be: Acon. Apis. Arn. *Ars.* Bar. Calc. *Cinch. Eup. perf.* Ferr. *Hep.* Iod. *Lach.* Lyc. Mur. ac. **Natr. m.** Nitr. ac. Op. *Petr.* **Puls.** Spig. Staph. Verat.

**Uncovering,** aversion to: *Apis.* Ars. *Bell.* Clem. Coff. Colch. Con. Hep. Ign. *Mag. c.* Mer. Nux m. **Nux v.** Phos. ac. Puls. Rhus. *Samb.* Stram. *Stront.*

——, chilliness when: Arn. *Cinch.* **Nux v.** Puls.

**Urinate,** after drinking, desire to: Cim. Eup. purp.

**Urinating,** frequent: Arg. Bell. Kreos. Lyc. Mer. Phos. ac. Rhus. Staph. Stram.

**Urine,** brick-dust sediment with: Lyc. Phos.

——, whitish sediment: Phos. Sep.

**Urine,** pale: **Ced. Cham.**
——, profuse: Ant. t. Arg. Ced. *Cham.* Dulc. *Eup. purp.* Mur. ac. *Phos.* Scill. Stram.
——, red: Nux v.
——, suppressed: Cac.
——, turbid: Berb. Phos.
**Urticaria:** Apis. **Ign.** *Rhus.*
——, during heat, disappearing with sweat: **Ign.**
**Uterus,** pain in the region of: Cac.
**Veins,** blood burns in: *Ars. Hyos.*
——, —— runs cold in: Verat.
——, as from hot water running through: **Rhus.**
——, distendend: *Agar. Bell.* **Camph.** *Chin. s.* **Cinch.** Croc. Cycl. Dig. **Hyos. Led.** *Mercurialis.* **Puls.**
**Vertigo:** Ars. Bell. Berb. *Carb. v.* Cocc. Eucalyp. Gels. Hep. Ign. Ipec. Laur. Mer. *Natr. m.* Nux v. Phos. Puls. *Sep. Stram.* Valer. Verat.
**Vomiting:** Alston. Ant. c. Ars. Bry. Cac. *Cham. Cina.* Con. Elat. **Eup. perf.** Eup. purp. Fer. Ign. *Ipec.* Lach. *Lyc.* **Natr. m.** Nux v. Puls. Stram. Thuja.
——, of bile: *Cham. Cina. Eup. perf. Natr. m.* Thuja.
——, bitter: Eup. perf.
——, after drinking: *Ars.*
——, after cold drinks: Lyc.
——, frothy: *Elat.*
——, of ingesta: Cina. *Eup. perf.* Fer. Ign. Nux v.
——, sour: **Lyc.** Rob.
——, of water: Alston. Ars.
**Voice,** weak: Hep.
**Wanting.** (See Absent.)
**Warmth** of bed, intolerable: Lach. **Led.** *Puls.*
——, external, intolerable: Apis. Ipec. **Puls. Sep.**
——, ——, pleasant: *Ign.*
**Weakness:** Anac. *Arn. Ars.* Bry. Calc. Carb. v. Cur. Eup. perf. Ign. Ipec. Lyc. Natr. c. **Natr. m.** Nux m. Phos. **Rob.** Sarr. Sulf.
**Weeping:** Spong.
**Yawning:** Æsc. Calc. **Chin. s.** Cin. Kali c. *Rhus.* Sabad.

## HEAT, FOLLOWED BY:

**Chill:** Cinch. Mer. Nux v. **Puls.**
**Chilliness:** Meny. Mer.
**Debility:** Hydr.
**Exhaustion:** Ars.
**Face,** paleness of: Scill.
——, —— —— and fainting when rising up: Acon.
——, redness of, worse on the right side: Lachn.
**Headache:** Ars. Calc. *Carb. v.* **Eup. perf. Natr. m.**
**Hunger:** *Cim.* Dulc. Eup. perf. Ign.
——, ravenous: **Cim.**
**Sleep:** Apis. *Eup. perf.* Lob. Op.
——, with snoring: **Op.**
**Thirst:** Anac. Amm. m. Cac. *Cinch.* Coff. Cycl. Nux v. Op. Puls. Stan. Stram.
**Thirstlessness:** Op.
**Vomiting:** Calc. *Eup. perf.*
——, bilious: *Eup. perf.*
**Weakness:** *Ars.* Dig. Natr. m.

## HEAT, CHARACTERISTICS OF:

**Anxious,** of whole body: Casc.
**Anticipating:** **Nux v.**
**Afternoon,** without chill: Anac.
**Ascends:** Alum. Ang. *Cina.* Hyos. *Natr. m. Phos.* **Sep.** *Verat.*
**Back,** over the: Bap. Cur. Dul. Hyos. Phos.
——, from small of, in all directions: **Bap.**
**Bed,** in: Hell. Kali c. Mag. m. Mag. s. Sulf. ac.
——, ——, chilly when not in: Mer.
**Body,** left side of: **Mez.** Rhus.
——, —— —— ——, coldness of right: *Rhus.*
——, right side of: *Alum.* Meny. **Puls.**
——, upper part of: Anac. **Puls.**
——, whole of: Æsc. Bap. Camph. Ipec. Ign. Kali b. Led. Meny. Nitr. ac. Nux v. Op. Petr. Samb.
**Burning:** *Acon. Arn.* Ant. t. **Apis. Ars.** Bar. *Bell.* Bry. Cac. Canth. Caps. Cham. Chel. Cur. Dul. *Elaps.* Hell. *Hep. Hyos.* Lach. Laur.

Led. Lyc. Mag. c. Mercurialis. Mer. Mosch. Nux v. **Op.** Phos. **Puls.**
Sabad. Sarr. Sec. c. Staph. Stan.
**Burning,** in the mouth: Æsc.
———, which he does not feel: Canth.
———, even when bathed in sweat: **Op.**
———, without external redness: Hyos.
———, interrupted by shaking chills: Sec. c.
**Chest,** in or on: **Apis.** Cic.
**Chills,** with shaking: **Sec. c.**
**Chilliness,** with: **Apis.** *Arn. Caust.* Cur. *Elaps.* **Kali b. Kali c.**
Kali iod. Lach. Lachn. Mer. *Nux v.* Petr. Phos. *Pod.* **Puls.** *Rhus.*
Sabad. Sab. Sec. c. *Sil.* Sulf.
———, alternating with, not perceptible to the touch: Mer.
———, ——— with coldness here and there over entire body: Arn.
———, during the day: **Dros.**
———, from putting the hands outside the bed covering: Arn. Bar.
**Nux v.** *Stram.*
**Coldness,** with, except the face and head: Bell. *Op.* Stram.
——— all over, to the touch: Carb. v. Fer.
**Day,** during the, periodically: Sil.
**Dry:** *Acon.* Æsc. *Apis.* Arn. **Ars.** Bar. *Bell.* **Bry.** Cac. Ced. Cocc.
Coff. Col. Con. Dul. Fer. Graph. Hell. *Hep.* Hyos. Natr. s. Nitr. ac.
**Nux v.** Op. *Phos.* Phos. ac. **Puls.** Rhus. *Samb.* Sarr. Sec. c. Sep.
Stram.
——— on covered parts: Thuja.
**Evening:** Alum. Amb. Ang. Aran. *Berb.* Carb. v. **Cinch.** Dros.
Fer. Hell. *Hep.* Hyos. Lach. Lyc. Mag. c. Mer. Mur. ac. Phos.
Phos. ac. *Psor.* Sars. **Sil.** *Sulf.* Thuja.
**Face,** on: Acon. Æsc. Amb. Cac. Cina. Dros. **Lyc.** Stram.
———, after eating, of the: Asaf.
———, flushes in or over: Amb. Amm. m. Arn. *Bap.* Bar. *Cac.* Calc.
Carb. an. Carb. v. Chel. Cinch. Graph. Hep. Ign. Iod. *Kali b.* **Kali c.**
**Kali iod.** Lach. Lyc. Mag. c. Meny. Natr. c. Natr. m. **Nitr. ac.**
Nux v. Petr. Phos. Puls. Sabad. Sab. Sep. Sil. Spig. Stan. **Sulf.**
Sulf. ac. Thuja. Valer.
———, always ending in sweat: *Amm. m.*
**Forenoon,** in: Eup. perf. Kali c. *Natr. m. Nux v.* Rhus. Sars. Thuja.
**Head,** mostly on the: Cina. Cur. Dros. Mer. Sabad.

**Hips,** burning in the: Cur.
**Hot water,** on arms, chest, ears and legs, sensation of: *Cic.*
——, as if dashed with, sensation: Puls. Rhus. Sep.
**Intense:** *Acon. Ant. t.* Arn. **Ars.** *Bell.* Bry. Cac. Canth. Caps. Chin. s. Colch. Dig. Hep. Kali iod. Lyc. Mag. c. Mercurialis. **Mez. Natr. m.** Nux m. *Nux v. Op.* Puls. **Rhus. Sec. c. Sil.** Staph. Stram.
**Internal:** *Acon. Arn.* Ars. **Bell.** *Bry.* Caps. Cham. Chel. Cic. Cinch. Con. Fer. Hell. Iod. Kali c. Mag. c. Nitr. ac. Nux v. Phos. Phos. ac. **Puls. Rhus.** *Sabad.* Sec. c. Sep. Spig. Stan. Verat.
—— with external coldness: Bell. Iod. Phos.
—— burning, external chilliness: **Mez.**
**Long-lasting:** **Ant. t.** Cac. Hep. *Sec. c.* Sil.
**Midnight,** at: Rhus. Stram. *Sulf.*
——, before: *Ant. c.* Calad. Laur.
——, after: **Ars.** Kali c. Thuja.
——, and noon: *Stram.*
**Morning:** Arn. Kali c. Mag. c. *Nux v.* Rhus. **Sulf.** Thuja.
——, towards: Caust.
**Night:** **Alum.** Ant. c. Ars. Bar. Bry. *Calc.* Carb. an. Carb. v. Caust. Ced. Cham. Cic. Cina. Cocc. Coff. Cur. **Dros.** Dul. Graph. Hep. Kali b. Lach. Laur. Mag. c. Mag. m. Mer. Natr. m. Nitr. ac. Petr. Phos. Phos. ac. Polyp. Psor. **Puls.** Rhus. Sab. Sarr. **Sil.** Staph. Stram. Sulf. Thuja.
**Noon:** Stram. *Sulph.*
**Parts affected,** of: Acon. Bry. Sulf.
—— covered, of: Thuja.
**Part,** heat of one, with chill of another at same time: Cinch.
**Predominating:** *Ant. t.* Bell. Cac. **Ipec.** Sec. c. Sil.
**Shiverings,** with: Acon. Anac. Ant. t. *Apis.* Arn. Calc. Carb. v. Caust. Cham. Cinch. *Cur. Elaps.* Eup. perf. *Gels.* Hep. Ign. Lach. Meny. **Nux v.** Petr. Phos. ac. Pod. Rhus. Sabad. **Sulf.**
——, alternating with: Caust. Cinch. Cycl. Elaps. Hep. Lach. Mer. Phos. ac. Sabad.
——, drinking from: *Caps.* Eup. perf. **Nux v.**
——, motion from: Apis. *Arn.* **Nux v.** Pod. Stram.
——, mingled with: Acon. Anac. Ant. t. Apis. Calc. **Caust.** Cham. Petr. Pod. Rhus.
—— uncovering from: **Arn.** Apis. *Bar.* **Nux v.**

**Short:** **Ant. t.** Aran. Nitr. ac.
**Slight:** Lob. Lyc. Nux m.
**Spine,** along the: Hyos.
**Spot,** in one, which is cold to the touch: *Arn.*
**Sweat,** with: **Alum.** Amm. m. **Ant. c.** Camph. Canch. Caps. Ced. Con. Eup. perf. Ipec. *Kali iod.* Mag. c. **Mez. Op.** Phos. Pod. Psor. Puls. *Rhus.* Sabad. Sep. Stram. **Verat.**

———, ——— on the face: Valer.
**Warmth,** over whole body, except the head: Ang.

## SWEAT AGGRAVATED.

**Air,** exercise in the: *Bry. Caust. Cinch.*

———, in open: *Bry.* Calc. *Carb. an. Caust. Cinch.* Ipec. *Psor.* Ruta.
**Bed,** getting out of: Lach.

———, in: *Nitr. ac.*
**Covered,** on being: **Bell. Cinch.** Nitr. ac.
**Drinking,** by: Cocc.
**Eating,** by: Bar. Bor. Calc. *Carb. an. Carb. v.* Cocc. Con. Graph. Ign. Laur. Lyc. Natr. m. Nitr. ac. Nux v. Phos. Sars. Sep. Sulf. ac.
**Exercise,** by: Bell. Berb. Brom. Bry. *Calc.* Canth. Carb. v Caust. Cinch. Cocc. Corn. f. *Fer. Graph. Hep. Kali c.* Led. Lyc. Mer. *Natr. c. Natr. m.* Op. *Phos. Psor. Stan.* Sulf. ac.
**Exertion,** mental: Hep. *Kali c. Psor. Sep. Sulf.*
**Eyes,** upon closing the: *Con.*
**Lying down,** after: Mag. s. Meny.
**Midnight,** after: Alum. Amb. Amm. m. Bar. Clem. Dros. Kali c. Mag. m. Nux. v. Phos. *Sil.*
**Morning,** in the: Amb. Puls.
**Motion:** Alum. Amm. m. Bell. Bry. Calc. Camph. Canth. *Carb. an. Caust.* Chin. s. *Cinch.* Cocc. Cur. Gels. Graph. **Hep.** Ipec. Kali b. Kali c. Mag. c. **Mer.** *Natr. m. Phos.* **Psor.** Sep. *Sil. Sulf.* Valer. *Verat.*
**Room,** in a: Fluor. ac.
**Side affected,** on: Amb.
**Sitting,** during: Anac. *Kali b.* Rhus. Sep. Staph.
**Sleep,** during: Ars. Bell. Camph. Cham. Chel. Cinch. **Con.** Hyos. *Mez. Phos.* **Thuja.**

———, commencing to, when: Amm. c. Ars. Con. Mur. ac. Tab. Thuja. Verat.

**Sleep, in first:** Calc.
**Smoking, by:** Cocc.
**Stool, after every:** **Verat.**
**Vomiting, after mucous:** *Verat.*
**Waking, on:** Canth. **Samb. Sep.** *Sulf.*
**Warmth of room:** Plant.
**Weather, in damp:** Cur.
**Wind, by cold:** Cur.
**Writing, by:** *Hep. Kali c.* **Sep.** *Sulf.*
**Weakness:** Apis. Ars. Bar. Camph. Fer. Iod. *Mer. Phos.* Psor. Puls.
**Yawning:** Caust.

## SWEAT AMELIORATED.

**Air, in open:** Alum. Graph.
**Bed, on getting out of:** Hell.
**Covered, by being:** Acon.
**Drinking, after:** Chin. s.
**Eating, after:** Cinch. Lach. Phos.
——, **by:** Anac. Cur.
**Food, after warm:** Kali c. Phos. Sulf. ac.
**Morning, in the:** Borax. Lachn.
**Motion, by:** **Caps.**
**Sleep, in:** Nux v. Rumex. *Samb.*
**Walking, on:** Cham. Chel. *Puls. Thuja.*

## SWEAT, FOLLOWED BY:

**Chill:** **Carb. v.** Corn. f.
**Cough:** Eup. perf. Sil.
**Diarrhœa:** Puls.
**Hunger:** **Cina.** Staph.
——, **canine:** **Cina.**
**Madness, paroxysms of:** Cup.
**Prostration:** Ars.
**Sleep:** Nux m.
**Thirst:** Bell. Bor. **Lyc.** Nux v. Sabad.
——, **much:** Lyc.
**Vomiting:** *Cina.*
**Weakness:** Ars.

## SWEAT ABSENT.

Acon. Alum. Amm. c. Apis. *Aran.* Arn. *Ars.* Bell. Bis. *Bov.* Bry. Calc. Cham. Cinch. Coff. Colch. Corn. f. Dulc. *Eup. perf.* Gels. *Graph.* Hyos. Ign. Iod. Ipec. Kali b. Kali c. Lach. Led. *Lyc.* Mag. c. Mer. Natr. c. Nitr. ac. Nux m. Nux v. Oleand. Op. Phel. Phos. Phos. ac. Plat. Psor. Puls. Rhus. Sabad. Sec. c. Seneg. Sil. Spong. Staph. Sulf. Verb.

## SWEAT, IN GENERAL.

*Acon.* Æsc. Æth. *Agar.* Alston. Alum. *Amb.* Amm. m. Anac. Ang. Ant. c. **Ant. t.** Apis. Arn. Ars. Asaf. Bap. **Bar.** *Bell.* **Benz.** *Bov.* **Bry.** Cac. Calad. **Calc.** *Camph.* Canch. *Canth.* *Caps.* **Carb. an.** *Carb. v.* **Caust. Ced.** Cham. Chel. **Chin. s.** Cic. Cim. Cina. **Cinch.** Cocc. Coff. Con. Corn. f. Cupr. Cur. Cycl. **Dig.** Dros. Dulc. *Elat. Elaps.* Eup. perf. *Eup. purp.* Euphor. **Fer.** Gamb. *Gels. Graph.* Hell. **Hep.** *Hyos.* Ign. *Iod.* **Ipec.** Kali b. *Kali c.* Kali iod. **Lach.** Lachn. Laur. Led. Lob. **Lyc.** Mar. **Mag. c.** Meny. Mercurialis. **Mer.** *Mez.* Natr. c. **Natr. m.** Nitr. ac. Nux m. **Nux v.** Op. Par. Petr. **Phos. ac. Phos.** Plant. *Pod. Polyp.* **Psor.** Puls. *Rhus. Rob.* Sabad. Sab. **Samb.** *Sarr.* **Sec. c. Sep. Sil.** Spong. Stan. *Staph.*

## SWEAT PREDOMINATES.

Benz. **Carb. an.** *Cinch.* Fer. Hep. Kali b. **Mer.** *Nitr. ac.* Nux v. Phos. ac. **Psor. Samb. Tarax.** *Thuja.*

**Day,** during the: Carb. an. Cinch. Con. **Fer.** Lyc. Natr. m. Sep. Stram.

**Evening,** in the: Bar. Samb. Sulf.

**Morning,** in the: Alum. Fer. **Mag. c.** Mer. Natr. m. *Nitr. ac.* **Phos.** Phos. ac. Rhus. Sep.

**Night,** at: Alum. Ars. **Carb. an.** *Carb. v.* Caust. *Cinch.* **Kali c. Mer.** *Nitr. ac.* Phos. Sep. **Sil.** Stram. **Sulf. Tarax. Thuja.** *Valer.* Verat.

## SWEAT, PRODUCED BY:

**Covering,** on slightest: **Cinch** *Spig.*
**Cramps:** Ced.
**Exertion,** least: Æth. Agar. Bry. Corn. f. Psor. Valer.

Headache: *Fer.*
Hunger: Staph.
Produced easily: Æth. Colch.
Sleep, on going to: Æth.
Thirst: Coff. Thuja.

## SWEAT, CHARACTER OF.

Acrid: *Caps.* Cham. Con. Graph. Iod. Rhus. Tarax.
Ascends: Arn. Bell.
Awake, profuse while: **Samb.** Sep.
——, —— ——, on going to sleep dry heat returns: **Samb.**
Bed, in: **Alum.** Ang.
——, when getting out of: Lach.
Bloody: Calc. Clem. *Crotal.* **Cur. Lach. Lyc.** *Nux m.* Nux v.
——, staining red: **Lach.**
Chill, after the: *Ant. c.* Caust.
——, ——, without previous heat: *Caps.*
——, alternating with: Ant. c. *Nux v.*
——, at the same time as (simultaneously): Ant. c.
Chilliness, with: Ant. c. Bry. **Eup. perf.** Eup. purp. *Natr. m.* Nux v. Petr. Phos.
——, ——, from bathing: Arn.
——, ——, from motion, or allowing the air to strike him: Eup. perf. Nux v.
Coldness, with, on motion: Eup. perf. **Nux v.**
——, ——, on uncovering: Eup. perf. **Nux v.**
Clammy: Acon. Anac. Ant. t. Arn. **Ars.** Calc. Camph. Cham. Cup. Dig. Elat. *Fer.* Hell. Hep. Iod. Lach. Lachn. Lyc. Mer. Nux. Op. Phos. ac. *Phos.* Spig. Verat.
Cold: Agar. Anac. **Ant. t.** Arn. **Ars.** Bar. Bry. Calad. **Camph.** Canth. Caps. *Cina.* Cinch. Cocc. Cup. *Cur.* Dig. Dulc. Dros. Elaps. Gels. **Hep.** Hyos. Iod. *Ipec.* Lach. Lachn. Lob. **Lyc.** Mer. Mez. Natr. c. Natr. m. Nux v. Op. Plant. Pod. Puls. Ruta. Sec. c. **Sep.** Sil. Spig. Stan. Staph. **Stram.** Sulf. Sulf. ac. Thuja. **Verat.**
——, all over body: Spig.
——, on forehead and limbs: Asaf.
Debility, not causing: Agar. Casc. Natr. s. **Rhus. Samb.** Valer.
Debilitating, from least movement: Stan. Tarax.

**Dryness**, alternating with: Apis. Natr. c.
**Exhausting: Benz. Cinch.** Kali b. Stan.
**Face**, cold on the: Cocc. Nux v.
**Feet**, beginning at the: Arn. Bell.
**Flies**, which attracts the: **Calad.** *Sumbul.*
**Heat**, with: Æsc. Ant. c. Apis. Bell. Hep. Kali b. Laur. Lob. Natr. c. Op. Phel. Samb. Staph. Valer.
——, dry remaining, sweat soon disappears: *Ant. c.*
——, with, during sleep: **Samb.**
——, ——, in flushes: Ant. c. Bell. **Hep.** Kali b. Op.
**Hot**: Æsc. **Op.**
**Linen**, making it stiff: Mer. Selen.
——, staining it bloody: **Lach.** *Nux m.*
——, —— —— red: Arn. Dulc. *Lach.* Nux v.
——, —— —— yellow: Bell. Bry. **Carb. an.** Cinch. *Fer. Graph.* Ipec. Lach. Mag. c. **Mer. Thuja.** *Verat.*
**Lying down**, after: Mag. s. Meny.
**Oily**: Agar. **Bry.** *Cinch. Mag. c.* **Mer.** Nux. v. Rob. **Stram. Thuja.**
**Oil**, as if mixed with: Cinch.
**Partial**: Cham. *Cinch.* Mer. Nux v. **Petr.** Stram. **Thuja.**
**Profuse**: Acon. Æsc. Agar. Amb. *Ant. t.* Bar. Bell. **Benz. Bry. Calc.** Camph. Canth. Caps. Carb. ac. **Carb. an.** Carb. v. *Casc. Caust.* **Ced. Chin. s. Cinch.** Colch. *Dig.* Elaps. Elat. Eup. perf. Eup. purp. *Fer.* Gels. Graph. **Hep.** Hyos. Iod. *Ipec. Kali b.* Kali br. Kali c. *Lach.* **Lyc.** Lob. *Mag. c.* **Mer.** Mez. **Natr. m.** *Nitr. ac. Nux v. Op.* Par. **Phos. ac.** *Phos.* Pod. *Polyp.* Petr. **Psor.** Rob. Rhus. Sabad. **Samb.** Sarr. *Sec. c. Sep.* **Sil.** Stan. Staph. Stram. *Sulf.* **Tarax.** *Thuja.* Valer. **Verat.**
——, after congestive chill: *Nux v.*
——, on covered parts: Cham. **Cinch.**
——, after light chill: **Eup. perf.**
——, on uncovered parts, except head: **Thuja.**
——, quinine, after abuse of: *Ipec.*
**Room**, in a: Ipec.
**Shivering**, with: Ced. Coff. Eup. perf. *Nux v.*
**Slight**: Ant. c. Apis. Cim. *Cina.* Casc. Croc. Cycl. Elaps. *Eup. perf.* Eup. purp. Ign. *Ipec.* Kali iod. Lach. Led. Nux m. Nux v. Phel. Sep. Sil.

**Smelling,** aromatic: Cop. Rhod.
——, bitter: Verat.
——, blood, like: Lyc.
——, camphor, like: Camph.
——, elder blossoms, like: Sep.
——, fetid: Æsc. Rob.
——, mouldy: Puls. Rhus. **Stan.**
——, musk, like: Puls. *Sulf.*
——, musty: Cim. Rhus. **Stan.**
——, offensive: **Arn.** Ars. *Bar.* Bell. **Carb. an.** *Carb v.* Cim. Con. Cycl. *Dulc.* Euph. Fer. **Graph.** Kali c. *Lach.* Led. **Lyc.** Mag. c. *Mercurialis.* **Mer.** *Nitr. ac. Nux. v.* Puls. *Rhus.* Rob. **Sep. Sil.** Spig. Stan. Staph. Sulf. Verat.
——, onions, like: *Bor. Lach. Lyc.*
——, ——, —— in axillæ: **Bov.**
——, putrid: **Carb. v.** Led. Rhus. Spig. **Staph.** Stram. Verat.
——, rhubarb, like: Rheum.
——, sour: Acon. **Arn.** Ars. Asar. **Bry.** Calc. Carb. v. *Caust.* **Cham.** Cim. *Colch.* Graph. *Hep.* Hyos. Iod. *Ipec.* Led. **Lyc.** *Mag. c.* Mer. Natr. m. *Nitr. ac.* Nux v. Rhus. *Sep. Sil. Sulf.* Thuja. Verat.
——, sourish, as in measles: Fer.
——, sulphur, like: *Phos.*
——, urine, like: Berb. **Canth.** Col. **Nitr. ac.**
——, ——, —— horses: **Nitr. ac.**
**Staining.** (See Linen.)
**Sticky:** Ant. t. Kali br. Lachn.
**Stool,** before: Mer.
**Sudden:** Ipec.
**Suppressed** or wanting: Colch.
**Talking,** when: Graph. Iod.
**Viscid,** profuse all over body: Kali br.
**Walking,** after: Sulf.
——, when: Agar. Amb. Casc. Cocc. Kali c. Led. Natr. m. Sil.
**Warm:** Acon. Ant. c. Benz. Camph. Cham. Cocc. Dros. Ign. Kali c. Lach. Led. Natr. m. Nux v. Op. Phos. Sep. Staph. Stram.
**Warmth,** easy sweating on exposure to: Carb. v.
**Wash off:** difficult to: *Mag. c.* **Mer.**

## SWEAT, TIME OF.

**Afternoon:** Berb. Mag. m. Mag. s. Natr. m. Nux v. Sil. Staph.
**Day,** during the: Agar. Amb. Amm. m. Anac. Ant. t. Bell. Bry. *Calc.* **Carb. an. Cinch. Con.** *Dulc.* **Fer.** *Graph. Hep.* Kali c. Lach. Laur. Led. *Lyc.* Natr. c. **Natr. m.** Nitr. ac. Phos. ac. Puls. **Sep.** Sil. *Staph.* **Stram.** Sulf. Sulf. ac. *Verat.* Zinc.
**Evening,** during the: Bar. Mur. ac. **Samb.** *Sulf.*
———, every other: Bar.
**Forenoon,** during the: **Fer.** Samb.
**Long lasting:** Fer. Kali br. Led.
**Midnight,** after: Alum. Amb. Amm. m. Bar. Clem. Dros. Lachn. Mag. m *Mercurialis.* Nux v. Par. Phos. *Polyp.* Stan.
———, before: Mur. ac.
**Morning,** in the: *Alum.* Ang. Ant. c. Arg. n. Aur. Benz. Bov. Bry. *Calc.* Carb. v. Caust. Chel. Chin. s. Cic. Clem. Cocc. Coff. Dulc. Dros. *Euphorb.* Euph. *Fer.* Graph. Hell. Hep. Iod. Kreos. Lachn. Lyc. **Mag. c.** Mag. m. Mag. s. Mercurialis. **Mer.** Mosch. Mur. ac. Natr. c. Natr. m. Natr. s. **Nitr. ac.** Nux v. Par. **Phos. Phos. ac.** Puls. **Rhus.** Sabad. *Sep.* Sil. Spong. **Stan.** Sulf. Sulf. ac.
———, every other, at precisely same hour: **Ant. c.**
**Night,** at: Acon. Agar. *Alum. Amb.* Amm. c. **Amm. m.** *Anac.* Ang. Ant. t. Arg. Arn. *Ars.* Aur. Bar. Bell. Benz. Bry. *Calc.* Camph. Casc. Carb. ac. **Carb. an. Carb. v.** Caust. Cham. Cic. Cinch. Cist. Cocc. *Coloc. Con.* Cup. Cur. Cycl. Dig. *Dros. Dulc.* Eup. perf. Euph. Fer. *Graph.* Gamb. Hell. **Hep.** Iod. Ipec. **Kali c.** Lach. Laur. Led. Lob. Lyc. *Mag. c.* Mag. m. Mag. s. Meny. Mercurialis. **Mer.** *Mur. ac.* Natr. c. *Natr. m.* Natr. s. **Nitr. ac.** Nux v. Petr. Phos. ac. **Phos.** Polyp. Puls. Rhus. Sabad. Samb. Sarr. **Sep. Sil.** Spong. *Staph.* Stram. *Stront.* **Sulf.** Tabac. *Tarax.* Thuja. Valer. Verat. Zinc.
———, ———, profuse, every other: **Nitr. ac.**
———, ———, putrid-smelling: Spig.
———, ———, on chest and abdomen: Anac. Benz. Thuja.
———, ———, only, then cold and debilitating: Croc.
———, ———, slight, over whole body on waking from sleep: Cycl.
**Noon,** at: Cinn.
**Several hours** after the heat: Ant. t. Ars.

**Sleep**, during: Æth. Agar. Ars. Bell. Camph. Cham. Chel. **Cinch.** Con. Hyos. Phos. Sabad. Thuja.
——, after restless: Lachn.

## SWEAT, LOCATION OF.

**Abdomen**: Amb. **Anac.** Cic. **Dros.** Staph.
**Arms**: Ipec. **Mercurialis.**
**Axilla**: *Benz. Bov.* Caps. Chin s. Dulc. **Kali** c. Lach. Nitr. ac. Petr.
**Back**: Casc. Chin. s. *Cinch.* Dulc. Hyos. Ipec. Lach. Petr. Plant. Puls. **Sep. Sulf.**
——, lumbar region: Plant.
——, sacral region: Plant.
**Body**, all over the: *Ant. t. Benz. Caust.* Cocc. Coff. Dulc. Elaps. Gamb. Hyos. Iod. Led. *Lyc. Mercurialis.* **Natr. m.** *Nitr. ac.* Op. *Phos.* Puls. Sec. c. Sep. **Sil. Stram.** Sulf. *Tarax.* Thuja.
——, —— ——, except the head: *Thuja.*
——, but not face: *Rhus.* Sec. c.
——, front of: Agar. Arg. *Calc.* Graph. Mer. Phos. *Sel.*
——, lower part of: Croc. Cycl. Euph.
——, not on the limbs: Lyc.
——, upper part of: Arg. Asar. *Cham.* Cina. Dulc. Eup. purp. Ipec. Kali c. Laur. Nux v. Op. *Rheum.* Sep. Spig. Sulf. ac. Valer. Verat.
**Chest**: *Agar. Anac. Benz.* Bov. Calc. Cim. Cocc. Graph. *Sep.*
**Face**: *Agar.* Alum. Coff. **Dros.** *Psor. Puls.* Rhus. Rob. Sabad. *Samb. Sil. Stram.*
——, all over excepting the: Rhus.
—— and head only: Æsc. Sil.
——, right side of: *Alum.* Puls.
**Feet**: Bell. Calc. Camph. Canth. *Carb. an.* Carb. v. Dros. Graph. Led. *Petr.* Phos. Puls. Sab. **Sil.** Staph.
——, soles of: **Nitr. ac.** Sabad.
——, from the, over the whole body: Euphor.
**Forehead**: *Cina.* Elaps. Eup. purp. Ipec. Kali b. Led. Op. Stan. Stram. **Verat.**
**Genitals**: Canth. Con. Gels. Staph.
——, male: Hydr. Petr. Psor. *Sep.*
——, profuse, offensive, of the: Hyd.
**Hand**, left: Anac.

**Hands:** Canth. *Cina.* Cocc. *Kali b.* Led. Phos. Sec. c. **Sticta.**
——, alternating on the: Cocc.
——, palms of: Calc. Coff. Dig. Dulc. Iod. Petr. *Psor.*
**Head:** Calc. Cim. Eup. purp. *Op.* Petr. Phos. Sabad. *Sil.*
——, occipital region: Sulf.
——, only: *Sil.*
—— and face: Æsc.
**Inflamed surfaces:** Graph.
**Joints:** Lyc.
**Knees:** Calc.
——, hollows of: *Carb. an.*
**Limbs:** Agar. Calc. Con. Euphor. Hyos. Petr. Sarr.
**Neck:** Agar. Elaps. Euphor. **Stan.**
**Nose:** *Cina.*
**Parts affected: Ant. t.** *Amb.* Cocc. Mer. Sep. Sil.
——, on affected side, worse: **Amb.**
——, covered: *Acon. Bell.* Cham.
——, pressed by clothing: *Chin. s.*
——, single: *Acon.* Bar. Bell. Bry. *Calc.* Caps. Caust. Cham. Cinch. Graph. Hell. Hep. Ign. Ipec. Led. *Lyc.* Mer. Nux v. Petr. Phos. Puls. Rhus. Sab. Samb. *Sel. Sep.* Sil. Spig. Spong. *Stan. Sulf. Thuja.*
——, uncovered: **Thuja.**
**Pelvis,** region of: Canth.
**Perinæum:** Chin. s. Con. *Hep. Kali c. Psor. Thuja.*
**Scalp:** Puls. Rob.
**Scrotum:** Natr. s. Petr. *Thuja.*
**Side, affected: Amb.** Nux v.
——, left: *Bar. Puls.* Phos.
——, not lain upon: *Benz.*
——, on one: *Amb.* Acon. *Bar.* Benz. Bry. Cham. Cinch. Lyc. Nux m. Nux v. **Puls.** Rhus. Sulf.
——, on which he lies: *Acon.* Bry. Cinch. *Nitr. ac.*
——, right: Nux v. *Puls.*
**Sides:** *Mercurialis.*
**Thighs:** Amb. *Carb. an.* Euphor. *Hep. Sep.*
——, inner surface of: *Thuja.*

## SWEAT, SYMPTOMS DURING.

**Abdomen,** distention of: Stram.
**Appetite good:** Stram.
**Anxiety:** Arn. Berb. Bry. Calc. Cocc. Fer. Natr. c. Nux v. Phos. Puls. Sep. Sulf.
——, relieved: Acon. Bar.
**Back,** pain in: Carb. v.
**Body,** lower part of, hot and dry: Op.
——, red, hot and dry: *Stram.*
——, hot and dry on going to sleep: Samb.
**Bones,** pains in: *Eup. perf.*
**Breathing,** stertorous: *Op.*
**Chest,** pain in: *Bry.*
**Colic:** Nux v. Stram.
**Convulsions:** Nux v.
**Cough:** *Ars.* Bry. **Dros.** Ipec.
——, spasmodic: *Dros.*
**Covered,** desire to be: *Acon.* Æth. Aur. Clem. Colch. Con. Nux m. Nux v. *Samb. Stram. Stront.*
**Debility:** Amb. *Benz.* Bry. Calc. Camph. Cocc. *Carb. an.* Chin. s. *Cinch.* Croc. Dig. *Fer.* Graph. Hyos. Ign. Iod. Lyc. *Mer.* Natr. m. Phos. Psor. Sep. Sil. *Stan.* Sulf. Tarax.
——, at night, causing biting of the skin: **Tarax.**
**Delirium:** Thuja.
——, relieves: Æth.
**Diarrhœa:** Acon. Chin. s. Stram. Sulf.
——, nightly: Chin. s.
**Dreams:** Puls.
**Dyspnœa:** Anac. Cac. Mer.
**Earache:** Ign.
**Ears,** roaring in: Ars. Ign.
**Eruption:** Con.
**Excitability,** nervous, relieved: Acon.
**Exhaustion:** *Benz. Camph.* **Carb. an. Cinch.** Ign.
**Extremities,** pain in: Ced.
**Eyes,** burning in: Stram.
**Face,** coldness of: Canch. Lach. Nux. v.

**Face,** dry: *Kali b.*
——, heat of: Bell. Nux v. Sabad.
——, paleness, deathly of: **Verat.**
——, red: Bell. Con. Sep.
**Fainting:** Anac. *Apis.* Ars. Cinch. Ign. Sulf.
**Feet,** cold: Ced. Iod.
——, cramps in: Puls.
——, pains in: *Nitr. ac.* Staph.
——, soreness of: Graph. **Sil.**
——, —— of the balls of: **Nitr. ac.**
**Fingers,** shriveling of, like a washer-woman's: *Ant. c.* **Canch.** *Mer.* Phos. ac. **Verat.**
**Hands,** cold: Canch. Ced. Kali b. **Nitr. ac.**
——, cramps in: Puls.
——, hot: Nux v.
**Head,** congestion of blood to the: Thuja.
——, heaviness of: Ars. Caust.
——, roaring in: Caust.
**Headache:** Arn. Eup. perf. Fer. Natr. m. Rhus. Thuja.
——, commencing with: Fer.
——, relieved gradually: **Natr. m.**
——, —— by thirst: Chin. s.
**Heart,** palpitation of: Ced. Mer.
**Hunger:** *Cimex.* **Cina.**
**Legs,** pain in: Carb. v.
——, weakness of: Ars. Iod.
**Limbs,** cold: *Sec. c.*
**Loquacity: Puls.**
**Mouth,** dry: Ced.
——, open: *Op.*
**Nails,** blueness of: **Nitr. ac.**
**Nausea:** *Dros. Ipec.* Mer. Thuja.
**Nervousness:** Coff.
**Odor,** smoky: Bell.
**Pain,** uncovering, on: Stram.
**Pains,** aggravated by coffee and tobacco: Ign.
——, continue: Eup. perf. Kali c. Lach. Mer. Natr. c. Natr. m. Nux v. Puls. Rhus. Tab.

**Pains,** relieved: *Arn.* Bry. Calad. Chel. *Lach. Natr. m. Nux v.* Sec. c.
——, ——, except headache, all: Eup. perf.
——, ——, gradually: Bell. **Natr. m.**
**Periosteum,** pain in: *Arn.*
**Pulse,** intermittent: Sec. c.
——, weak: Chin. s. Sec. c.
**Respiration,** hurried: Ced.
**Restlessness:** Bry. Lachn.
**Sighing:** Bry.
**Side,** stitches in: Mer.
**Skin,** biting of: Tarax.
——, biting-itching, that compels scratching: Par.
——, burning of: Mer. Op.
——, itching of: Apis. Col. Mang. Par. Rhod. Rhus.
——, parboiled: **Canch.** *Cinch.* Mer.
——, smarting of: Caps. Cham. Con.
**Sleep:** Arn. Ars. Bell. Carb. an. Chel. Cic. Cina. Cinch. Cycl. Euph. Fer. Hyos. Ign. Kali c. Lob. Mez. Mur. ac. Nitr. ac. Nux m. **Op.** Phos. Phos. ac. Plat. **Pod.** Psor. *Puls.* **Rhus.** Sabad. Sulf.
——, deep, snoring: **Op.**
——, restless: *Sulf.*
**Spleen,** pain in: Tarax.
**Spine,** irritation of: Agar.
——, painful to pressure: *Chin. s.*
——, irritation of: Agar. Zinc.
——, sensitive to touch: Agar.
——, weakness of: Agar.
**Stretching:** Caust.
**Symptoms,** aggravated while sweating: *Fer.* **Ipec.** *Mer.* **Op.**
——, cessation of previous: Æsc. Ars. Calad. Cim. Elat. Gels. *Natr. m.* Samb. Sec. c.
——, ——, gradual: **Natr. m.**
**Tenesmus:** Sulf.
**Thirst:** Acon. Anac. **Ars.** Cac. Ced. **Cinch.** *Chin. s. Coff.* Con. Hep. Iod. Mercurialis. **Natr. m.** Phos. ac. Rhus. Sec. c. **Stram.** Tarax. Thuja.
——, commencing with: Coff. Thuja.
——, wanting: *Apis.* Bar. *Calc. Caps.* Caust. *Cim. Cina.* Eup. perf. Euph. Hell. *Ign.* Natr. s. *Nux v. Samb.* Staph. Stram. *Verat.*

**Toes,** soreness of: **Nitr. ac.**
**Toothache:** Carb. v. Cinch. *Coff.*
———, relieved by holding cold water in the mouth, but returns when the water is warm: **Bry.** *Coff.*
**Trembling:** Apis. Ars. Nux v. Rhus.
**Uncovered,** desire to be: *Acon.* Calc. *Eup. perf.* Fer. Iod. Led. Mur. ac. *Natr. m. Op.* Spig. Staph. Verat.
———, cannot bear to be: Æth.
**Uncovering,** pain upon: Stram.
**Urine,** copious: Acon. Dulc. Phos.
———, high colored: Ced.
———, increased amount of: Ant. t. Dulc.
———, milky: Phos.
———, scanty: Ced.
———, transparent: Dulc.
———, turbid: *Ipec.* Phos.
**Urticaria:** *Apis. Rhus.*
**Veins,** swelling of: *Agar.*
**Vertigo:** Lachn.
**Vision,** dimness of: Stram.
**Vomiting:** *Ars.* Camph. Cina. Cinch. *Dros. Eup. perf.* Ipec. Sulf.
———, bitter: **Eup. perf.**
———, drinks, after cold: *Ars.* Cinch.
———, face cold, when: Camph.
———, ingesta, of: Cina. *Eup. perf.*
**Waking up,** when: Anac. Natr. m. Nitr. ac. Par.
**Weakness:** Apis. Ars. Bar. Camph. Fer. Iod. **Mer.** *Phos.* **Psor.** Puls.
**Yawning:** Caust.

### TONGUE, APPETITE, TASTE, ETC.
#### Symptoms of the:

**Appetite,** good: Alum. Caps.
———, ———, as soon as paroxysm is over: Canch.
———, complete loss of: Apis. Lob. Op. Petr. Polyp. Sarr. Sil.
———, unimpaired: Caps.
———, voracious: *Verat.*

**Appetite,** want of: Apis. Dig. Lob.
—, between paroxysms of vomiting: *Verat.*
**Aversion to** alcoholic liquors: Rhus.
—— bread: Natr. m. Nitr. ac. *Nux v.*
—— coffee: **Nux v.**
—— fat: Hep. **Petr.** Sec. c.
———— pork: **Puls.**
———— things: Carb. v. Hep. *Puls.*
—— fish: Graph.
————, smell of cooking: *Colch.*
—— food: Ars. Bry. Op. Sec. c.
————, cooked: Graph. Petr.
———— and drink: Bry. Colch.
————, warm boiled: Lyc. Petr. Sil.
————, —— things: Petr. **Verat.**
————, with loathing when looking at it and still more when smelling it: Colch.
—— milk, which causes flatulence: Carb. v. Puls.
—— meat: Alum. **Arn.** Carb. v. Graph. Kali b. Nitr. ac. Petr. Rhus. Sec. c. Sep. Sil. Sulf.
—— salt: Graph.
—— sweet things: Ars. Caust. Graph. Mer. Nitr. ac. Phos. Sulf.
———— ——, which disagree: **Caust.**
—— sour things: Cocc.
—— tobacco: *Ign.* Lyc. **Nux v.**
—— water: **Nux v.**
**Breath,** sour: **Arn.**
—, fetid: **Arn.** Gels. Nitr. ac.
—, ——, if tongue coated thickly: Gels.
—, offensive: Plant. Pod. Psor.
—, ——, objectively: Pod.
—, putrid: Plant.
—, cadaverous: Nitr. ac.
—, urine, smells like: Graph.
**Choke,** when eating or drinking, apt to: *Anac.*
**Cough,** caused by irritating things—salt, vinegar, pepper, etc.: **Alum.**
**Cracking,** in maxillary articulation when chewing or eating: Nitr. ac.

**Desire for,** apples: **Ant. t.** (See Longing for.)
———, acids: Ant. c. Sec. c.
———, alcoholic drinks: Spig.
———, beer: Caust. Kali b. Puls. Rhus.
———, bitter food: Dig.
———, brandy: Ars. Nux v.
———, coffee, but it nauseates: Caps.
———, cold drinks: *Dulc.* Phos. Sil. *Verat.*
———, ——— food: *Phos.* **Verat.** Sil.
———, ——— milk: **Rhus.**
———, ——— water: Rhus. *Verat.*
———, ——— fruits: **Verat.**
———, fruit, juicy: Ant. t. Phos. ac. Verat.
———, everything cold: Phos. **Verat.** *Sil.*
———, food, juicy, refreshing: Phos. ac. Puls. **Verat.**
———, lemonade: Eup. purp. Sec. c.
———, ice cream: *Eup. perf.* Phos.
———, ——— water: *Phos.* Rhus. **Verat.**
———, pickles: **Ant. c.** Ars.
———, smoked meat: Caust.
———, sour things: Ant. c. Ant. t. Ars. Eup. purp. Polyp. *Puls.* Sec. c.
———, ——— ———, which always relieved: Polyp.
———, things, which are refused when offered: Bry.
**Eating,** better while, worse after: Caps.
**Eructations,** sour: **Lyc.**
———, sulfur, tasting of, lasting all day: Plant.
**Faint,** smell of fish, eggs, fat meat, makes him: **Colch.**
———, feels: Phos.
**Food,** cannot digest: Bap.
———, no desire for: Apis. Colch.
———, disgust for: Cycl.
———, disgust for, sudden, while at meals: Bar. Fer.
———, straw, tastes like: **Stram.**
———, dry, woody, tastes: Fer.
———, indifference to all, even when thinking of it: *Cinch.*
———, highly seasoned, can only digest: Nux m.
———, repugnance to: *Arn.*
———, regurgitation of, in mouthfuls, without nausea: Alum. Phos.

**Food,** tasteless: *Ant. t.* Dros. *Eup. perf.* **Ign.** *Natr. m.* Plant.
——, scarcely swallowed, comes up again: Phos.
——, sweet, wants: Sulf.
**Gums,** loose and spongy: Dulc. **Mer.** Staph.
——, pale: Fer. Staph.
——, ulcerated, bleed when touched: **Staph.**
——, white: *Staph.*
**Hunger:** Dig.
——, canine: Eup. perf.
——, ——, after quinine: *Nux v.* Phos. Staph.
——, must eat before he can get up: Phos.
——, eating does not relieve: Ant. c.
—— and appetite between paroxysms of vomiting: Verat.
——, ravenous: Carb. an. **Meny.** Petr. Verat.
——, ——, with nausea and thirst: Spig.
——, great, without appetite: **Psor.** Rhus.
**Hungry,** but cannot eat: Bar.
——, head aches if he does not eat: *Lyc.*
**Lips,** dry, peeling off: Bry.
——, ——: Nitr. ac. *Nux. m.*
——, ——, without actual dryness or real thirst: Nux m.
——, cracked: Ars. Hep. Natr. m.
——, —— at commissures: Eup. perf. Natr. m.
——, —— and sore, as from cold: Graph.
——, pale: Eup. perf. **Fer. Sec. c.**
——, —— and bloodless: **Fer.**
——, sticky, dry: *Nux m.*
**Longing for,** acids: Alum. Ant. t. Arn. Hep. Kali b. Mag. c.
——, acid drinks: **Eup. purp.** *Mag. c.*
——, alcohol: *Arn.* Ars. *Puls.* Spig.
——, beer: Nux v. *Sulf.*
——, bitter things: Natr. m.
——, brandy: Nux. v. Sulf.
——, chalk: Alum.
——, charcoal: Alum.
——, clean rags: Alum.
——, coffee: Caps. Coff.
——, —— grounds: Alum.

**Longing for,** dainties: Ipec.
——, fat: Nitr. ac.
——, —— food: Nux v.
——, food, refreshing, juicy: Phos. ac.
——, meat: **Canth.** Mag. c. **Meny.**
——, milk, which agrees: Apis. Chel.
——, ——, —— disagrees: Carb. v.
——, indigestible things: Alum.
——, oysters, which disagree: **Lyc.**
——, tea grounds: Alum.
——, salt: Calc. **Natr. m.**
——, strong tasting things: Hep.
——, sour things: Con. Dig.
——, spirituous liquors: Op. Puls.
——, stimulants: Puls.
——, sweets: Ipec. Lyc. Mag. m. Sulf.
**Milk,** disagrees, causes sour taste, sour eructations: Sulf.
**Mouth,** bitter when not eating: *Bry.*
——, rawness of: Carb. an.
——, —— ——, relieved by eating: Carb. an.
——, odor rotten from the: Graph.
——, offensive objective odor from the: Hep.
—— —— odor: Petr. Pod. Psor.
——, sore and ulcerated, corners of: Natr. m. Nitr. ac.
——, rinse the, must: **Nux v.**
——, —— ——, must get up in the night to: Thuja.
**Nausea,** with restlessness: Colch.
**Nauseates,** the smell of broth: *Colch.*
**Papillæ,** red: *Ant. t.* Bell. Mez. Nux m. Stram.
——, —— and elevated: Acon. *Ant. t.*
——, —— bright and raised: **Bell.**
——, —— large and elevated: *Mez.*
——, —— —— —— —— as in scarlatina: Ant. t. Bell. Mez.
**Potatoes:** disagree, cause colic: Alum.
**Salivation:** Dig. Dul. *Iod.* **Mer.** Pod.
——, constant: Dig.
**Saliva,** blood-colored: Gels.
——, acrid: Nitr. ac.

**Saliva,** "cotton:" Nux m.
———, fetid: **Mer.** *Nitr. ac.*
———, iron, tastes of: Cim. **Mer.**
———, metallic: **Mer.**
———, on middle of tongue: Cim.
———, profuse: Ipec. Mer. Nitr. ac. Pod.
———, salty: Ant. c. Iod.
———, soapy: Dul.
———, sour: Ign.
———, stringy, ropy: **Kali b.**
———, tastes bitter in the mouth: Chel.
———, tenacious: Dul. **Kali b.**
———, thready: Con.
**Satiety:** Carb. v. Lyc.
———, a few mouthfuls fill him up: Lyc.
**Stomach,** deranged: Cac. Hep.
**Taste,** acute, too: Cinch.
———, bad: Hyos. Kali c. Sarr.
———, bitter: Ant. c. Aran. Arn. Bap. Bov. **Bry.** Calc. Carb. v. Cham. Chin. s. Cinch. Con. Dul. Elat. *Eup. perf.* Eup. purp. Gels. Graph. Hep. Ipec. Kali c. Lyc. Mag. c. Natr. m. **Nux v.** Polyp. *Psor.* **Puls.** Sulf. Thuja. Staph.
———, ———, bread, after eating: Rhus.
———, ———, goes off after eating or drinking: **Psor.**
———, ———, after smoking: **Anac.** Puls.
———, ———, ——— eating: Nitr. ac. Puls.
———, bitter, before and after eating: Carb. v. Puls.
———, ———, in morning, food tastes natural: Sulf.
———, ———, with clean tongue: Chin. s.
———, ———, bread tastes: Dig. Dros.
———, ——— sweetish: Meny.
———, ———, everything tastes: **Bry.**
———, ——— water: *Ars.*
———, ———, all food tastes: Fer.
———, blood of: Sil.
———, coppery: Æsc. Kali b. Polyp.
———, disgusting: **Puls.**
———, fatty: Lyc.

**Taste**, flat: Anac. Bap. Kali c. Cycl.
——, foul: Calc. Gels. Pod. **Psor. Puls.**
——, fruit juicy, tastes dry: Stram.
——, herring brine, like: Anac.
——, ink, like: Calc.
——, insipid: Eup. perf. Fer.
——, iron, like: Calc.
——, —— with salivation: Æsc.
——, lost: Canth. **Pod.** Sil.
——, metallic: Æsc. Cocc. Hep.
——, nauseous, relieved by smoking: Aran.
——, oil, of: Sil.
——, offensive: Anac. *Bell*. Calc. Cycl. Hyos. Plant. Puls.
——, —— in throat when eating and drinking, although food tastes natural: **Bell.**
——, of rotten eggs: **Arn.** Fer. Graph. Sil.
——, pappy: Eup. perf. Petr. Pod.
——, pasty: Pod.
——, putrid: **Arn.** *Bell*. Bov. Cham. Cycl. Hep. Hyos. **Nux v.** Petr. Plant.
——, qualmish: Cycl.
——, ——, water has a: Caps. Natr. m. Spig.
——, ——, food, after eating: Rhus.
——, rancid oil, like: Ipec.
——, salt, too: Sep.
——, salty: Graph. Iod. **Natr. m.**
——, slimy: Petr. **Puls.**
——, soapy: Cocc.
——, soap-suds: Sil.
——, sour: Caps. Cham. Graph. Ign. Iod. *Lach.* **Lyc.** Mag. c. Mag. m. Natr. m. **Nux. v.** Pod. Thuja.
——, —— at night: Mag. m.
——, ——, everything turns: *Lach.*
——, ——, —— tastes: Pod.
——, sweetish: Ipec.
——, too fresh: Calc.
**Thirst:** Æsc. Eup. perf. Cic. Cim.
——, with inability to swallow: Æsc. Cic. Cim.

**Tip,** burning on the: Carb. an.
——, —— ——, relieved by eating: Carb. an.
——, bluish and sore: Sabad.
——, dry: Rhus. Thuja.
——, painfully sore to touch: **Thuja.**
——, red: Ars. Rhus. Verat.
——, ——, brown in centre: Lach.
——, ——, dry, triangular: **Rhus.**
——, sore: *Æsc.* Kali c. **Thuja.** Sabad.
——, ——, as if full of blisters: Sabad.
——, ——, as if ulcerated: Æsc. Kali c.
——, —— and painful: Hep. Thuja.
——, and edges red: **Verat.** Sec. c.
**Tongue,** adhering to roof of mouth: **Nux m.**
——, bleeding: Cur.
——, bluish: **Ars.** Carb. v.
——, broad, with indented edges: *Kali b.* **Mer.** Pod. Rhus.
——, ——, too: Puls.
——, burnt, tip feels, as far as middle: Psor.
——, clean: *Alum.* Cac. Caust. **Cina.** Dig. Gels. Dros. Elaps. Ign. Ipec. Mag. c. Sil. Stram.
——, ——, with dry, red tip: Sec. c.
——, —— on left, coated on right: Lob.
——, —— —— one side: Rhus.
——, ——, but dry: Lyc.
——, ——, in old cases: Apis.
——, ——, never: **Arn.**
——, coated, back of, like dry clay: Hep.
——, —— brown: Ars. Hyos. Lyc.
——, —— ——, mucous: Sil.
——, —— dirty: Elat.
——, —— —— brown fur: Elat.
——, —— brown streak down the middle: Arn. Bap. Eup. purp. Iod.
——, —— brownish-white: Sarr.
——, —— in centre: Sabad. Sec. c.
——, —— white: *Acon.* Æsc. Anac. Bar. Calc. Carb. v. Chin. s. Cinch. Cocc. Cycl. Dig. *Eup. perf.* Fer. Graph. Ipec. Kali c. Lob. Mag. c. Nux m. Plant. Pod. Polyp. Psor. *Puls.* Rhus. Sep. Spig. Staph. Sulf. Verat.

**Tongue,** coated white, edges dry: Cocc.
——, —— thickly, milky white: **Ant. c.**
——, —— white or yellowish-brown: Verat.
——, —— —— thick: **Mez.** Pod.
——, —— with tough, yellow mucus: Camph.
——, —— —— white pasty fur: Ant. t. Cinch. Pod.
——, —— dirty white: Arn. Cinch. Pod.
——, —— —— yellow: Op.
——, —— downy white: **Colch.**
——, —— —— —— which wears off during the day and becomes red and clean in evening: **Sulf.**
——, —— white or yellow: Æsc. Arn. *Nitr. ac.* Nux v. Psor. *Puls. Sulf.*
——, —— —— in centre, dark streak on sides: Petr.
——, —— —— on sides, red in middle: Caust. Cham.
——, —— —— in A.M., tip and edges clean: Mag. m.
——, —— —— on edges, brown in centre: Iod. Phos.
——, —— —— in middle, edges red: Bap. Bell. Gels.
——, —— —— or brown, red edges, dark in centre: Phos.
——, —— —— or yellow in centre, pale on sides: Chin. s.
——, —— —— fuzzy: Bar.
——, —— heavily: Bry. Canth. Nux v.
——, —— —— brown along the centre: Bap. Eup. purp.
——, —— only in the middle: Phos.
——, —— slightly: Aran.
——, —— thick: Bry. Canth. Polyp.
——, —— —— fur: Phos.
——, —— —— yellow: Kali b. Pod. Polyp. Spig.
——, —— —— ——, with red tip: Polyp.
——, —— yellow: Bov. Ced. Cham. Cinch. Eup. perf. *Kali b.* **Pod.** Polyp. Sec. c.
——, —— yellowish-white: Ars. Cham. Cycl. Gels. Ipec. Natr. m.
——, cracked: Cur. Lyc. Spig.
——, dry: Arn. Carb. v. Caust. Dul. Lach. Lyc. Pod. Rhus. Stram.
——, —— and sticky: *Con.*
——, —— on waking in morning: Calc. Nitr. ac.
——, blisters, burning pain, on: Caps. Carb. an.

**Tongue**, blisters on sides, pain as if burnt: Carb. an.
——, —— on: Cham.
——, fissured: Carb. v. Cur.
——, flabby: Camph. Chin. s.
——, insensible: Colch.
——, itching: Ced. •
——, large, too: Puls.
——, painful: Apis.
——, mapped: Lach. Natr. m. Ran. b. Tarax.
——, pale: **Fer.** *Ipec.* **Sec. c.**
——, paralyzed, partially: Hyos.
——, pricking: Ced.
——, —— in early morning, goes off after eating: Ced.
——, protrudes it with difficulty: Hyos. Lach. Stram.
——, —— —— —— ——, catches behind the teeth: Lach.
——, quivering: Op.
——, raw: Apis.
——, red and white in alternate streaks: *Ant. t.*
——, —— dry: Bell. Lach.
——, red: Lyc. *Rhus.* Stram. **Thuja.**
——, —— bright: Colch. Lyc.
——, —— deep: Cur. Elaps. Hyos.
——, red streaks down the middle: *Ars.* Phos. ac.
——, rough and white: Anac.
——, scalded, feels as if: *Æsc.* Cim.
——, —— gums and palate feel as if: Cim.
——, sensation of a hair on forepart of: Sil.
——, sensitive: Graph.
——, sore: Apis.
——, ——, does not care to talk or protrude it: Apis.
——, spongy: Camph.
——, sticky, yellow: Sec. c.
——, stiff: Colch. Con. Lyc. **Verat.**
——, —— and painful: Con.
——, strawberry: Acon.
——, swelling of: Cic. Dul. Thuja.
——, swollen and black: Elaps.

**Tongue,** swollen: **Thuja.** Verat. Stram.
———, ———, as if paralyzed with cold: Dul.
———, tender: Apis. Graph.
———, trembles: Camph. Canth. Lyc.
———, ——— when protruded: Lach.
———, very thick: Bar.
**Tobacco,** has no taste: Ant. t.
———, tastes bitter: Cocc.
**Toothache,** when infant nurses: Cinch.
**Throat,** dry: Æsc. Cim.
———, ———, causing drinking: Cim.
**Ulcers,** flat: Caps.
———, irregular: **Mer.**
———, lardaceous: Caps. **Mer.**
———, ———, base surrounded with dark halo: **Mer.**
———, apt to run together: *Mer.*
———, have a dirty look: Mer.
———, on gums, tongue, cheeks, throat: **Mer.**
———, spreading: Caps. **Mer.**
———, with undefined edges: **Mer.**
**Water,** dread of: Hyos.
**Vesicles,** painful burning, on sides and tip: Carb. v. Thuja.
———, on tip: Carb. an. Lyc.
———, ——— margin: Carb. an. Sep. Thuja.
**Vomiting,** on assuming the upright position: Colch.

### APYREXIA.

#### Apyrexia, Symptoms During.

**Abdomen,** bloated: *Ars.* Cinch. Graph. Natr. m. Sil.
———, cramps in: Verat.
———, distended after eating: Carb. v. *Kali c.* Lyc.
———, pain in: Ant. t. Led. Petros. Polyp. Ran. b. Sulf.
**Acids,** longing for: Ant. c. Arn. Ars. Dig. Eup. purp. Kali b. Polyp. Puls. Sec. c.
———, ——— ———, especially pickles: **Ant. c.**
**Air,** sensitiveness to cold: Bar. *Hep.* Nux m.
**Alone,** cannot bear to be left: Bis. *Kali c.* **Lyc.**

**Alone,** wants to be: **Cinch.** Ign. Nux v.
——, dreads being, but avoids society: Con.
**Anæmia,** with: **Ars.** Carb. v. **Cinch. Fer.** Eup. perf.
**Anasarca,** after ague: Dul.
**Anxiety,** with: Acon. Camph.
**Appetite,** good: Alum. **Canch.** Caps.
——, loss of: Acon. *Ant. c.* Apis. Arn. Ars. Bry. Caps. Carb. v. Cocc. Cinch. *Corn. fl.* Cycl. Dig. Graph. Ign. Ipec. Kali c. Lob. Natr. m. **Nux v.** Petr. Pod. Polyp. Puls. Rhus. Sabad.
**Bed,** must be in: Canth.
**Beer,** desire for: *Nux v.* Puls.
**Black,** everything looks: *Nux v.*
**Bladder,** pain in, from drinking: Canth.
**Body,** every spot of, painful to pressure: *Bap.* **Bry.**
**Bones,** pain in: Aran. **Arn.** Bry. Caust. **Eup. perf.** Nux v. *Rhus.*
**Bowels,** rumbling in: Carb. v. **Lyc.** Pod.
**Brain,** symptoms of congestion of: Acon. **Arn.** Cinch. Lyc. **Nux v.** *Op.* Phos. Sep. Sulf.
**Brandy,** desire for: Nux v. Puls.
**Bread,** aversion to: Bell. Con. Cycl. Ign. Kali c. Lyc. Natr. m. Nitr. ac. Nux v. Phos. ac. Phos. Puls. Rhus.
**Breath,** fœtid: Gels. **Pod.** Psor.
——, offensive: **Pod.** Psor.
——, ——, which he notices: Hep.
——, ——, —— —— does not notice: Puls. Pod.
——, shortness of: *Calc.*
——, smelling like urine: Graph.
——, sour: *Arn.* Rob.
**Bruised,** feeling as though: *Arn.* Bap.
**Carried,** desire to be: **Cham.** Cina.
**Cerebral congestion,** symptoms of: Laur. *Op.*
**Chest,** constricted feeling of: Ars. Caps. Carb. v. Cocc. Ign. Kali c. Natr. m. Puls. Sabad. Samb. Spig. Stan. Stram. Sulf. Verat.
——, pain in: Sabad.
——, pressure on, cannot bear: Lach.
——, weakness of: Dig. **Stan.**
**Chilly,** constantly: Anac. **Ars.** Bry. Caps. Cocc. Dig. **Hep.** Led. Natr. m. Puls. Sabad. Sil. Verat.

22

**Clear:** Caps. Dros. Ign. Sabad.
——, not: *Acon.* Calc. Carb. an. Chel. *Cina. Colch.* **Eup. perf. Gels.** Ipec. **Natr. m.**
**Coffee,** aversion to: Nux v.
**Cold,** easily takes: Bar. Calc. Caust. Dulc. Hep. Psor.
**Colic:** Cham. Col. Nux v. Petros. Pod.
**Conjunctiva,** jaundiced: **Eup. perf.** Fer. Lyc. Pod. Sabad.
**Convulsions:** Alum. Ars. Bell. Calc. Camph. Caust. **Cham.** Cina. Dig. Dros. Hyos. Ign. Mer. *Nux v.* **Op.** Phos. ac. Stan. Stram. Valer. Verat.
**Constipation:** Æsc. Alum. Anac. Ant. c. **Bry.** Calc. *Canch.* Carb. v. Cinch. Cocc. Con. Fer. Graph. Ign. Led. *Lyc.* Mag. m. **Natr. m.** Nux v. **Op.** *Phos.* Polyp. Sabad. Sil. Staph. Stram. **Sulf.** *Verat.*
**Cough:** Ant. t. Apis. Arn. Ars. Bell. Bry. Cinch. **Cina.** Cocc. Con. Dros. **Eup. perf.** Hep. Hyos. Ign. Ipec. Lyc. Mer. Natr. m. Nux m. Nux v. Op. Phos. *Puls.* Sep. Sil. Spong. Stan. Sulf.
**Countenance,** sallow: Eup. perf. *Iod.* Lyc. *Natr. m.*
**Covered,** must be: **Hep.**
**Covering,** aversion to: Camph. *Sec. c.*
**Debility: Ced. Cinch.** *Eup. perf.* Eup. purp. *Lob.* **Natr. m.**
**Diarrhœa:** Ant. c. Ant. t. *Ars.* Calc. Caps. Carb. an. Cham. Cina. Cinch. Corn. fl. Dig. Dros. Dulc. Gels. Ign. **Iod.** Mer. Mag. c. Nitr. ac. Nux v. Phos. ac. *Phos.* Puls. Rhus. Sab. Sil. **Sulf.** Valer. Verat.
——, early morning: Pod. **Sulf.**
——, exhausting: **Carb. an.**
——, from taking cold; in damp weather: Dulc.
——, painful: Corn. fl.
**Drinks,** cold, desire for: Dulc.
**Dropsy:** Ars. Apis. Cinch. Fer. Eup. perf.
——, from suppressed sweat or eruptions: Dulc.
**Dyspepsia,** intermittent, every other day: Ipec.
**Ears,** ringing in: **Cinch.** Chin. s.
**Emaciation:** Ars. Carb. v. Cinch. Fer. Iod. Mer. **Natr. m.** Nux v. Op. Phos. ac.
**Eructations:** *Alum.* Ant. c. Ant. t. *Arn.* Cinch. Corn. fl. Lyc. Petros. Puls. Sabad.
**Eyeballs,** sore to touch; as if drawn back into head: Hep. Oleand. Paris.

**Eyelids,** agglutination of: Graph. Kali c.
——, half open: *Pod.* Stram. *Sulf.*
——, swelling of upper: Apis. **Kali c.**
——, —— —— lower: **Apis.**
**Eyes,** pupils dilated: Bell. Laur. Stram.
**Face,** bloated: *Ars.* Eup. perf. Fer.
——, clay-colored: *Ars.*
——, flushed after exertion: *Fer.*
**Face,** pale: Anac. Ars. Camph. Carb. v. Cina. Cinch. **Fer.** Ign. Lyc. Mez. Nux v. Petr. Phos. Puls. Sec. c. Spong. Stan. Sulf. Verat.
——, sunken: *Ars. Camph. Sec. c.* Verat.
——, yellow: **Arn. Ars.** Caps. *Cinch.* **Eup. perf.** Fer. **Natr. m. Nux v.** Petr. Rhus. *Sep.*
——, —— spots on: Fer. **Sep.**
**Faintness:** Arn. **Ars.** Bry. Calc. *Carb. v.* Caust. Cina. Cinch. Cocc. Con. Dig. Ign. Ipec. Lyc. Natr. m. Nitr. ac. Nux v. Op. Puls. Sabad. Sulf. *Verat.*
**Fats,** aversion to: Carb. v. *Cycl.* Hell. Hep. Natr. m. Petr. **Puls.** Sec. c.
——, longing for: Nitr. ac. Nux v.
**Feet,** coldness of: Carb. v. Graph. Hyos. Lyc. Rhus. Sep. Sil.
——, dampness about: **Calc.**
——, heaviness of: Canth.
——, sensitive to touch, especially soles: Kali c.
——, swelling of: Bry. Caps. Caust. Cinch. Fer. Lyc. Nux v. Puls. Sep. Sil.
**Flatulency:** Carb. v. Cinch. **Kali c.** Lyc. Petros. Polyp.
**Food,** aversion to: **Ant. c.** Ars. Ipec. Kali c.
——, cold, desire for: Phos. Verat.
——, ——, aggravates: Lyc.
——, juicy, craves: *Phos. ac.* Verat.
——, desire for, changeable: Bry.
——, fluid, desire for: Staph.
——, little, satisfies: Cinch. Lyc.
——, tasteless: Ant. t. Canth. **Dros.** Plant. Sil.
——, warm and cooked, aversion to: Colch. **Petr.** Sec. c.
**Fretting:** Ant. c. Ant. t. *Cham.* **Cina.** *Gels.* Sil.
**Fruit,** longing for: Alum. Ant. t. *Phos. ac.* Verat.

**Fruit**, longing for apples: **Ant. t.**
**Gastric symptoms**: *Ant. c.* Ant. t. Bry. **Carb. v.** Colch. *Cycl.* Dros. Ipec. **Puls.**
——— ———, predominate: Acon. **Ant. c.** Ant. t. Bell. Bry. Carb. v. Cham. Coff. **Colch.** Corn. fl. *Cycl.* Dig. Ign. **Ipec. Nux v.** Petros. **Puls.** Rhus.
**Glands**, affections of: Apis. *Bar.* Bell. *Calc.* Carb. an. Cina. Cocc. Con. Iod. Spong. Staph. *Sulf.*
**Grief**, bad effects of: Ign. Lach. Op. Staph.
**Gums**, bleed when touched: Carb. v. Staph.
———, feeling as though scalded: Cim.
———, scorbutic condition of: Natr. m. *Nitr. ac.*
———, spongy: Staph.
———, white: Fer. Staph.
**Hæmorrhage**: Cac. **Cinch.** Fer. *Ipec.* Nitr. ac. **Phos.**
———, labor-pains cease from: Cinch.
———, from bowels: Ipec. Nitr. ac. Rhus.
**Hæmorrhoids**: Æsc. Natr. m. *Nux v.* **Sulf.**
**Head**, vertex, burning heat in: Calc. Graph. Lach. **Sulf.**
———, ———, coldness of: Sep. Verat.
———, ———, tightness over: Cinch.
**Headache**: Arn. Ars. Bell. Bry. Caps. Carb. v. Cinch. Cocc. Dros. Fer. Gels. Ign. Mez. **Natr. m. Nux v.** *Op.* Phos. ac. Polyp. Puls. Rhus. Sep. Spong. Stan. Valer.
———, menstrual: **Natr. m.** *Puls.*
**Heart**, palpitation of: Acon. Cinch. Ign. Lach. Mer. Natr. m. Sep. Spig. Sulf. Verat.
———, pulsations of, shake the body: **Natr. m.**
———, sensation as if it would stop beating if she moved: Dig.
———, ——— ——— ——— ——— ——— ——— unless constantly on the move: Gels.
**Heat**, aversion to: Apis. Puls. Sec. c.
———, when asleep: *Samb.*
**Hunger**: Ant. c. Arn. Bar. *Carb. an.* Carb. v. **Cina.** Cinch. Dig. Graph. Ign. **Iod.** Lyc. *Meny.* Nux. Petr. Rhus. Sep. **Staph.** Stan. Sulf. Verat.
———, but cannot eat: Bar. Elaps. Ign.
———, which eating does not relieve: Ant. c.

**Hypochondrium**, right, tender to the touch: *Eup. perf.* **Kali** c.
**Hypochondria**, painful, swollen, sensitive: **Cinch.** Chin. s.
**Ice cream**, desire for: Eup. perf.
**Irritability**: Acon. *Anac.* Bell. *Bry. Cham.* Cina. Cinch. Coff. Gels. Ign. Mer. *Nux v.* Puls. Sil. Valer.
——, excessive physical: Nitr. ac.
**Joints**, pain in: Apis. Arn. Ars. Bry. Caust. Cham. Cinch. Cocc. Ign. Ipec. Phos. ac. *Pod.* Puls. Rhus. Sab. Sulf.
——, soreness of: Apis.
**Labiæ**, ulceration of commissures of: **Natr. m.** Nitr. ac.
**Leucorrhœa**, staining the linen yellow: *Carb. an.*
——, exhausting: Carb. an.
**Light**, aversion to bright: Nux v.
**Limbs**, cramps in: Cup. Sulf. Verat.
——, pain in: Calc. Caps. Carb. v. Caust. Cinch. Dros. *Eup. perf.* Graph. Lyc. Natr. m. Nitr. ac. Nux v. Puls. Sab.
——, paralytic immobility of: Canth.
——, soreness of: Apis. Arn.
**Limbs**, weakness of: Bar. Nux v.
**Lips**, burning of: Apis. Ars.
——, cracked: Graph. Ign.
——, dry: Ars. Bry. *Con.* Ign. *Nux m.* Rhus.
——, eruption on: Hep. Ign. **Natr. m. Nux v.** *Rhus.*
**Liver**, pain in: Ars. Bell. *Bry.* Cham. Dulc. *Chel.* Cinch. **Kali c.** Lyc. *Mer.* **Natr. m. Nux.** Polyp. Pod. Puls.
——, sensation as if swollen: Cinch.
**Love**, disappointed, bad effects of: Calc. p. Hyos. **Ign.** Staph.
**Meat**, aversion to: Alum. **Arn.** Ars. Bell. Calc. Carb. v. Cham. Fer. Graph. Ign. Lyc. Mer. Nitr. ac. Op. Petr. Puls. Rhus. Sabad. Sec. c. Sep. Sil. Sulf.
——, desire for: **Canth.** *Mag. c.* **Meny.**
**Menses**, suppression of: Ars. Calc. Cham. Cinch. Con. Fer. Graph. Kali c. Lyc. Mer. Nux v. Puls. Sep. Sil. Sulf.
——, too early: Acon. Alum. Aran. Ars. Bar. Bell. Bry. **Calc.** Carb. v. Cham. Cocc. Fer. Hyos. Ign. Iod. Kali c. Led. Lyc. Mer. Nux v. Petr. Phos. Rhus. Sab. Sep. Spong. Staph. Sulf. Verat.
——, too late: Bell. Caust. Cinch. Con. Fer. Graph. Hyos. Ign. Ipec. Kali c. Lyc. Natr. m. Puls. Sabad. Sil. Sulf.

**Menses,** too profuse: Acon. Aran. Ars. Bar. Bell. *Calc.* Cham. Cina. Cinch. Fer. Hyos. Ign. Ipec. Led. Lyc. Mer. Natr. m. Nux v. Op. Phos. Sab. Sep. Sil. Spong. Stan. Stram. Sulf.
——, too scanty: Alum. Con. Cycl. Graph. Lyc. Natr. m. Phos. Puls. Sabad. Sil. Sulf. Verat.
——, exhausting: Carb. an.
——, flow intermits: Fer. Sulf.
——, morning sickness during: Graph.
**Metrorrhagia** between the periods at every little accident: Amb.
**Milk,** aversion to: Puls. Sil.
——, desire for: Apis. Chel.
——, —— ——, but causes flatulence: Carb. v.
**Mouth,** corners of, eruptions at: Hep. *Ign.* **Natr. m. Nux v.** *Rhus.*
——, —— ——, sore and ulcerated: Natr. m. Nitr. ac.
——, desire to rinse the: **Nux v.** *Thuja.*
——, mucous membrane of, pale: *Eup. perf.* **Fer.**
——, rawness of: Carb. an.
**Muscles,** feeling as though bruised: Arn. Bap. Nux m.
**Nausea:** Ant. c. Ant. t. Arn. Ars. Caps. Dros. Eup. perf. Graph. Hep. Hyos. Ipec. *Nux v.* Petros. Rhus. Sabad. Sil.
——, relieved by drinking: **Lob.**
**Neck,** pain in back of: Fer.
**Nervousness:** Ced. *Cham.* Cinch. Coff. *Gels.* Ign. Nux v. Puls. Rhus. Valer.
**Night-sweats:** Cinch. Kali c. Natr. m. Stan. Tarax.
**Œdema:** Apis. Ars. Cinch. Fer. Eup. perf.
**Pain,** sensitive to: Cham. Cinch. Coff. Ign.
——, better while thinking of it: Camph.
**Palate,** scalded, feeling as though: Æsc. Cim.
**Perspiration:** Ars. Cinch. Lach. Sulf.
**Pickles,** desire for: *Ant. c.*
**Prolapsus ani: Ign.** *Lach. Lyc.* Mer. Nitr. ac. Plumb. **Pod.** *Sep. Sulf.*
——, from moderate straining: **Ign.**
——, —— overlifting or straining; after parturition: Pod.
**Pulse,** accelerated by motion: Ant. t. *Dig.* Gels.
——, full: Acon. Bell. Bry. Dig. Fer. Gels. Hyos. Lach. Op. Stram.
——, rapid, then slow: Ant. c.

**Pulse**, slow: Chel. Cinch. **Dig.** Sec. c. **Verat.**
——, third, fifth, or seventh beat intermits: *Dig.*
——, thread-like: Acon. Gels. Lach.
——, weak: *Acon.* Ars. *Carb. v.* Cinch. Cup. Fer. Gels. Lach. *Laur.* Op. *Sil. Stram. Verat.*
**Remission**, slight: Bap. **Eup. perf.** Gels.
**Restless**, continually moving from place to place: Bap. Rhus.
**Restlessness**: Apis. Ars. Bap. Ced. Colch. Iod. Rhus.
**Rheumatism**: *Acon.* Ant. t. Arn. *Bell. Bry.* Carb. v. *Caust.* Cham. Colch. Nux v. *Puls. Rhus.* Thuja. Valer. Verat.
**Saliva**, acrid: Nitr. ac.
——, bitter, collection of, in the mouth: Chel.
——, bloody: Gels.
——, cotton, like: Nux v.
——, saltish: Ant. c. Iod.
——, secretion of, profuse: Ipec. Pod.
——, sticky: *Nux m.*
——, sour: Ign.
——, thready: Con. Hydr. *Kali b.*
**Salivation**: Æsc. Iod. Mer. Pod.
**Scapula**, pain under inferior angle of right: Chel.
——, —— —— —— —— of left: Sang.
**Sick** feeling all over, indescribable: Bap.
**Side**, better when lying on painful: *Bry.*
——, left, pain in: Apis.
**Sighing**: Ign. Verat.
**Sinking**: *Camph. Carb. v.*
**Skin**, blueness of: **Verat.**
**Skin**, itching of: Hep. Ign. Rhus.
——, yellow: Acon. Arn. Ars. Bell. Cham. Cinch. Dig. *Eup. perf.* Fer. Natr. m. *Nux v.* Polyp. Puls. Rhus. Sulf.
**Sleep**, dreams with: Acon. Ign. Natr. m. Stram.
——, restless: Acon. Bap. Cina. Fer. Ign. Rhus. Stram.
——, snoring with: Ign. *Op.*
**Sleepiness**: Acon. Bell. Bry. Calc. Carb. v. Hyos. Mer. Op. Sabad. Spig. Stan. Stram. Sulf. Valer.
**Sleeplessness**: Ars. Bell. Bry. Carb. v. Cinch. Cina. Coff. Hyos. Ipec. Led. Mer. Natr. m. Nitr. ac. Op. Puls. Ran. b. Rhus. Sil. Spig.

**Somnolence:** *Ant. t.* Bell. Cham. Cocc. Hyos. **Op.** Puls. Rhus.
**Sour things,** aversion to: Cocc.
——— ———, desire for: Ant. c. Arn. Ars. Cocc. Dig. Eup. perf. Hep. Kali b. Polyp. Puls. Sec. c.
**Spine,** irritation of: **Agar.** Ang. Gels. **Zinc.**
**Spleen,** enlarged: Aran. Ars. Bell. *Cinch. Eup. perf.* Fer. **Iod.** Mer. Mez. Nitr. ac. Pod. Puls.
———, pain in region of: Apis. Ars. Chel. Cinch. Fer. **Natr. m. Nux v.** Pod. Tarax.
———, region of, sensitive to pressure: Apis. Ars. *Chel.* Cinch. Chin. s. Fer. **Iod.** *Nux v.* Pod. Puls.
**Sputum bloody:** Nux m.
**Stomach,** cramps in: Cup. Verat.
———, distention of: Nux v. Petros. Sabad.
———, fulness of, sense of: Carb. v. Lob. *Lyc.* **Natr. m.** Pod. Rhus.
———, oppression at pit of: Lob.
———, pain in: Acon. Arn. Ars. Calc. Caust. *Chel.* Cocc. Con. Fer. Ign. Lyc. Natr. m. Nux v. Petros. Puls. Rhus. Sabad. Sep. Sil. Stan. Verat.
———, pressure in the region of: Ant. c. Rhus.
———, relaxed, as if hanging down: Ipec. Staph.
———, spasms in: Ars. Bell. Bry. Carb. v. Cham. Cocc. Fer. Ign. Natr. m. Nux v. Puls. Sil. Stan. Sulf. Valer. Verat.
———, weak sensation in: Lob. Phos.
**Sweat,** debilitating: **Cinch.** Eup. perf. Tarax.
———, not debilitating: **Samb.**
———, profuse when awake: **Samb.**
———, ———, of head: Calc. Mag. m. Sil.
**Sweating:** **Cinch.** Nux v. **Samb.** Sil. *Verat.*
**Taste,** acute: Cinch.
———, bitter: Ant. c. Aran. **Arn.** Ars. *Bry.* Calc. Carb. v. Cham. Chel. *Chin. s.* **Cinch.** Con. Dros. Dulc. Eup. perf. Fer. Gels. Graph. Hep. Ipec. Lach. Lyc. Mag. c. Mer. Natr. m. Nitr. ac. **Nux v.** Phos. ac. Polyp. Psor. Puls. Rhus. Sab. Staph. Sulf. Tarax. Thuja.
———, ———, everything except water: **Acon.**
———, ———, sweet: *Meny.*
———, ——— of tobacco: *Cocc.* Puls.
———, coppery: Kali b. Mer.

**Taste,** herring brine, like: Anac.
——, iron, like: Cim.
——, lost: Canth. Natr. m. Pod. Sil.
——, metallic: Cocc. Mer. Nux v. Polyp. Rhus.
——, putrid: **Arn.** Bell. Caps. Cham. *Fer. Graph.* Hep. Hyos. Mer. Natr. m. Nitr. ac. **Nux v.** Petr. Plant. **Pod.** *Psor. Puls.* Rhus. Sil. Staph.
——, salt: Ars. *Carb. v.* Cinch. Mer. Natr. m. **Sep.**
——, soapy: Cac.
——, sour: Calc. Caps. Cham. Graph. Ign. Iod. Lach. **Lyc.** Mag. c. *Nux v.* Petr. Phos. Pod. Rob. Sep. Thuja.
**Things,** wants, which he repels when offered: Bry. *Cham.* Cina. Iod.
**Thirst:** Canth. Cic. Cim. **Cinch.** Dulc. Sulf. Verat.
——, but disgust for all kinds of drink: **Canth.**
**Thirstlessness,** with nearly all complaints: Apis. Puls.
**Throat,** liability to sore: Bar.
——, dry, painful, sore: Æsc.
——, sore, during menses: Mag. c.
**Tobacco,** aversion to: Alum. Arn. Bell. Calc. Cinch. **Ign.** Led. Natr. m. Nux. Phos. Rhus. Sep. Spig. Stan.
——, cannot bear: **Ign.**
——, has no taste: Ant. t.
**Tongue black:** Elaps.
——, blistered: Caps. *Carb. an.* Carb. v. Cham. **Natr. m.** Thuja.
——, broad, red with indented edges: Kali b. Mer. Pod. Rhus.
——, brown: Ars. Carb. v. Elat. Hyos. Iod. Lyc. Phos. Verat.
——, —— in centre, edges white: *Iod.*
——, —— streak down the middle: *Arn.* Eup. purp. Iod. Lach. Phos.
——, burning: Carb. an. Carb. v. Cim. Sang.
——, burnt, feeling as though: Psor.
——, catches behind the teeth: Lach.
——, clean: Alum. Apis. Cact. Caust. Chin. s. **Cina.** Dig. Dros. Elaps. Gels. Ign. Ipec. Lyc. Mag. c. Puls. Sec. c. Stram. Sulf. *Thuja.*
——, coated thickly: **Ant. c.** Arn. Bar. *Bry.* Canth. Chel. Cinch. Iod. Kali b. Mez. **Nux v.** Phos. Polyp.
——, cold: **Camph.** Carb. v. *Verat.*
——, contracted: Carb. v.
——, cracked: Cur. Lyc.

22

**Tongue**, dry: Arn. **Bell.** *Calc. Carb. v.* Caust. Dulc. Lach. Lyc. *Natr. m.* **Nux m.** Pod. Puls. *Stram.*
——, —— at the back of: Hep.
——, —— at the edges: Cocc.
——, edges red: **Ant. t.** Bell. Canth. Gels. Phos. Sec. c. *Verat.*
——, —— ——, white in the middle: Bell.
——, furred, with red streak down the middle: *Ars.* Verat.
——, too large: Puls. Stram.
——, lead-colored: Camph. **Carb. v.** Verat.
——, mapped: Lach. **Natr. m.** *Ran. b.* **Tarax.**
——, —— like herpes (ringworm) on the sides: **Natr. m.**
——, mucus, covered with: **Puls.**
——, —— yellowish on: Camph.
——, painful: Con. Graph. Hep.
——, pale: **Eup. perf. Fer.** Ipec. Kali c. *Sec. c.*
——, papillæ elevated: Acon. **Ant. t.** *Bell.* Mez. Nux m.
——, —— red: *Acon.* **Apis.** *Bell.* Mez. Nux v. *Stram.*
——, protrude cannot: Apis. *Lach.* Stram.
——, red: *Ant. t. Apis.* **Bell.** Cur. Elaps. Hyos. Kali b. Lyc. Sulf. *Thuja.*
——, —— and white in streaks: **Ant. t.**
——, —— streak in centre: Phos. ac.
——, rough: Anac.
——, sore: *Apis.* Tarax.
——, spots on dark, red and sensitive: **Tarax.**
——, stiff: Con. Dulc. Lyc.
——, strawberry: *Acon.* Ant. t. **Apis. Bell.**
——, swelling of: Dulc. Cic. Elaps. Mer. *Thuja.* Verat.
——, tip blue: Sabad.
——, —— dry: Psor. *Rhus.* Sec. c.
——, —— —— and red: *Ars.* Lach. Nux v. Polyp. **Rhus.** Sec. c. Verat.
——, —— sore: Carb. v. *Hep.* Kali c. Sabad. *Thuja.* Tarax.
——, —— red, triangular: **Rhus.**
——, shows imprint of teeth: Chel. **Mer. Pod.** Rhus.
——, trembling: Camph. Canth. Lach. *Lyc.* **Op.**
——, ulcers on: Caps. Carb. an.
——, vesicles on sides and tip: Carb. an. Caust. Lyc. Sep. Thuja.

Tongue, white: Anac. *Ant. c.* Arn. Ars. Bar. Calc. Carb. v. Chel. Cinch. Cina. Cocc. Dig. Eup. perf. **Fer.** Graph. Ipec. Kali c. Lach. Mag. c. Mez. Natr. m. Nitr. ac. Nux m. Nux v. Phos. Plant. Pod. Polyp. Psor. **Puls.** Rhus. Sabad. Sarr. Sep. Staph. Stram. Sulf. Verat.
——, white in centre, dark streak along sides: Petr.
——, —— milky: **Ant. c.**
——, —— at sides, middle red: Cham.
——, ——, or yellow in centre, margin pale: Chin. s.
——, ——, —— with margin red: Chel. Gels.
——, yellow: Arn. Ars. Bov. *Bry.* Canth. Carb. v. Ced. Cham. Chel. Cinch. Eup. perf. Fer. Gels. Ipec. Kali b. *Mer.* Natr. m. Nitr. ac. *Nux v.* Op. **Pod.** Polyp. Psor. *Puls.* Sec. c. Sulf.
Tonsils, induration of: **Bar.** Lach. Mer. iod.
Touch, sensitive to: *Apis.* Bell. **Cinch.** Kali c. *Lach.*
Urinary organs, irritation of: Canth. Dulc. *Petr.* Petros. Sars.
Urination, difficult: *Canth.* Sars.
——, frequent: Canth. Cham. *Eup. perf.* Phos. ac. Plant.
——, —— at night: *Phos. ac.*
——, ——, flow intermits: **Con.**
——, painful: Canth. *Eup. purp.*
——, profuse: Canth. **Eup. purp.** Phos. ac.
——, —— but pale, clear as water at night: **Phos. ac.**
Urine, black: Canth.
——, brick-dust sediment: Chin. s. Cinch. **Lyc.** Natr. m. Sars.
——, brown: Camph. Cim.
——, fatty: Chin. s.
——, green: Camph. *Plant.*
——, horses, smelling like: **Nitr. ac.**
——, hot: Cim.
——, incontinence of: Caust. Dulc. Nitr. ac. Puls. Rhus. Sulf.
——, milky, turning so after standing: *Cina.* Dulc.
——, offensive: **Nitr. ac.** Nux v.
——, pale: Cham. **Eup. perf. Phos. ac.** Thuja.
——, red: Bry. Camph. **Lyc.** Nux v.
——, red, yellow: Kali c.
——, retained, bladder full: **Op.**
——, scanty: **Apis.** Bry. Cinch. Lyc. *Natr. m.*
——, —— and painful: **Apis.** Canth.

**Urine,** suppressed: Stram.
—, turbid: Ant. t. Berb. Camph. Cina. Cinch. Dulc. Graph. Ipec. **Lyc.** Mer. *Natr. m. Nitr. ac.*
—, white sediment, with: Berb. Graph.
—, yellowish: Camph.
**Urticaria: Apis.** Elat. **Hep.** *Ign.* **Rhus.**
**Walk,** desire to slowly, which gives relief: *Fer.*
**Vegetables,** longing for: Alum.
**Veins distended:** Fer.
**Vertigo:** Acon. Arn. Ars. Bell. Calc. Caust. Cham. Cocc. Con. **Eup. perf.** Fer. Hyos. Lyc. Nitr. ac. Nux. Op. Petr. Phos. Polyp. Puls. Sep. Sil.
—, in occiput: Petr.
—, with sensation of falling to the left: Eup. perf. **Eup. purp.**
**Vomiting:** Ant. c. Ant. t. Cina. Cinch. *Eup. perf. Fer.* Hyos. Ipec. Lyc. Mer. Nux v. Petros. Sep. Sil. Verat.
—, bitter: Cinch. Eup. perf.
—, bile, of: Ars. **Eup. perf.** Ipec. Mer. Nux v. Stram. Verat.
—, ingesta, of: Ars. Cham. **Eup. perf. Fer.** *Ipec.* Nux v. Puls.
—, mucus, of: Mer. Nux v. *Puls.*
—, sour: **Lyc.** *Rob.*
**Weakness:** Acon. *Alum.* Apis. Arn. **Ars.** Bap. Bar. Calc. Camph. **Carb. an. Carb. v. Ced.** Chin. s. **Cinch.** Corn. fl. Dig. Eup. purp. Fer. *Gels.* Ign. Iod. Ipec. Lyc. **Natr. m.** Nitr. ac. Nux v. Polyp. Sulf. Verat.
—, in stomach and abdomen: Chel. **Phos.** *Sep.*
—, on going up stairs: Calc. Iod.
**Weep,** disposition to: *Cina.* Puls. Nux v.
**Worms,** with symptoms of: *Cina.* Spig. Stan. Sulf.

# ABBREVIATIONS AND REMEDIES.

Acon.—Aconitum napellus.
Æsc.—Æsculus hippocastanum.
Æth.—Æthusa cynapium.
Agar.—Agaricus muscarius.
Alum.—Alumina.
Alston.—Alstonia (constricta?).
Amb.—Ambra grisea.
Amm. c.—Ammonium carbonicum.
Amm. m.—Ammonium muriaticum.
Anac.—Anacardium orientale.
Ang.—Angustura.
Ant. c.—Antimonium crudum.
Ant. t.—Antimonium tartaricum.
Apis.—Apium virus.
Aran.—Aranea diadema.
Arg. n.—Argentum nitricum.
Arn.—Arnica montana.
Ars.—Arsenicum album.
Asaf.—Asafœtida.
Asar.—Asarum europeum.
Aur.—Aurum.
Bap.—Baptisia tinctoria.
Bar.—Baryta carbonica.
Bell.—Belladonna.
Benz.—Benzinum.
Berb.—Berberis vulgaris.
Bov.—Bovista.
Brom.—Bromium.
Bry.—Bryonia alba.
Cac.—Cactus grandiflorus.
Calad.—Caladium.
Calc.—Calcarea ostrearum.
Camph.—Camphora.
Canch.—Canchalagua.
Canth.—Cantharis.
Caps.—Capsicum.

Carb. ac.—Carbolic acid.
Carb. an.—Carbo animalis.
Carb. v.—Carbo vegetabilis.
Casc.—Cascarilla.
Caust.—Causticum.
Ced.—Cedron.
Cham.—Chamomilla.
Chel.—Chelidonium.
Chin. s.—Chininum sulfuricum.
Cinch.—Cinchona.
Cic.—Cicuta virosa.
Cim.—Cimex lectularis.
Cina.—Cina.
Clem.—Clematis erecta.
Cocc.—Cocculus.
Coff.—Coffea.
Colch.—Colchicum.
Col.—Colocynth.
Con.—Conium.
Corn. fl.—Cornus florida.
Crot.—Crotalus.
Croc.—Crocus sativa.
Cup.—Cuprum met.
Cur.—Curare.
Cycl.—Cyclamen europeum.
Dig —Digitalis purpurea.
Dros.—Drosera.
Dulc.—Dulcamara.
Elaps.—Elaps corallinus.
Elat.—Elaterium.
Eucalyp.—Eucalyptus.
Eup. perf.—Eupatorium perfoliatum.
Eup. purp.—Eupatorium purpureum.
Euphor.—Euphorbium.
Fer.—Ferrum.
Gamb.—Gambogia.

Gels.—Gelsemium.
Graph.—Graphites.
Hell.—Helleborus niger.
Hep.—Hepar sulfuris calcareum.
Hyd.—Hydrastis canadensis.
Hyos.—Hyoscyamus.
Ign.—Ignatia (strychnos).
Iod.—Iodum.
Ipec.—Ipecacuanha.
Kali b.—Kali bichromicum.
Kali br.—Kali bromatum.
Kali c.—Kali carbonicum.
Kali iod.—Kali iodatum.
Lach.—Lachesis.
Lachn.—Lachnanthes tinctoria.
Led.—Ledum palustre.
Lob.—Lobelia inflata.
Lyc.—Lycopodium clavatum.
Mag. c.—Magnesia carbonica.
Mag. m.—Magnesia muriatica.
Mar.—Marum verum.
Meny.—Menyanthes.
Mercurialis perennis.
Mer.—Mercurius.
Mez.—Mezereum.
Mur. ac.—Muriatic acid.
Natr. c.—Natrum carbonicum.
Natr. m.—Natrum muriaticum.
Natr. s.—Natrum sulfuricum.
Nitr. ac.—Nitric acid.
Nux m.—Nux moschata.
Nux v.—Nux vomica.
Oleand.—Oleander.
Op.—Opium.
Par.—Paris quadrifolia.
Petr.—Petroleum.
Petros.—Petroselinum.
Phel.—Phellandrium aquaticum.

Phos. ac.—Phosphoric acid.
Phos.—Phosphorus.
Plant.—Plantago majus.
Plat.—Platinum.
Pod.—Podophyllum peltatum.
Polyp.—Polyporus officinalis.
Psor.—Psorinum.
Puls.—Pulsatilla.
Ran. b.—Ranunculus bulbosa.
Rob.—Robinia.
Rhod.—Rhododendron.
Rhus.—Rhus toxicodendron.
Ruta.—Ruta graveolens.
Sabad.—Sabadilla.
Sab.—Sabina.
Samb.—Sambucus nigra.
Sang.—Sanguinaria canadensis.
Sarr.—Sarracenia purpurea.
Sars.—Sarsaparilla.
Sec. c.—Secale cornutum.
Sel.—Selenium.
Sep.—Sepia.
Sil.—Silicea.
Spig.—Spigelia anthelmia.
Spong.—Spongia tosta.
Stan.—Stannum.
Staph.—Staphisagria.
Stram.—Stramonium.
Stron.—Strontiana carbonica.
Sulf.—Sulfur.
Sum.—Sumbul.
Tab.—Tabacum.
Tarax.—Taraxacum.
Thuja.—Thuja occidentalis.
Valer.—Valeriana officinalis.
Verat.—Veratrum album.
Zinc.—Zincum.